Clinical Rheumatology

Rohini Handa

Clinical Rheumatology

Springer

Rohini Handa
Department of Rheumatology
Indraprastha Apollo Hospital
New Delhi
India

ISBN 978-981-33-4884-4 ISBN 978-981-33-4885-1 (eBook)
https://doi.org/10.1007/978-981-33-4885-1

This Springer imprint is published by the registered company Springer Nature Singapore Pte Ltd.
The registered company address is: 152 Beach Road, #21-01/04 Gateway East, Singapore 189721, Singapore

This book is dedicated to my patients who, through their suffering, fortitude, and even death taught me rheumatology.

Preface

Science changes perennially and perpetually and the much-feted concepts of today become the antiquated discards of tomorrow. Nothing exemplifies this better than rheumatology, a subject that has metamorphosed from a *passive discipline* to a *happening subspecialty* at the intersection of immunology, molecular biology, and clinical medicine. Autoimmune rheumatic diseases, viewed through the prism of the uninitiated, may seem esoteric but exotic they are not.

The increasing importance of rheumatology has to be viewed in the context of a transformed medical landscape—shifting demographics with the aging of the population, ever-burgeoning environmental triggers of autoimmunity, and dominance of non-communicable diseases over communicable diseases—all of which have translated into an increased incidence of rheumatic diseases. At the same time, the narrowing of the gap between the bench and bedside has led to an exponential increase in path-breaking discoveries and game-changing treatments. While catapulting rheumatology to new heights, the knowledge explosion has generated a voluminous amount of literature. Words like conventional synthetic DMARDs, targeted synthetic DMARDs, bio-originators, and bio-similars have entered the lexicon of rheumatologists in the last decade. Pari passu the size of the average rheumatology textbook has increased manifold.

Despite the commonality of rheumatic diseases, the teaching of rheumatology is often marginalized in undergraduate and postgraduate medical curricula in many developing countries. The situation is slightly better in the developed world but does not come anywhere near the more visible medical subspecialties like cardiology, pulmonology, nephrology, and neurology. The curriculum in internal medicine is dominated by these subspecialties. This leaves the young doctors inadequately trained and poorly prepared for the avalanche of cases with musculoskeletal problems that await them as they step out of medical school. The undergraduate books offer sketchy information, while the voluminous reference books can be quite daunting for the non-rheumatologists seeking to find precise and concise evidence-based information that will equip them to handle real-life clinical situations. ***Clinical Rheumatology*** aims to fill this gap without intimidating the reader by the quantum of information.

An aphorism prevalent among clinicians is "those who see patients hardly get the time to write books and those who write books hardly see patients." ***Clinical Rheumatology*** bridges this seeming dichotomy. Written by a clinician for clinicians, the thrust is on practical insight into rheumatic diseases while pruning unnecessary detail. It is meant to be a complement to and not a substitute for the several excellent rheumatology textbooks already available. While some may criticize the book for its oversimplification of complex disorders, I have tried to forsake complexity for simplicity. As Denis Waitley has said "Never become so much of an expert that you stop gaining expertise."

"No man is an island, entire of itself" wrote the seventeenth-century English poet John Donne. In the same context, a single-author book like ***Clinical Rheumatology*** may seem somewhat of an anachronism in this current era of multi-author texts. This might be a perceived weakness but may well prove to be an inherent strength of the book—uniformity of style and consistency of concepts possible only with a single author.

I do hope this compact book shall prove relevant for both beginners and experienced clinicians.

New Delhi, India Rohini Handa

Acknowledgments

My father, Prof. F. Handa, an astute clinician and a much loved teacher, who always believed that "there is no profession better than teaching, and arguably, no teacher better than a medical teacher."

My mother, Late Dr. Kumud Handa who inculcated in me the value of thrift and hard work.

My wife Madhu, for enduring my unreasonableness while being a constant pillar of support and encouragement.

My children, Praerna and Prateek, for making everything worthwhile.

Contents

About the Author

Rohini Handa is currently working as Senior Consultant Rheumatologist at the Apollo Hospitals, New Delhi. He has earlier served on the faculty of the All India Institute of Medical Sciences, New Delhi, for over two decades. Prof. Handa's contributions to rheumatology have been recognized by several awards and citations by the Indian Council of Medical Research (MN Sen Oration Award and Shakuntala Amir Chand Prize), the Indian Rheumatology Association (IRA Oration), the Association of Physicians of India (Netaji Oration, Searle Oration, JC Patel and BC Mehta Prize, Pawan Kumari Jain Oration and Dr. JN Berry Award), and the Indian Academy of Clinical Medicine (Dr. GB Jain Oration and Dr. Sukumar Mukherjee Honor Lecture) among others. Prof. Handa was conferred the Distinguished Academician Award by the Apollo Hospitals in 2018.

In an illustrious career spanning four decades, Prof. Handa has held several leadership positions: Chair of the International League of Associations for Rheumatology, President of the Asia Pacific League of Associations for Rheumatology, President of the Indian Rheumatology Association, Dean of the Indian College of Physicians, Distinguished Clinical Tutor Apollo Hospitals Educational and Research Foundation, Honorary Consultant Armed Forces Medical Services, and President of the Delhi Rheumatology Association. Prof. Handa has served/serves on the editorial board of reputed medical journals including Rheumatology Oxford, Current Rheumatology Reports, Best Practice and Research Clinical Rheumatology, Clinical Rheumatology, Indian Journal of Rheumatology, African Journal of Rheumatology, Indonesian Journal of Rheumatology, and Journal of Association of Physicians of India.

1 Bedside Approach to Musculoskeletal Complaints

1.1 Introduction

Musculoskeletal (MSK) pain is common in clinical practice. It may originate from the joints or the surrounding structures like bone, ligaments, tendons, etc. It is important to differentiate arthralgias from arthritis. Arthralgias are joint pains without obvious inflammation. Often nonspecific, arthralgias are encountered in several non-rheumatological conditions like hematological diseases, post-viral fever, hypothyroidism, statin use, etc. Arthritis, on the other hand, is associated with demonstrable features of inflammation like joint swelling and tenderness. Raised temperature and visible redness are usually not seen in chronic arthritides like rheumatoid arthritis (RA) or spondarthritides (SpA). These are more a feature of acute conditions like gout or septic arthritis.

Patient history is the single most important source of diagnostic information in MSK complaints, followed by a careful physical examination and judicious use of laboratory investigations. Screening questions in history include *P*ain, *A*ctivity limitation, *S*tiffness, and *S*welling in joints or soft tissues, easily remembered by the acronym "PASS."

1.2 Bedside Approach

The approach revolves around three key points:

1. Origin of pain
2. Nature of the disease: Inflammatory or noninflammatory
3. Pattern recognition

1.2.1 Origin of Pain (Articular or Nonarticular)

Not all pains around a joint originate in the joint itself. Adjacent periarticular structures such as bone, ligaments, tendons, bursae, or muscles may be responsible (Table 1.1). History and examination go a long way in ascertaining the exact source of pain. In general, articular pains tend to be diffuse and deep-seated. In contrast, the pain of bursitis is characterized by localized point tenderness away from the joint line. Active (patient moves the joint himself/herself) and passive (physician puts the patient's joint through range of motion) movements also help in making this distinction at the bedside. Articular pain is aggravated by both active and passive movements in

R. Handa, *Clinical Rheumatology*, https://doi.org/10.1007/978-981-33-4885-1_1

contradistinction to periarticular pain, which is more aggravated by active than passive movements. Mechanical symptoms like locking, instability, or "giving way" point to an articular origin of pain. The clinician also has to be alive to the possibility of "referred pain." For example, hip pain may be referred to the knee.

Table 1.1 Identifying the site of musculoskeletal pain

Disease	Distinguishing characteristics
Arthritis	Joint swelling and tenderness. Pain often diffuse, deep-seated. Pain increases on both active and passive movements
Bursitis	Point tenderness over the anatomical site. Pain more on active than passive movements
Tendinitis	Linear, tender swelling of the tendon sheath. Stretching the tendon induces pain. Tendon rub may be palpable/audible
Enthesitis	Pain at the tendon insertion site. A characteristic feature of spondarthritides
Bone pains	Deep-seated. Tenderness can be elicited by pressing bones
Muscle pains	Diffuse, not well localized. Tenderness on squeezing muscles
Fibromyalgia	Diffuse pain with characteristic tender points
Growing pains	Benign leg pains, typically bilateral, in children 8–12 years. Usually, a diagnosis of exclusion.

1.2.2 Inflammatory or Noninflammatory?

One of the fundamental concepts in Rheumatology is to differentiate inflammatory rheumatic diseases like RA, SpA, lupus, etc. from noninflammatory disorders like osteoarthritis (OA) since the management is radically different (Fig. 1.1). Inflamed joints stiffen or "gel" after periods of inactivity and tend to loosen with use. In contrast, noninflammatory or mechanical joint pain improves with rest and is typically associated with use-related pain. Table 1.2 outlines the points that help in clinical differentiation. Even patients with inflammatory joint disease can develop mechanical symptoms, for example, secondary OA of knees in a patient with RA.

1.2.3 Pattern Recognition

Joint pains are a near-universal feature of rheumatic or MSK diseases. However, other features outlined in Fig. 1.2 like chronology, number/

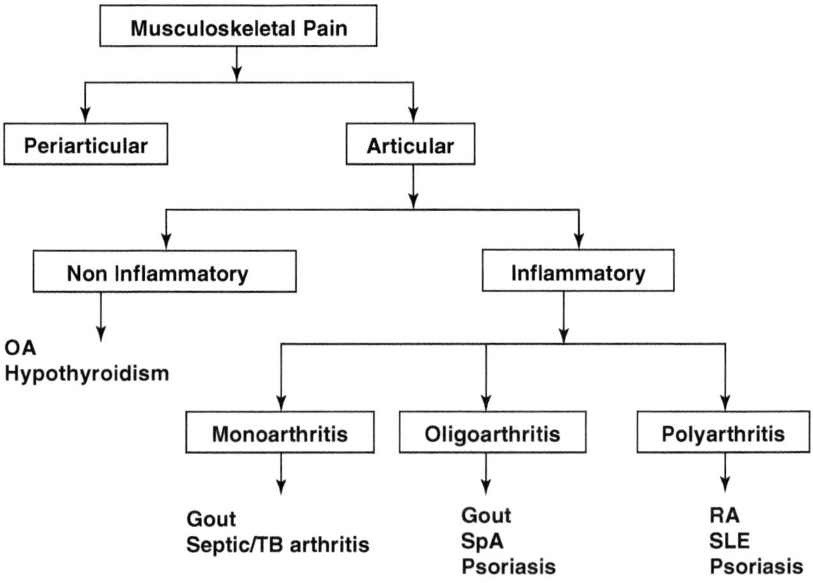

Fig. 1.1 Approach to a patient with musculoskeletal pain. *SpA* spondarthritides, *RA* rheumatoid arthritis, *TB* tuberculosis, *SLE* systemic lupus erythematosus

Table 1.2 Differentiating inflammatory from noninflammatory arthritis

	Inflammatory arthritis	Noninflammatory arthritis
Examples	RA, SpA, SLE	OA, trauma, hypothyroidism
Morning stiffness	>30 min	<30 min
Pain aggravation	On resting the joint	On moving the joint
Spontaneous flares	Common	Uncommon
Acute phase reactants like ESR, CRP	Increased	Normal

RA rheumatoid arthritis, *SpA* spondarthritides, *SLE* systemic lupus erythematosus, *OA* osteoarthritis, *ESR* erythrocyte sedimentation rate, *CRP* C reactive protein

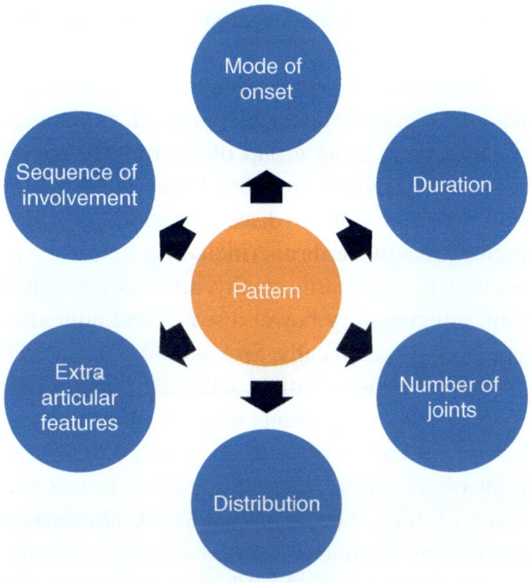

Fig. 1.2 Key features that aid pattern recognition

type/sequence of joints affected, symmetry, presence or absence of fever, extra-articular involvement, etc. give rise to a distinctive pattern that helps in making a diagnosis (Table 1.3). For example, an inflammatory polyarthritis in a young woman that is associated with fever and malar rash is highly likely to be lupus. Similarly, an insidiously developing arthritis associated with Raynaud's phenomenon and skin thickening and tightening suggests a diagnosis of systemic sclerosis (SSc). On occasions, especially at disease onset, the symptoms and signs may not fit into any one pattern, when the term "undifferentiated" arthritis is used. Over a period of time, the disease may resolve, evolve into a definitive entity, or stay "undifferentiated." It is because of this reason that management decisions in Rheumatology are based on organ involvement rather than diagnostic labels. Often, features of two or more MSK diseases may be present in the same patient when the term "overlap syndrome" is employed. The various features that aid pattern recognition are discussed in the below paragraphs (Table 1.3)

Table 1.3 Pattern recognition in arthritis

Mode of onset Acute Insidious
Duration Acute or self-limited Chronic
Number of affected joints Monoarthritis Oligoarthritis Polyarthritis
Distribution Symmetrical or asymmetrical Lower limbs versus upper limbs Small versus large joints Specific joints
Extra-articular features Fever Mucocutaneous lesions Eye Nodules
Sequence of involvement Intermittent Migratory Additive

1.2.3.1 Chronology

The mode of onset and duration of symptoms help in the differential diagnosis. Acute onset is seen with septic arthritis, reactive arthritis, viral arthritis, gout, or trauma. On the other hand, conditions like RA, SpA, and OA tend to be insidious in onset. Based upon duration, MSK complaints may be classified into acute (lasting <6 weeks) or chronic (lasting >6 weeks). Patients with acute, self-limited conditions like viral arthritis may require only a limited evaluation and follow-up. However, patients with symptoms lasting >6 weeks need detailed evaluation. Other groups of patients who merit detailed evaluation irrespective of symptom duration are patients with prominent constitutional/systemic symptoms, e.g., fever, weight loss, etc., older patients, and patients who exhibit multiple organ involvement. Deviations from the textbook picture like acute onset of RA are uncommon, but not unknown! As is said, exceptions prove the rule.

1.2.3.2 Number of Joints Affected

Arthritides are divided into monoarthritis (single joint involvement), oligoarthritis (affecting 2, 3, or 4 joints) [also known as pauciarticular disease], and polyarthritis (affecting ≥5 joints). The important conditions in each category are listed in Table 1.4. It is important to know the number of joints affected because it narrows down the diagnostic possibilities and helps the clinician in embarking upon investigations in a planned manner. The involvement of a single joint should prompt the clinician to consider crystal arthropathy (like gout) or septic arthritis. *A good rule of the thumb is to consider every case of monoarthritis as* ***infection*** *of the joint unless proven otherwise.* Joint aspiration and synovial fluid analysis are mandated in most such instances because overlooking septic arthritis is a serious error. Delay in treatment of infection can result in rapid joint destruction. Synovial fluid (SF) should be subjected to gross examination, total and differential leukocyte counts, Gram and Ziehl Neelsen staining, culture, and crystal studies. Protein and sugar estimations in synovial fluid, unlike CSF or pleural/peritoneal fluids, are of no value. Tests for mucin clot and viscosity are no longer performed. Polymerase chain reaction (PCR) for *Mycobacterium tuberculosis* in synovial specimens can be associated with false positives and should never be interpreted in isolation from clinical findings. The normal SF has a cell count of <200 WBC/mm^3, mostly mononuclear. The cell count in noninflammatory conditions like osteoarthritis is <2000 WBCs/mm^3 while the count in inflammatory conditions like RA and gout is >2000 WBCs/mm^3. Septic arthritis is associated with very high counts in the range of 100,000/mm^3 with >90% polymorphonuclear neutrophils. Crystal identification in SF is the gold standard for the diagnosis of gout and other crystal arthropathies.

The spondarthritides constitute the vast majority of oligoarthritides encountered in clinical practice. It is a big group of interrelated conditions where ankylosing spondylitis is the prototypic illness. Other disease entities in SpA include reactive arthritis (including Reiter's syndrome), psoriatic arthropathy, arthritis associated with inflammatory bowel disease, and nonradiographic SpA. Clinically, SpA should be suspected whenever a young patient <40 years (males outnumber females) presents with inflammatory low back pain and asymmetrical, lower limb, large joint oligoarthritis, that is, asymmetric involvement of hips, knees, or ankles. Enthesopathy (pain along tendinous insertion sites) is a characteristic feature of SpA. While dealing with low

Table 1.4 Differential diagnosis based on number of joints affected

Monoarthritis	Oligoarthritis	Polyarthritis
• Septic arthritis • Tuberculous arthritis • Gout and other crystal deposition diseases • Spondarthritides • Monoarticular onset of polyarticular disease[a]	• Gout • Juvenile idiopathic arthritis • Psoriatic arthropathy • Spondarthritides	• Rheumatoid arthritis • Psoriatic arthropathy • SLE • Systemic sclerosis • Juvenile idiopathic arthritis • Adult-onset Still's disease • Inflammatory bowel disease • Gout (rarely)

Gout presents most often as monoarthritis, less commonly as oligoarthritis, and rarely as polyarthritis. Juvenile idiopathic arthritis and psoriasis can cause both oligoarticular and polyarticular joint disease. Spondarthritides are characterized by inflammatory low back pain in addition to arthritis. *SLE* systemic lupus erythematosus

[a]Polyarticular nature of disease becomes apparent over time

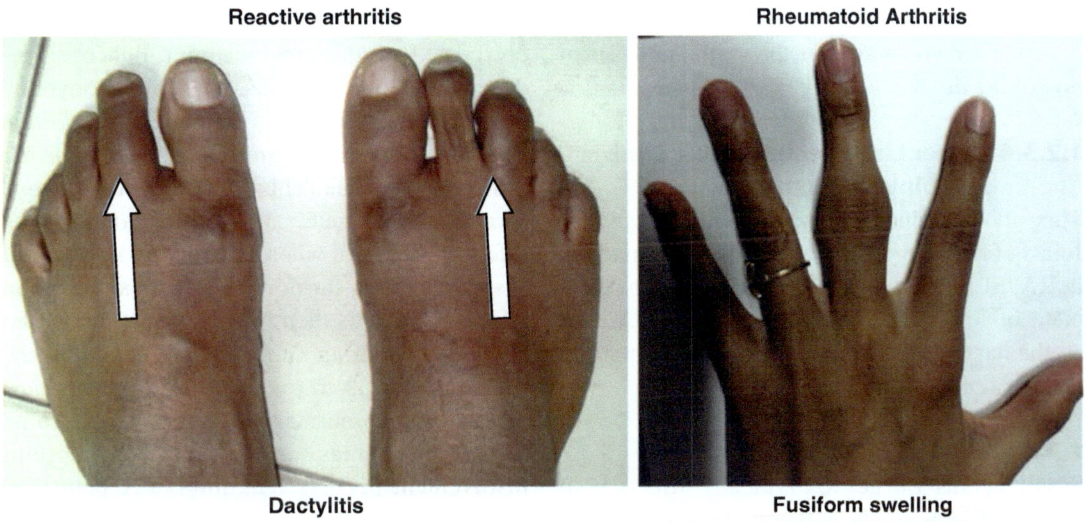

Fig. 1.3 Dactylitis in reactive arthritis versus fusiform swelling in rheumatoid arthritis

backache (LBA), it is clinically helpful to differentiate between mechanical and inflammatory low backache. Mechanical causes comprise more than 90% of cases of LBA. Inflammatory LBA, a typical feature of SpA, worsens after rest or prolonged sitting in the same posture, in contrast to mechanical causes like a prolapsed intervertebral disc, which improves on rest. Early morning stiffness, buttock ache, enthesitis, dactylitis, peripheral joint synovitis, and eye involvement, if present, support the diagnosis of SpA. Sacroiliitis is the characteristic radiologic hallmark of SpA. HLA B27 is present in a varying proportion of patients with SpA depending on the underlying condition. However, HLA B27 can be present in healthy individuals also. The presence of HLA B27 does not mean SpA, and conversely, the absence of HLA B27 does not rule out SpA. Nonradiographic SpA refers to patients where plain x-rays are normal, and the MRI reveals acute sacroiliitis in the form of bone marrow edema.

Another clinical feature with discriminant value is *sausage digit* or dactylitis seen in reactive arthritis or psoriatic arthropathy. Herein, the entire digit is diffusely swollen. This is clinically a very important point of distinction from joint diseases like RA, where only the joint gets swollen (fusiform or spindle-shaped swelling) and not the entire digit (Fig. 1.3).

The term polyarthritis refers to the involvement of more than four joints. It may be due to inflammatory causes like RA, SLE, psoriasis, SSc, JIA, rheumatic fever, adult-onset Still's disease, etc., or noninflammatory causes like OA. Hand examination is crucial in patients with polyarthritis, as explained below.

1.2.3.3 Symmetry

Symmetrical involvement refers to the affliction of the same joints on the right and left sides. Even in symmetrical involvement, mirror-image symmetry is not required. To clarify things, the involvement of right fourth, fifth, and left second metacarpophalangeal (MP) joints is deemed symmetrical involvement of MP joints. RA, SLE, SSc, and nodular osteoarthritis of hands are typical examples of symmetric polyarthritis. Gout and SpA are typically asymmetric oligoarthritides. Psoriasis can cause either asymmetric oligoarthritis or symmetric polyarthritis. The most important practical point is that a clinician should hesitate to give a diagnosis of RA if the disease is persistently asymmetrical. One important caveat is that treatment instituted early, as is done these days, may alter the textbook description of the disease.

1.2.3.4 Upper Limb Versus Lower Limb Joint Involvement

This offers a clue to the differential diagnosis. Joints of both upper and lower limbs are involved in RA, SLE, and psoriasis. Predominant involvement of lower limbs is seen in gout, SpA, and erythema nodosum, whereas, hemochromatosis preferentially affects joints of upper limbs.

1.2.3.5 Type of Joints Affected

Small Versus Large RA typically affects both small and large joints. Inflammatory, symmetric polyarthritis of small joints of hands like MP joints and proximal interphalangeal (PIP) joints is a characteristic feature of RA. Similarly, psoriasis, lupus, and SSc affect both small and large joints. In contrast, SpA affects large joints much more than smaller joints. Therefore, the typical pattern of joint involvement in SpA is asymmetric oligoarthritis of large joints of lower limbs. Thus, the pattern in RA and SpA is quite different but distinctive, permitting bedside recognition.

Specific Joints These can point toward the nature of arthritic illness, e.g., distal interphalangeal (DIP) joint involvement is characteristic of OA, while DIP joints are spared in RA. Other conditions that give rise to DIP joint involvement are psoriasis and scleroderma (SSc). The involvement of the first carpometacarpal joint is typical of OA, while the ankle and shoulder are rarely involved in primary OA.

Spine Spinal involvement other than the cervical spine is rare in RA. In contrast, inflammatory low back pain is a characteristic feature of SpA.

1.2.3.6 Sequence or Pattern of Involvement

The three common patterns of joint involvement are intermittent, additive, and migratory. *Intermittent arthritis* is episodic, and the patient may be totally asymptomatic in between the episodes. Examples include gout, Behcet's syndrome, Reactive arthritis, intermittent hydrarthrosis, and palindromic rheumatism. *Additive arthritis* is one where more and more joints are afflicted with time. This is seen with RA, SpA, psoriasis, OA, etc. *Migratory polyarthritis* refers to a pattern wherein pain and swelling in a specific joint starts rapidly and subsides in 24–36 h; arthritis then picks up new joints. The difference from an *additive pattern* is that the previously involved joints in the *migratory pattern* return to normal as new joints become involved, whereas, in the former, the joint involvement persists. The migratory pattern is seen in rheumatic fever, gonococcal arthritis, viral disease, sarcoidosis, and bacterial endocarditis. Palindromic rheumatism refers to a pattern where attacks of arthritis remit and recur. The patient is normal in between these attacks. The arthritic and remission phases last for a variable period of time. Some patients with palindromic rheumatism may evolve, over a period of time, into RA.

These patterns may not be seen in the classical form due to treatment received by the patient. Also, these patterns may coexist in the same patient. However, when one pattern dominates, it may suggest a particular diagnosis.

One of the commonly overlooked diagnoses in India is juvenile idiopathic arthritis (JIA), formerly known as juvenile rheumatoid arthritis (JRA) or juvenile chronic arthritis (JCA), in children below the age of 16 years. There is a tendency to label all joint pains in children as rheumatic fever with undue reliance on one laboratory marker, that is, elevated ASO (antistreptolysin O) titers. The joint pains in rheumatic fever (RF) are migratory, affect large joints, and tend to subside over 6–12 weeks, with or without treatment. The major brunt is borne by the heart. In contrast, arthritis in JIA tends to be additive, persistent, and may involve small or large joints. The presence of fixed deformities and erosions strongly militates against a diagnosis of rheumatic fever since arthritis in RF is most often nondeforming.

1.2.3.7 Extra-Articular Features

Features that may be associated with joint involvement like fever, skin lesions, Raynaud's, nodules, etc. play a role in the differential diagnosis (Tables 1.5, 1.6, 1.7 and 1.8). Fever, along with arthritis, narrows down the diagnostic possibilities to SLE, systemic-onset JIA (Still's disease), vasculitis, infective endocarditis, rheumatic fever, and adult-onset Still's disease. Although malaise is very common in RA, fever of moderate to high grade is not seen with RA and should necessitate a search for other causes.

Table 1.5 Differential diagnosis of joint pains associated with fever

• SLE
• JIA (systemic-onset type)—Still's disease
• Infective endocarditis
• Rheumatic fever
• Vasculitis
• Adult-onset Still's disease

SLE systemic lupus erythematosus, *JIA* juvenile idiopathic arthritis

Table 1.6 Differential diagnosis of joint pains associated with nodules

• Rheumatoid arthritis
• Tophaceous gout
• Rheumatic fever
• Multicentric reticulohistiocytosis
• Sarcoidosis
• Erythema nodosum
• Vasculitides
• Infective endocarditis

Table 1.7 Arthritides associated with Mucocutaneous lesions

• SLE
• Gonococcal arthritis
• Reactive arthritis (including Reiter's syndrome)
• Behcet's syndrome
• Erythema nodosum
• Psoriasis
• Vasculitides
• Systemic sclerosis

Table 1.8 Rheumatic conditions associated with Raynaud's phenomenon

• Systemic sclerosis (commonest)
• Mixed connective tissue disease
• Systemic lupus erythematosus
• Sjogren's syndrome
• Rheumatoid Arthritis
• Cryoglobulinemia
• Dermatomyositis
• Antiphospholipid syndrome

Mucosal or cutaneous lesions are seen in SLE, psoriasis, Behcet's syndrome, reactive arthritis, SSc, erythema nodosum, vasculitides, gonococcal arthritis, etc. The malar rash of SLE is characteristic and can be appreciated even in dark-skinned individuals. Gonococcal infection usually occurs in young, sexually active adults, and the skin lesions comprise a pustule with an erythematous base. Psoriasis has a spectrum of skin changes. Occasionally, these are confined to hidden areas like the umbilicus or natal cleft. Nail changes of psoriasis can easily be masked by nail paint in female patients.

The type of eye involvement may also vary with different eye diseases. RA usually causes keratitis or scleritis in contrast to uveitis seen in SpA. Conditions causing nodules in a patient with arthritis include RA, OA (Heberden and Bouchard nodes), tophaceous gout, rheumatic fever, multicentric reticulohistiocytosis, sarcoidosis, erythema nodosum, vasculitides, etc. (Fig. 1.4). However, the associated features make the pattern recognition possible. For example, carditis, migratory polyarthritis, erythema marginatum, and chorea in RF hold the clue to the diagnosis. Rheumatoid nodules are uncommon in Indian patients with RA when compared to western patients. Similarly, nodular OA of hands is less often encountered in India as compared to Caucasians.

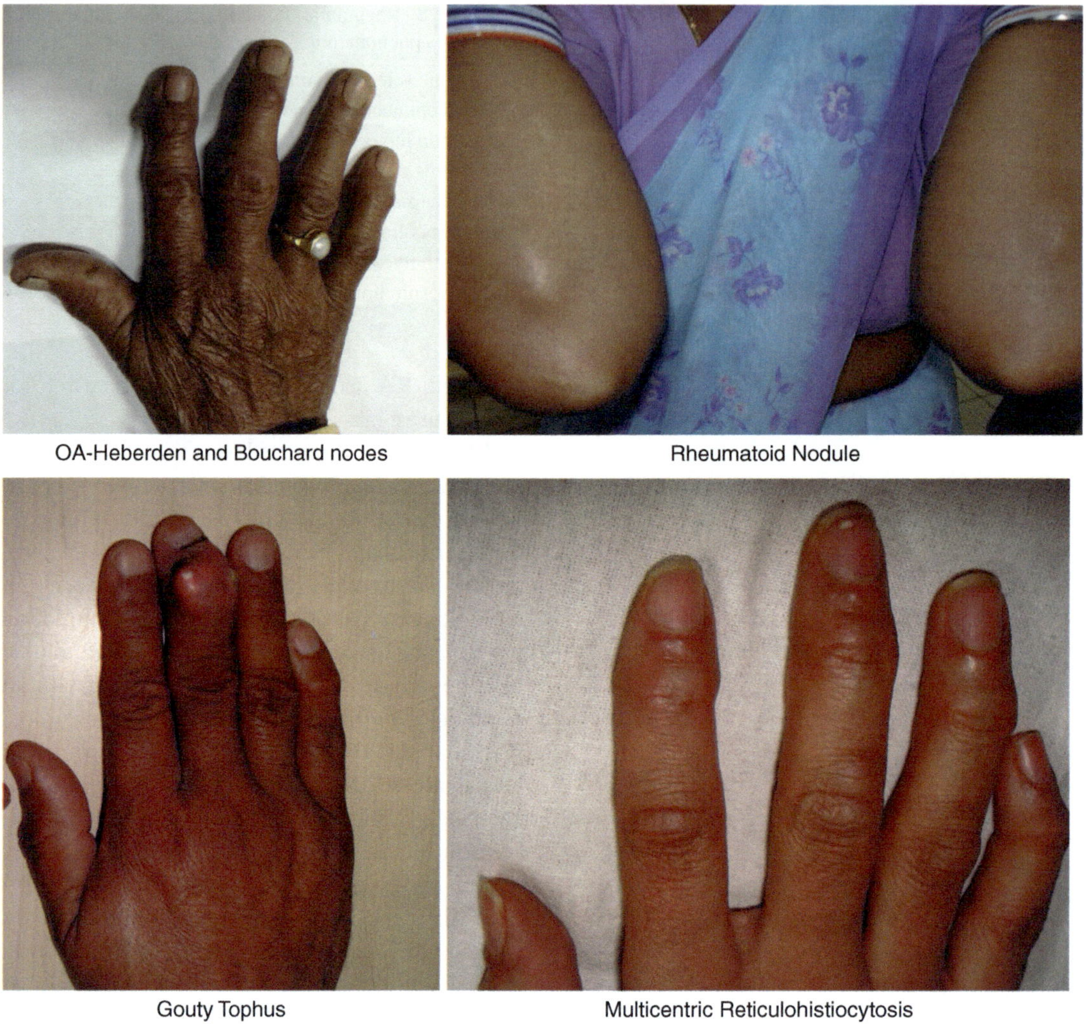

Fig. 1.4 Arthritis with nodules

1.3 Conclusions

The approach to MSK complaints is predominantly clinical and relies on pattern recognition. A good history provides as much as 80% of diagnostic information, with physical examination and investigations contributing only 15% and 5%, respectively. The evolution of distinct patterns may take time, and periodic reassessment can be rewarding. Rheumatology is "high touch," not "high tech."

Suggested Reading

1. Handa R. Basic considerations of rheumatology. In: Kamath SA, Ed-in-chief. API textbook of medicine. 11th ed. Mumbai: Association of Physicians of India; 2019. p. 485–488

2 Laboratory Investigations in Rheumatology

2.1 Introduction

Rheumatology is primarily a clinical subspecialty. A good history and thorough physical examination enable the physician to make a correct diagnosis in most, if not all, instances. Laboratory tests serve only as adjuncts. However, it is not uncommon to come across physicians ordering so-called "arthritis/autoimmune panels" only to be baffled by results, like the absence of rheumatoid factor in a patient with suspected rheumatoid arthritis. This chapter provides an overview of common lab investigations in *Rheumatology*. Some other laboratory investigations are dealt with in the respective chapters.

2.2 Acute Phase Reactants (APRs)

These investigations play an important role in differentiating inflammatory from noninflammatory rheumatic diseases. Commonly employed acute phase reactants include erythrocyte sedimentation rate (ESR) and C-reactive protein (CRP). Platelet elevation and reversal of albumin globulin ratio are also frequently encountered as a part of the acute phase response. Plasma viscosity, another parameter, is less commonly utilized.

2.2.1 Erythrocyte Sedimentation Rate (ESR)

ESR measures the rate of fall of red blood cells (RBCs) in a vertical column of anticoagulated blood over 1 h. Inflammation induces overproduction of plasma proteins like fibrinogen, immunoglobulins, etc. which react with the RBC membrane causing them to stick together in stacks (*rouleaux*). Stacks of RBCs, being heavier than individual RBCs, fall rapidly to the bottom of the column. ESR is influenced by many conditions like age, fasting, smoking, infections, anemia, pregnancy, etc. In men, the upper limit of ESR can be obtained by dividing age in years by 2. For women, it is age+10 divided by 2. Some individuals may demonstrate a high ESR without any obvious reason. Others may exhibit normal or modestly increased ESR despite active inflammatory disease. ESR may decrease in conditions like congestive heart failure, cryoglobulinemia, hypofibrinogenemia, macrophage activation syndrome, etc. The preferred method for ESR measurement is Westergren. ESR rise is slow compared to CRP, and the normalization may take weeks, unlike CRP.

2.2.2 C-Reactive Protein (CRP)

C-reactive protein (CRP) is an acute-phase protein produced by the liver. It is a member of the pentraxin family of proteins. It reacts with the

R. Handa, *Clinical Rheumatology*, https://doi.org/10.1007/978-981-33-4885-1_2

capsular polysaccharide (C-polysaccharide) of pneumococcus, and hence the name. It is widely employed as a marker of inflammation. It also shows a rise in infection, trauma, necrosis, malignancy, and allergic reactions. Unlike ESR, levels of CRP are not influenced by age, gender, fasting, anemia, plasma proteins, smoking, or diurnal variations. CRP rises within 4–6 h of the stimulus, peaks in 36–48 h, and returns to baseline in 3–7 days. ESR, on the other hand, rises slowly and normalizes slowly.

The high-sensitivity C-reactive protein (hs-CRP) test is more sensitive than a standard test. Conventional CRP measures concentrations of 3–5 mg/L, whereas hs-CRP measures levels around 0.3 mg/L. In clinical practice, hs-CRP is largely employed to define an increased risk of cardiovascular disease. Low-risk, average-risk, and high-risk cutoffs are <1, 1–3, and >3 mg/L. Indians may have higher basal hs-CRP levels. The use of hs-CRP in rheumatology practice tends to reveal inordinately high levels in patients with an inflammatory disease. Even patients in clinical remission with normal CRP levels may have hs-CRP levels that are way above normal. Thus, the routine use of hs-CRP in rheumatology practice is not recommended at this point in time.

2.2.3 Other Acute Phase Reactants

Platelets may rise as part of acute-phase response-reactive thrombocytosis due to IL-6 stimulating megakaryocytopoiesis in the bone marrow. Other acute phase reactants include ferritin (very high levels are seen in Adult Still's disease), alkaline phosphatase, and serum amyloid-A protein. Some proteins like albumin decrease in concentration during inflammation. This leads to the reversal of albumin to globulin (A/G) ratio to <1 (normal A/G ratio is 1 or >1).

2.3 Autoantibodies

Several rheumatic diseases are associated with the production of antibodies to intrinsic antigens (autoantibodies). Some autoantibodies, like antinuclear antibodies (ANA), have high sensitivity making than a valuable screening test for connective tissue disease (CTD). Others, like antibodies to double-stranded deoxyribonucleic acid (ds DNA), are highly specific and used for disease confirmation rather than detection. Of note, several infections may trigger transient autoantibodies of no clinical significance. It is important to appreciate that the mere presence of autoantibodies does not translate into the diagnosis of an autoimmune disease. Clinical correlation is mandatory.

2.3.1 Rheumatoid Factor (RF)

Rheumatoid factor is one of the most frequently ordered tests in the workup of a patient with joint symptoms. However, it is imperative to point out that rheumatoid arthritis (RA) is purely a clinical diagnosis. RA and RF can exist independently of one another. One does not require the presence of RF to make a diagnosis of RA since as many as 15–20% of patients with RA are seronegative, that is, RF is absent. Seronegative RA is diagnosed only on clinical grounds. RF can be present in a variety of conditions other than RA and, therefore, RF performs poorly as a screening test for RA due to the high frequency of false-positive results. Some of the other conditions associated with a positive RF include old age (RF is present in ~5% healthy elderly people), tuberculosis, infective endocarditis, viral hepatitis, sarcoidosis, systemic lupus erythematosus (SLE), scleroderma, etc. (Table 2.1).

RA is a diagnosis that should be considered in patients presenting with bilateral, symmetrical, inflammatory, polyarthritis affecting hand joints, and where the duration of symptoms exceeds 6 weeks. Careful attention to this definition helps the clinician to avoid mistakes. Duration exceeding 6 weeks enables the exclusion of viral arthritides, which are self-limited. The current 2010 classification criteria of RA have done away with the insistence of 6 weeks provided the score is ≥6/10, and there is no better explanation for the synovitis. A duration >6 weeks fetches a score of 1 while a shorter duration does not exclude clas-

Table 2.1 Diseases associated with a positive RF

Condition
• RA
• Elderly people
• Other chronic inflammatory rheumatic diseases
– Primary Sjogren's syndrome
– Mixed cryoglobulinemia
– SLE
– Systemic sclerosis
– Mixed connective tissue disease
• Infections
– Infective endocarditis
– Tuberculosis
– Viral hepatitis
• Miscellaneous conditions
– Sarcoidosis
– Idiopathic interstitial fibrosis
– Autoimmune hepatitis

sification as RA. At the bedside, the thumb rule of 6 weeks is a sturdy tool to prevent overdiagnosis despite not being sacrosanct anymore. In the absence of clinical involvement of small joints of hands, one should be extremely reluctant to make a diagnosis of RA.

The commonly available tests detect IgM rheumatoid factor (RF is an autoantibody directed against Fc of IgG). Detection of IgG or IgA rheumatoid factors is seldom required in clinical practice. Common test methodologies include latex agglutination, enzyme-linked immunosorbent assay (ELISA), and nephelometry. In the latex agglutination method, latex beads are coated with human IgG and mixed with test serum. RF, if present, will cause agglutination. In the original Rose-Waaler test, sheep RBCs coated with rabbit IgG were used. Since rabbit IgG bears fewer reactive epitopes, the sensitivity was lower while the specificity was higher. Rose-Waaler is not employed these days. Nephelometry and ELISA are more sensitive but expensive. This explains why in patients with low titers of RF, some labs give a positive result while others, using latex agglutination, give a negative result. Awareness of test methodology is vital for correct interpretation.

There is no inviolable "cutoff" or titer of RF above which a patient is deemed to have RA. The cutoff above which a sample is positive for a test like RF is generally one that should give negative results in at least 95% of healthy normal controls. In other words, no more than 5% of the healthy population should exhibit RF titers above this level. More important than the absolute cutoff is the clinical context. RF should always be interpreted in light of the clinical picture. While higher titers constitute one of the poor prognostic factors, titers of RF do not parallel response to treatment. Repeated measurements give no meaningful information and should not be obtained.

Occasionally, the clinician is confronted by an asymptomatic individual carrying a report positive for RF. Such individuals should be assessed clinically, and treatment instituted only if there is evidence of active RA at the bedside. Individuals negative for clinical arthritis should be followed up for the development of RA since serology may precede clinical disease by months to years. Intervention based only on serologic evidence sans clinical disease is not recommended.

2.3.2 Antibodies to Cyclic Citrullinated Peptide (Anti-CCP Antibodies)

Antibodies to cyclic citrullinated peptide (CCP), also abbreviated as ACPA (anti-citrullinated peptide antibodies) have emerged as an important marker for RA. The earlier tests for antifilaggrin antibodies (filaggrin contains a large amount of citrulline) like antiperinuclear factor (APF) using human buccal mucosa cells and antikeratin antibodies (AKA) using rat esophagus sections were cumbersome and have been replaced by ELISA to detect anti-CCP antibodies.

Anti-CCP antibodies are more specific than RF for the detection of RA. These should not be employed for screening since the specificity is far higher than sensitivity. A recent meta-analysis reported that the pooled sensitivity, specificity, and positive and negative likelihood ratios for anti-CCP antibody were 67% (95% CI 62%–72%), 95% (CI, 94%–97%), 12.46 (CI, 9.72–15.98), and 0.36 (CI, 0.31–0.42), respectively. For IgM RF, the values were 69% (CI, 65%–73%),

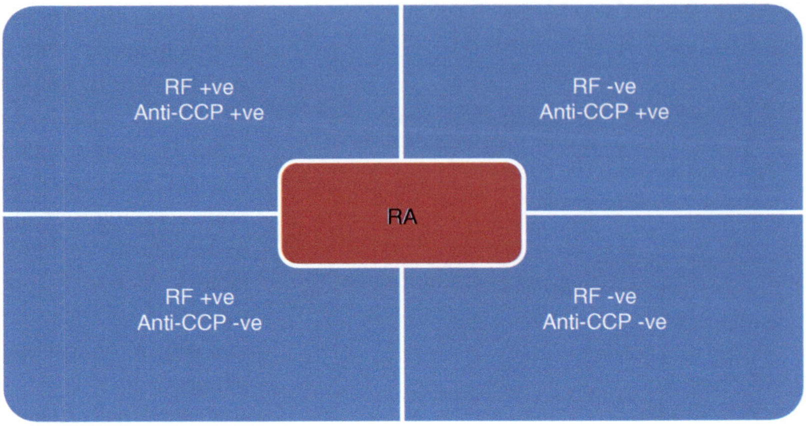

Fig. 2.1 Serologic subsets of rheumatoid arthritis. *RF* rheumatoid factor, *anti-CCP* antibody to cyclic citrullinated peptide, *+ve* positive, *−ve* negative

85% (CI, 82%–88%), 4.86 (CI, 3.95–5.97), and 0.38 (CI, 0.33–0.44). Anti-CCP antibodies are also a predictor of erosive disease and portend a poor prognosis.

Patients with RA may be positive for both RA and anti-CCP, negative for both, or show the presence of one of these antibodies (Fig. 2.1). Serologic status does not influence treatment.

2.3.3 Antinuclear Antibodies (ANA)

The detection of ANA has replaced the "LE cell" test, which is now only of historical importance. ANA testing is used primarily to screen for connective tissue diseases. It is also one of the entry points for the 2019 classification criteria for lupus. The diagnosis of SLE is based on the presence of several clinical and laboratory features, not just ANA. Many conditions apart from SLE can be associated with positive ANA like systemic sclerosis (SSc), MCTD (mixed connective tissue disease), polymyositis, etc. (Table 2.2). Low titer ANA may be seen in healthy young women and relatives of patients with lupus. The sensitivity of ANA for the diagnosis of SLE is 99% and specificity 90%. In an unselected population, the positive predictive value of ANA for the detection of SLE is only 30–40%, while the negative predictive value is greater than 99%. Thus, about two-thirds of patients with positive ANA test results will not have SLE. A negative ANA virtually rules out SLE because ANA-negative SLE is very rare in clinical practice (less than 5% of patients with SLE are negative for ANA on indirect immunofluorescence). With the use of HEp-2000® cells that are transfected to hyper express the 60kD SS-A/Ro antigen, the frequency of ANA-negative SLE is even lower. Rarely, SLE patients, after years of treatment, become seronegative.

Table 2.2 Conditions associated with positive ANA

Autoimmune rheumatic diseases	Non-rheumatic diseases
SLE	Autoimmune hepatitis
SSc	Primary biliary cirrhosis
Sjogren's	Myasthenia gravis
MCTD	Infectious mononucleosis
Inflammatory myositis	5% healthy young women
RA	Infections (transient positivity)
Pauciarticular JIA	Drugs like procainamide, hydralazine, penicillamine, isoniazid, anti-TNF drugs like infliximab and etanercept, chlorpromazine, methyldopa, anticonvulsants, etc.

20–30% of first-degree relatives of patients with SLE may show low titer ANA

ANA should be ordered in patients (especially females) with multisystem illness with features like photosensitive skin rash, alopecia, joint pains, and fever. The test is not useful for evaluating the course of SLE, and titers do not reflect changes in disease activity. Certain ANA subsets such as dsDNA (sensitivity 50–60%) and Sm (sensitivity 30%) are highly specific for SLE.

There are two common methods of doing ANA-Indirect immunofluorescence (IIF) and ELISA. While ELISA offers the ease of automated assay with little interobserver difference, IIF is far more sensitive. This is because the ELISA systems identify only some of the several antigen–antibody specificities known. With IIF, all nuclear and cytoplasmic antigens in a cell, characterized and not so well characterized, are targeted. With the refinement of ELISA techniques, this might change in the future. This is in contrast to the situation in antineutrophil cytoplasmic antibody (ANCA) testing, where ELISA is now recommended over IIF.

The ANA report by IIF includes both a titer and a pattern. Most labs screen samples at a starting dilution of 1:40 or 1:80. Samples identified as positive at the screening dilution are titered out to endpoint dilution. The results are generally reported in serial doubling dilutions like 1:40, 1:80, 1:160. 1:320, 1:640, 1:1280, etc. The screening dilution of ANA that should be considered for cutoff is a matter of debate. It has been recommended that the screening dilution be defined by a cutoff at the 95th percentile, that is, 95% of healthy individuals should be negative at that dilution. Raising the cutoff improves specificity but lowers sensitivity. The 2019 classification criteria of SLE require ANA at a titer of ≥1:80. The titers of ANA, unlike dsDNA, do not correlate with disease activity. Repeat estimations do not confer any meaningful information.

The pattern refers to the visual characteristics of the fluorescence. These give some idea about the target antigen and the underlying disease. Although patterns may add to the specificity of the test, they possess variable and usually limited sensitivity. The classical patterns include homogeneous, speckled, nucleolar, and centromere (Fig. 2.2 and Table 2.3). It is now apparent that this is a gross oversimplification (vide infra). The association between HEp-2 IIFA patterns and the distinct diseases should be tempered by the clinical context. The pattern of ANA on IIF does not affect clinical decision-making.

Automated systems that incorporate slide processing and reading are now available. These obviate the need for a darkroom. Digital images from different areas of the slide are acquired, and the fluorescence intensity is measured. The pre-programmed computer algorithm reads the pattern and interprets the fluorescence intensities in the context of known ANA patterns. Ideally, a trained laboratory person should confirm the computer-generated result.

2.3.4 ANA or Anti-cellular Antibodies (ACA)?

The introduction of Human epithelial type 2 (HEp-2) cells as the substrate for ANA IIF led to the recognition that IIF reveals patterns other than nuclear. The two additional patterns are called cytoplasmic and mitotic. Many of the laboratories in the past were omitting to mention anything other than nuclear. The cytoplasmic staining would get reported as negative ANA. It became increasingly evident that the term ANA is actually a misnomer and restrictive where the dichotomous outcome negative or positive may be an oversimplification that overlooks other cellular compartments—cytoplasm and mitotic apparatus. To reflect this changed thinking, it has been suggested that the term anti-cellular antibodies replace ANA to encompass the wider spectrum of these autoantibodies. However, a change in the acronym ANA that has been in usage for more than six decades has implications like a rewording of the existing guidelines, criteria, and coding/reimbursement issues and is difficult to implement.

The International Consensus on ANA Patterns (ICAP) initiative started in 2014 as a workshop

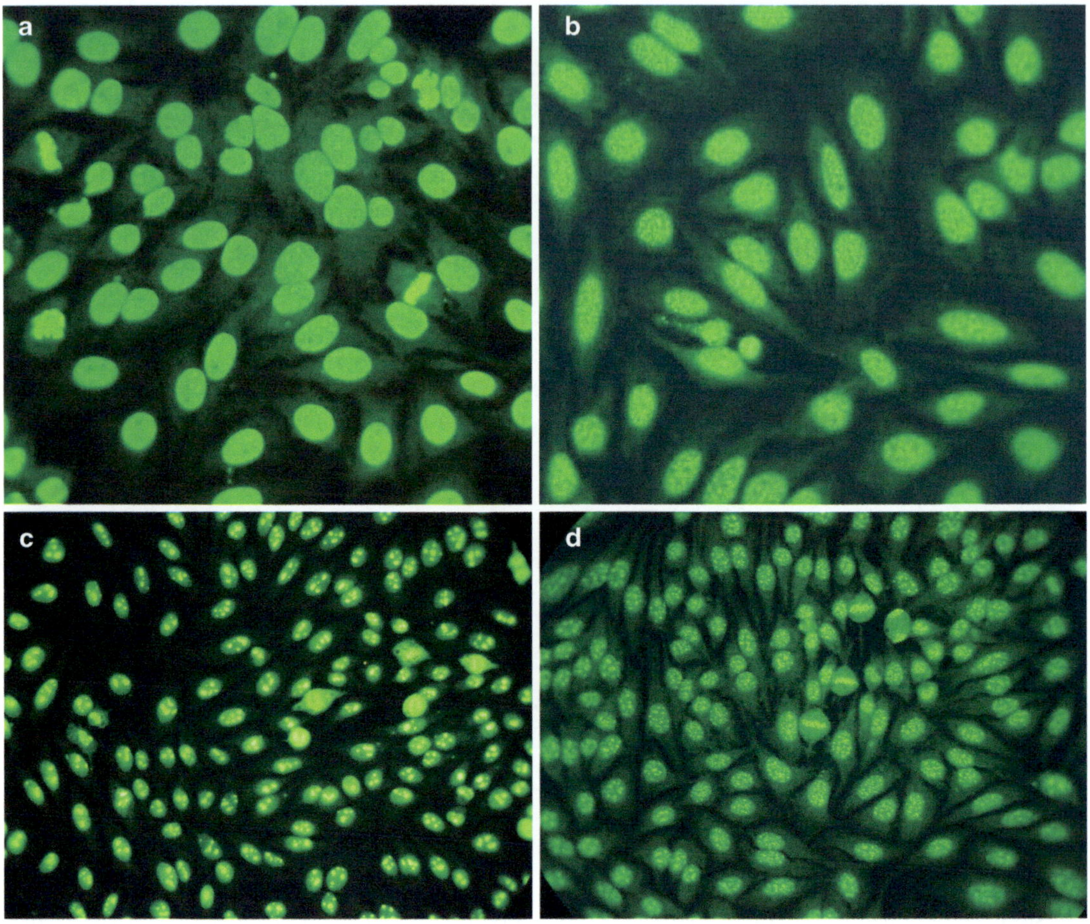

Fig. 2.2 (**a**) Homogeneous pattern, (**b**) speckled pattern, (**c**) nucleolar pattern, (**d**) centromere pattern. Courtesy: Dr. Pravin Hissaria, Adelaide

Table 2.3 Classical ANA patterns

Pattern	Characteristic	Target antigens	Disease association
Homogeneous	Diffuse uniform staining of entire nucleus	dsDNA, histone	SLE, drug induced lupus, JIA
Speckled	Fine and coarse speckles of staining scattered throughout nucleus	Extractable nuclear antigens	SLE, Sjogren's syndrome, MCTD, Polymyositis/dermatomyositis, SSc /PM overlap
Nucleolar	Staining of nucleoles inside the nucleus	RNA polymerase III, PM-Scl	Diffuse SSc, SSc/PM overlap
Centromere	Staining along the chromosomes	Centromere proteins A, B, C	Limited SSc, Primary biliary cirrhosis

parallel to the 12th International Workshop on Autoimmunity and Autoantibodies (IWAA) in Sao Paulo, Brazil. The ICAP initiative, in its last publication, has listed 29 distinct patterns on IIF assay (IIFA) (Fig. 2.3). All patterns are assigned an alphanumeric AC code (anti-cellular pattern):

(A) Nuclear HEp-2 IIFA patterns: 15 patterns viz. AC 1-14 and AC 29
(B) Cytoplasmic HEp-2 IIFA patterns: 9 patterns viz. AC-15–AC-23
(C) Mitotic HEp-2 IIFA patterns: 5 patterns viz. AC 24-28

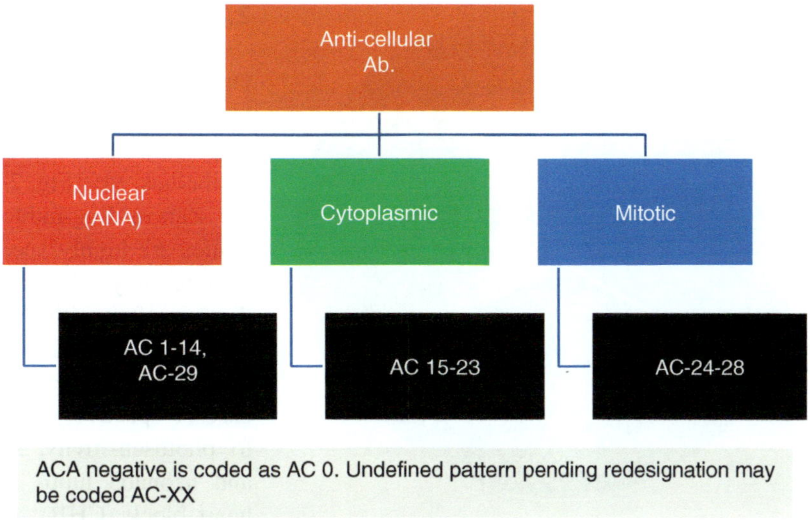

Fig. 2.3 Changing concepts of ANA

An interim category has been proposed AC-XX (a pattern not yet defined by any of the current ICAP AC patterns as a transitional solution to accommodate undefined HEp-2 IIFA patterns that will eventually get redesignated.

Some healthy individuals may have autoantibodies on HEp-2 IIFA. The pattern best associated with apparently healthy individuals is the nuclear-dense, fine-speckled pattern (AC-2) if the specificity is confirmed as monospecific for DFS70.

The IIFA patterns are not mutually exclusive. Mixed patterns may be encountered. In the case of mixed patterns, the reporting mentions nuclear patterns first followed by cytoplasmic and then mitotic patterns. Each pattern is directly followed by the respective titer. According to this nomenclature, the nuclear pattern is mentioned first even when the antibody level of the cytoplasmic pattern is higher. Alternate nomenclature systems suggest that within each category, i.e., nuclear, cytoplasmic, and mitotic, the pattern with the highest titer be mentioned first. This is an evolving field.

Many smaller laboratories doing clinical work may not be able to achieve this degree of sophistication. Also, it may not be required in routine clinical practice. Because of this, ICAP has differentiated basic "competent-level" reporting from more comprehensive "expert-level" reporting.

2.3.5 Antibodies to ENA (Extractable Nuclear Antigens)

ANA is a generic term for antibodies that target a variety of nuclear (cellular) antigens. ANA-positive individuals may need confirmation of the antigen type by determination of antibodies to ENA—"extractable nuclear antigens." These proteins are known as "extractable" because they can be removed from cell nuclei using saline. The important ones include Ro, La, Sm, RNP, Scl-70, and Jo1. Anti-ENA should be ordered only in ANA-positive individuals. ELISA-based kits are widely used for anti-ENA antibody testing. Several companies also offer line immunoblot tests where as many as 15–20 antigens like RNP/Sm, Sm, SS-A, Ro-52, SS-B, Scl-70, PM-Scl, Jo-1, centromere protein B, PCNA, dsDNA, nucleosomes, histones, ribosomal P-proteins, AMA M2, etc. can be detected conveniently in one go. The purified antigens are deposited as bands onto nitrocellulose strips, and the bound antibodies are detected after staining by an enzyme-catalyzed substrate reaction

2.3.6 Antibodies to Double Stranded Deoxyribonucleic Acid (dsDNA)

The sensitivity of this test in the diagnosis of SLE is only about 60%, while the specificity

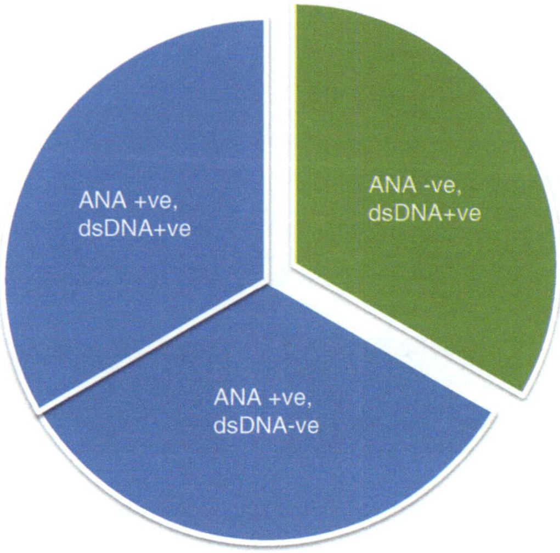

Fig. 2.4 Clinical scenarios of ANA and dsDNA. The scenarios in blue are plausible, the scenario in green is likely false positive

is very high (>99%). It should not be used as a screening test for the diagnosis of SLE. The major utility is in confirmation of the diagnosis of lupus in ANA-positive individuals. Unlike ANA, dsDNA levels generally correlate with disease activity, especially in lupus nephritis. In some patients, the dsDNA levels may not parallel disease activity, the so-called "clinico-serologic discordance." In such cases, the dictum is to treat the patient and not chase the dsDNA levels. While asking for dsDNA levels, one should be aware of the laboratory cutoff because different ELISA kits have different cutoff values and results from different kits are not comparable. Apart from ELISA, dsDNA antibodies can be detected by Farr assay and Crithidia lucilae assay. ELISA may give false-positive results due to contamination by single-stranded (ss) DNA. Three scenarios are encountered in clinical practice (Fig. 2.4). One should be extremely reluctant to accept a diagnosis of SLE when ANA on IIF is negative, and dsDNA is positive by ELISA—likely a false-positive.

2.3.7 Other Autoantibodies

Other autoantibodies seen in lupus include anti-histone antibodies, anti-Smith antibodies, anti-Ro, anti-La antibodies, antinucleosome antibodies, etc. (Fig. 2.5). Antihistone antibodies are seen in drug-induced SLE. Anti-Smith antibodies are highly specific but seen in ~30% of patients only. These correlate with more severe disease, often with CNS involvement and vasculitis. Anti-Ro (anti-SSA) and anti-La (anti-SSB) antibodies are seen in ~40% and ~15% of SLE cases, respectively. Anti-Ro antibodies are linked to photosensitivity, subacute cutaneous lupus, and neonatal lupus syndrome with congenital heart block (CHB). Anti-La antibodies too are seen in CHB. Anti-Ro and Anti-La antibodies are also seen in Sjogren's syndrome. Anti-U1-RNP antibodies are seen in ~30% of SLE patients, correlate with Raynaud's phenomenon, swollen fingers, arthritis, and myositis. Anti-U1-RNP antibodies are the defining feature of MCTD.

Recent data reveal that antinucleosome antibodies can serve as a useful parameter for the assessment of disease activity or renal involvement in SLE. The nucleosome is the structural unit of chromatin and consists of a segment of dsDNA coiled around a histone core. There is evidence to suggest that nucleosomes play an important role as the driving autoantigen in SLE. Serologically active, clinically quiescent patients with renal flares may demonstrate high antinucleosome antibody titers.

2.3.8 Antibody Subsets in Systemic Sclerosis (SSc)

ANA is seen in more than 95% of patients with systemic sclerosis. Several scleroderma-specific antibodies have been described. Antibodies specific to limited SSc include anticentromere (ACA), Th/To, Pm/Scl, and U1-RNP antibodies. Antibodies specific to diffuse SSc include

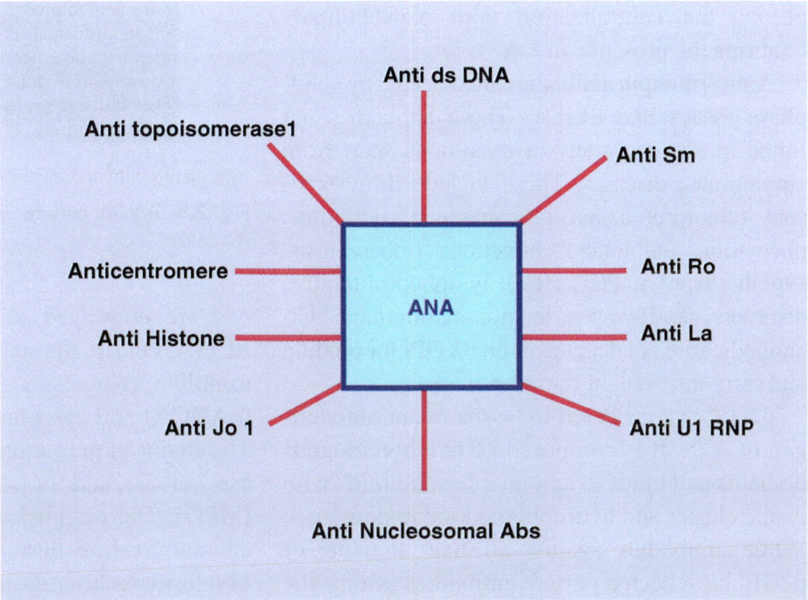

Fig. 2.5 Clinically important ANA subsets

anti-topoisomerase 1 (Scl 70), anti-RNA polymerase III, anti-U3 RNP (anti-fibrillarin) antibodies. These antibodies are usually present at the onset of symptoms and switch from one antibody to a different one during the course of the disease is rare. The distribution of these antibodies varies in different population groups. The frequency and severity of organ involvement in different antibody subsets are different. The scleroderma-specific antibodies are, in general, infrequent in other connective tissue diseases. ACA is directed against protein antigens in the kinetochore region of the chromosomes and is present in 60–80% of patients with limited cutaneous SSc and <5% of patients with diffuse cutaneous SSc. Anti-topoisomerase 1 antibodies are seen in nearly 40% of patients with diffuse cutaneous SSc and <10% of patients with limited cutaneous SSc. Anti-RNA polymerase III is seen in 4–20% of patients with diffuse cutaneous SSc. Anti-U1-RNP antibodies are seen in 5–10% of patients with limited cutaneous SSc and almost all patients with MCTD.

2.3.9 Antiphospholipid Antibodies (aPL)

This is a vast and heterogeneous family of autoantibodies, formerly believed to be directed against anionic phospholipids. In recent years they have been shown to be directed at plasma proteins bound to the phospholipid anionic surface. aPL often correlates with an increased risk of thrombosis, spontaneous miscarriage, or livedo reticularis. They are detected by several tests:

1. Lupus anticoagulant (LA) test
2. Anticardiolipin (aCL) assays (IgG and IgM, rarely IgA)
3. Anti-ß2 glycoprotein-I (GPI) antibodies

There is no gold standard screening test for LA, which can be determined by several methods. The activated partial thromboplastin time (aPTT) was for several years used as the standard screening test for LA. However, now it has been replaced by more sensitive tests, which include Dilute Russell Viper Venom time (DRVVT) and Kaolin Clotting time (KCT). Because lupus anticoagulants are heterogeneous, multiple screening assays are the preferable method of detection. A positive screening test, that is, prolonged clotting assay, does not mean LA. It should be followed by mixing studies that are done to differentiate antiphospholipid syndrome (APS) from clotting factor deficiency. Test normalization on the addition of pooled plasma indicates the latter condition. In APS, failure to correct with pooled plasma but neutralization with phospholipids confirms the presence of LA.

Anticardiolipin antibodies are detected by solid-phase assays like ELISA. These antibodies are found in a wide variety of conditions apart from autoimmune diseases. These include drug exposure (chlorpromazine, procainamide, quinidine, phenytoin, antibiotics); infections (tuberculosis, syphilis, leprosy, PCP, HIV); lymphoproliferative disorders, etc. However, the non-autoimmune aCL antibodies are not dependent on ß2 GPI for binding and carry little risk of thrombosis.

β2GPI is considered to be the major autoantigen in APS. It is composed of five homologous domains and binds to anionic phospholipids with lysine cluster and hydrophobic loop in domain 5. While antibodies against all five domains of β2GPI have been reported, antibodies against the first domain (DI) strongly correlate with thrombosis and obstetric complications. ß2 glycoprotein-I antibodies are also detected by ELISA.

Patients can have acL, β-2 GPI, LA in all combinations (single positive, double positive, or triple positive). Multiple aPL positivity confers a higher risk. "Triple-positive" patients are at the highest risk for thrombosis or abnormal pregnancy. LA activity may be abolished by steroid administration, whereas aCL and β-2 GPI levels remain unaffected. LA testing, unlike aCL or β-2 GPI, cannot be performed if a patient is on anticoagulants.

The laboratory criteria of APS require demonstration of LA in plasma on two or more occasions at least 12 weeks apart. Similarly, aCL antibodies of IgG and/or IgM isotype should be present in medium or high titer (i.e., >40 GPL or MPL, or >the 99th percentile), on two or more occasions, at least 12 weeks apart. The revised criteria also incorporate anti-ß2 glycoprotein-I antibody of IgG and/or IgM isotype in serum or plasma (in titer >the 99th percentile), present on two or more occasions, at least 12 weeks apart.

2.3.10 Antineutrophil Cytoplasmic Antibodies (ANCA)

These are a marker for vasculitis, first described in Wegener's Granulomatosis (WG). Two methods are employed to detect ANCA—IIF and ELISA. On IIF, the staining of ethanol-fixed neutrophils assumes two patterns: perinuclear (pANCA) and cytoplasmic (cANCA) (Fig. 2.6). The major target antigen for cANCA is proteinase-3 (Pr-3), and for pANCA is myeloperoxidase (MPO). The perinuclear pattern is an artifact of ethanol fixation during the staining procedure. Myeloperoxidase, the target antigen, is a highly cationic protein that moves and attaches to the negatively charged nuclear membrane during the fixation procedure. With the use of cross-linking fixatives (e.g., formaldehyde), pANCA pattern changes to a cytoplasmic pattern.

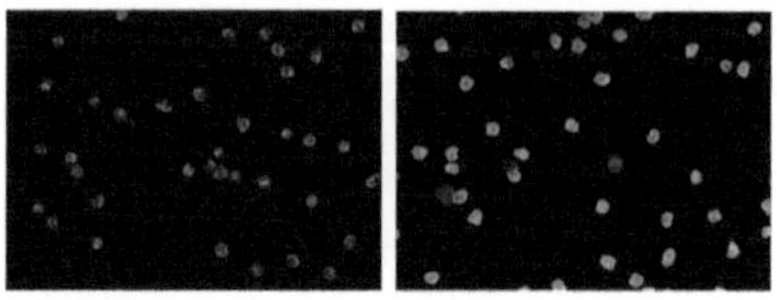

Fig. 2.6 ANCA patterns. Courtesy: Dr Pravin Hissaria, Adelaide

Patients with positive ANCA have specificity for either Pr-3 or MPO. Dual positivity is almost unknown except in one situation—exposure to levamisole-contaminated cocaine. The distinction between Granulomatosis with polyangiitis (GPA) and Microscopic polyangiitis (MPA) cannot be based on ANCA specificity. A negative ANCA does not rule out vasculitis, and conversely, a positive ANCA does not mean vasculitis. Apart from vasculitides, non-MPO pANCA has been reported in other conditions like ulcerative colitis (60%), primary sclerosing cholangitis (60%), RA (20%), and SLE (20%) (Table 2.4). Drug-induced ANCA-associated vasculitis may be seen with propylthiouracil, hydralazine, methimazole, etc.

ANCA should not be used as a screening test. Since vasculitides are rare, the positive predictive value of ANCA is quite low. This underscores the importance of ordering the investigation only in patients with a moderate to high clinical suspicion of vasculitis. The most important utility of ANCA for a clinician is in a patient with suggestive clinical features of Wegener's Granulomatosis, where the presence of positive cANCA or Pr-3 ELISA may help avoid the need

Table 2.4 Antineutrophil cytoplasmic autoantibodies (ANCA) in different conditions

Condition	Comment
Granulomatosis with polyangiitis (GPA)—Wegener's	Active, generalized GPA ~90%, Limited GPA ~60%. ANCA levels may vary according to disease activity. Pr-3 ANCA in 80–90% and MPO-ANCA in 10–20% of patients.
Microscopic polyangiitis (MPA)	~90% are ANCA positive with >95% MPO positivity.
Eosinophilic Granulomatosis with polyangiitis (EGPA)—Churg–Strauss syndrome	~50% are ANCA positive with ~80% MPO positivity
Renal limited vasculitis	~90% are ANCA positive with 75–80% MPO positivity.
Anti-glomerular basement membrane (GBM) disease	~10–40% are ANCA positive, with majority showing MPO positivity.
Gastrointestinal disorders	Aberrant pANCA pattern termed atypical pANCA or xANCA. Ulcerative colitis 50–67%, Crohn's disease 6–15%. Anti-Saccharomyces cerevisiae antibody (ASCA) combined with pANCA to help in the differential diagnosis. Crohn's is ASCA-positive and pANCA negative while ulcerative colitis is ASCA-negative and pANCA positive test. Pr-3 and MPO conspicuous by absence. Antigen specificities variable and include lactoferrin, bactericidal/permeability-increasing protein, cathepsin G, elastase, lysozyme, β-glucuronidase, etc.
Drugs	Variable frequency mostly MPO-ANCA. Sometimes antibodies to elastase or lactoferrin. Pr-3 rare.
Miscellaneous	~15% of patients with infective endocarditis (mainly Pr-3). Other conditions include leprosy, tuberculosis, autoimmune hepatitis. Variable frequency and variable specificity.

to obtain invasive biopsies. The other clinical setting is in patients with nephritis without any other explanation and in patients with pulmonary–renal syndromes. Histopathology continues to be the gold standard for the diagnosis of vasculitis.

The earlier recommendations advised the use of both IIF and ELISA to detect ANCA. The approach followed was to screen for ANCA by IIF and subsequently test for Pr-3 and MPO in IIF-positive samples. However, the current recommendations advocate the use of high-quality immunoassays as the preferred first screening method for ANCA detection in patients being worked up for the ANCA-associated vasculitides. A second PR3-MPO-ANCA or IIF can be considered for negative results in patients with a high clinical suspicion (to increase sensitivity) or in case of low antibody levels (to increase specificity). Antibody levels are taken into consideration. It is pertinent to note that ANCA detection for non-ANCA-associated vasculitis conditions is not included in this consensus proposed in 2017.

2.4 Serum Uric Acid (SUA)

Serum uric acid is another commonly ordered test in Rheumatology. The traditional utility has been in the diagnosis of gout. However, the sine qua non for the diagnosis of gout is a demonstration of monosodium urate (MSU) crystals in synovial fluid. The major clinical utility of SUA is not as much in the diagnosis of gout as in monitoring the treatment efficacy of xanthine oxidase inhibitors like allopurinol.

SUA may occasionally be normal in cases of acute gout, and a normal SUA by no means excludes the diagnosis of gout. Conversely, hyperuricemia may be seen in several conditions other than gout, and patients with hyperuricemia may have arthritis due to a cause other than gout. Hyperuricemia and gout are not synonymous in clinical terms. The vast majority of patients with hyperuricemia do not go on to develop gout, and the treatment of asymptomatic hyperuricemia with urate lowering therapies is not recommended.

The diagnosis of gout should be entertained in a patient presenting with monoarticular or oligoarticular joint disease. Polyarticular gout, though well known, is rare in clinical practice. Also, gout is exceedingly uncommon in prepubertal boys and premenopausal females. It is, therefore, not rational to order serum uric acid in females of childbearing age with polyarticular disease.

2.5 Antistreptolysin O (ASO)

Rheumatic fever is endemic in India. One of the common referrals to a rheumatologist is a young child with joint pains. Here the major task is differentiating rheumatic fever from juvenile idiopathic arthritis (JIA) (age of onset <16 years), formerly known as juvenile rheumatoid arthritis (JRA).

ASO is an antibody directed against streptolysin O, a toxic enzyme produced by group A Streptococci. The normal cutoff is <200 Todd units in adults and < 333 Todd units in children. ASO titers, interpreted in isolation, may be misleading. Rather than give a label of rheumatic fever based solely on elevated ASO titers, clinicians should be alive to the possibility of other inflammatory arthritides in children—notably JIA. In JIA, the pattern of arthritis is additive, with several joints being simultaneously involved at the same time (cf. Rheumatic fever, where joint involvement is migratory). Echocardiography can help pick up subtle cardiac involvement not evident clinically, and thus lend support to the diagnosis of Rheumatic fever. The presence of persistent, deforming arthritis in a child strongly militates against the diagnosis of rheumatic fever. Given the fact that rheumatic fever occurs in the age group of 5–15 years, ordering ASO in adults with joint pains is seldom warranted.

2.6 Complement

Low levels of components within the classical pathway of complement, especially C1q, C4, and C3, are seen with active SLE, particularly nephritis. Serum complement split products like C4d and Bb may be helpful in patients whose C3 and C4 levels remain normal despite evidence of clinical disease activity. Urinary C3d is also utilized to measure complement activation in lupus nephritis.

2.7 Synovial Fluid

It is an important, yet often neglected, laboratory test in Rheumatology. It is the only way to definitively diagnose gout and to "rule in" or "rule out" septic arthritis. Synoviocentesis and synovial fluid (SF) examination are mandatory in every patient presenting with monoarthritis. Its value is rather limited in patients who present with polyarticular disease. The synovial fluid should be subjected to white cell counts (total and differential), culture and Gram staining, and crystal studies, preferably under polarized light microscopy. Additional microbiologic testing like ZN staining, fungal cultures, mycobacterial cultures, etc. may be carried out if appropriate.

The key points about synovial fluid are summarized in Box 2.1 and Table 2.5.

Table 2.6 lists tests that are mentioned for historical reasons, offer no major diagnostic information and can be omitted. Viscosity is ascertained by expelling the synovial fluid from the syringe. The normal fluid will form a string 4–6 cm in length before breaking. In inflammatory conditions, the viscosity is low, and the fluid does not form a string but falls like drops. The mucin clot test is performed by adding acetic acid to the synovial fluid. A good mucin clot reflects the normal integrity of synovial fluid hyaluronate. A poor clot or friable clot is seen in conditions like septic arthritis, gouty arthritis, and rheumatoid arthritis. These tests have been abandoned because of poor reproducibility and observer bias. Traditionally, fluids like pleural, peritoneal, or cerebrospinal are subjected to sugar and protein estimations. In synovial fluid, these tests have limited utility and little discriminant value. Normal SF glucose is similar to serum. SF glucose is reduced in RA, gout, septic arthritis but permits no definite distinction between these diseases. SF protein is lower than serum (usually one-third of that in serum). This increases in inflammatory diseases. Again, this test does not reliably differentiate between various disorders.

Box 2.1 Key Points About Synovial Fluid Examination

- The sample should be anticoagulated with heparin or liquid EDTA. Powder EDTA may cause confusion in crystal identification.
- Synovial fluid viscosity, mucin clot, protein, glucose, ANA, LE cell, and RF do not confer any meaningful information and need not be done.
- Total and differential cell counts and crystal studies should be performed on all fluids. Gram stain and other microbiologic studies may be done in suspected septic arthritis.
- Cell count should be done normally using saline as a diluent. Acid diluents cause mucin to clot.
- The cell count of normal synovial fluid is <200/mm^3.
- A white count of 2000/mm^3 is used as a cutoff to differentiate inflammatory from noninflammatory fluids.
- A noninflammatory fluid generally has <50% neutrophils while infected fluids (septic arthritis) have >90% neutrophils.
- Polarized light microscopy is ideal for crystal identification. However, useful information can also be obtained on light microscopy.

2.8 HLA-B27

HLA-B27 is a MHC class I molecule comprising of an alpha chain that is encoded in the MHC region on chromosome 6 and a non-MHC encoded beta chain, β_2 microglobulin. HLA-B27 exhibits a high degree of genetic polymorphism with 105 known subtypes, named from HLA-B*27:01 to HLA-B*27:106, that are encoded by 132 allelic variants. These allotypes differ from one another by a few amino acid substitutions. Not every allelic variant is associated with the disease. Notably, HLA-B*27:06 and HLA-B*27:09 have been reported not to be associated with ankylosing spondylitis (AS).

HLA-B27 can be detected by serological techniques such as microlymphocytotoxicity (MLCT) or flow cytometry. In MLCT assay, lymphocytes are tested with a panel of sera containing well-characterized HLA-specific alloantibodies. The lysis of the lymphocytes by a serum containing anti-HLA B27 antibodies denotes the HLA-B27 positivity of the sample. In flow cytometry, HLA-B27 on the T cell surface is detected using a specific monoclonal antibody. Since serological techniques such as MLCT and flow cytometry require viable cells that adequately express HLA-B27, these techniques give false-negative results if HLA-B27 is downregulated or masked due to the blocking of an epitope on HLA-B27 by a cross-reacting antibody. False positivity can also occur on flow cytometry due to cross-reactivity of HLA-B27 monoclonal antibodies with other

Table 2.6 Synovial fluid tests of limited/no utility

• Proteins
• Sugar
• Viscosity
• Mucin clot
• ANA, LE Cell, RF

Table 2.5 Synovial fluid cell counts

Condition	Count (cells/mm^3)	Count per hpf (high power field)	Differential count
Normal	<200	Occasional mononuclear cell	<10% neutrophils
Noninflammatory	200–2000	0–2 wbc/hpf	<50% neutrophils
Inflammatory	2000–30,000	2–10 wbcs/hpf	>50% neutrophils
Septic	100,000	>15 wbc/hpf	>90% neutrophils

HLA-B antigens such as HLA-B7 and HLA-B37. Flowcytometry, being rapid, high-throughput, and relatively inexpensive, was widely used earlier. It is now being replaced by molecular typing methods like sequence-specific primer polymerase chain reaction (SSP-PCR), sequence-specific oligonucleotides probes (SSOP-PCR), or real-time (RT-PCR). Molecular typing of HLA-B27 relies on the detection of the HLA-B27-specific DNA sequence for the identification of B27 alleles and is not influenced by conformational antigenic changes. Analysis of HLA-B27 subtypes is possible only through molecular typing.

The Indian population demonstrates a variable frequency of HLA-B27 from the north (2.7–29%) to south (0.9–2.1%) of the country. HLA-B*27:05 is the most common subtype followed by HLA-B*27:04 in the Indian population. Other common alleles reported from India are HLA-B*27:07, HLA-B*27:02, and HLA-B*27:10. North Indian patients with spondyloarthritis have B*27:04 and B*27:05 as the most common HLA-B27 subtypes.

It is to be noted that HLA-B27 is present in a significant proportion of healthy individuals. For example, nearly 6% of healthy north Indians exhibit the presence of HLA B27, of whom only 10% develop SpA, while about 90% will never develop this disease. However, the risk for SpA among HLA-B27-positive persons with a first-degree relative with AS is increased threefold (30% instead of 10%).

2.9 Other Investigations

Table 2.7 summarizes the radiologic findings in some common rheumatic diseases. A detailed exposition of imaging modalities is beyond the scope of this chapter.

Table 2.7 Radiologic findings in some common rheumatic diseases

Condition	Which x-ray to order for diagnosis	Typical findings	Comments
Osteoarthritis knee	Knees AP and lateral (weight-bearing)	Joint space (inter-bone distance) narrowing, osteophytes, subchondral sclerosis, subchondral cysts.	Other sites: hips, cervical spine, lumbar spine. Nodular OA is less common in Indians.
Rheumatoid arthritis	X-ray hands and wrists-PA view X-ray bilateral feet-AP view	Soft tissue swelling, periarticular osteopenia, joint space narrowing, erosions	Radiographs of joints other than hands and feet may be obtained if symptomatic. Radiographs of bilateral joints should be obtained to compare the diseases with the unaffected side.
Ankylosing spondylitis	X-ray pelvis AP view (Oblique views have been abandoned)	Sacroiliitis	Offers information on hip joints and symphysis pubis in addition to SI joints. May show features of enthesitis
Gout	Feet, hands, other affected joints	Radiographs normal in early gout except for soft tissue swelling, which may be seen in some patients. Patients with chronic gout may show punched-out erosions with overhanging edges. The erosions may be in the joint or away from the joint.	The joint space in gout is preserved till late, and periarticular osteopenia is absent or minimal (cf. RA)
Tuberculosis	X-ray of affected joint	"Phemister's triad" typical of joint tuberculosis: (1) juxta-articular osteoporosis; (2) peripherally located osseous erosions; (3) gradual narrowing of the joint space.	Large weight-bearing joints like hip, knee, and shoulder are affected more commonly.

2.10 Conclusions

Laboratory evaluation employed for differential diagnosis of rheumatic complaints is most useful when the clinical suspicion is moderately high. There is no substitute for a careful clinical examination, and seldom can the diagnosis be based on any one single test. Some clinicians order RF, ANA, ESR, and SUA in every patient with joint pains, which is not cost-effective. The most powerful tests in Rheumatology are still the history and physical examination. The astute clinician should refrain from ordering autoimmune panels. For example, if ANA is negative, there are limited reasons to order additional tests such as anti-dsDNA, anti-Ro, anti-La, anti-Sm, etc.

Suggested Reading

1. Kamath DY, Xavier D, Sigamani A, Pais P. High sensitivity C-reactive protein (hsCRP) & cardiovascular disease: an Indian perspective. Indian J Med Res. 2015;142:261–8.
2. Damoiseaux J, Andrade LEC, Carballo OG, Conrad K, Francescantonio PLC, Fritzler MJ, et al. Clinical relevance of HEp-2 indirect immunofluorescent patterns: the International Consensus on ANA patterns (ICAP) perspective. Ann Rheum Dis. 2019;78:879–89.
3. Bossuyt X, Cohen Tervaert J, Arimura Y, Blockmans D, Flores-Suárez LF, Guillevin F, et al. Revised 2017 international consensus on testing of ANCAs in granulomatosis with polyangiitis and microscopic polyangiitis. Nat Rev Rheumatol. 2017;13:683–92.
4. Dhurandhar PS, Shankarkumar U. HLA association in seronegative spondyloarthritis patients from Mumbai, India. Int J Hum Genet. 2007;7:235–9.

3 Low Back Pain

3.1 Introduction

Low Back Pain (LBP) is an everyday clinical problem in outpatient practice. LBP, osteoarthritis, soft tissue rheumatism, and inflammatory rheumatic diseases, together constitute the "Big 4" of rheumatology—four musculoskeletal conditions most frequently encountered in the community (Fig. 3.1). The importance of LBP can also be gauged by the following facts: nearly 75% of the population experiences back pain at some time in their life, back symptoms are the most important cause of disability in the young and middle-aged, back pain is the commonest occupational injury, and also, LBP is associated with a substantial economic burden. Even though only a tiny minority of patients require surgical intervention, LBP has traditionally been considered the domain of orthopedic surgeons. This chapter outlines the current evidence-based approach to LBP.

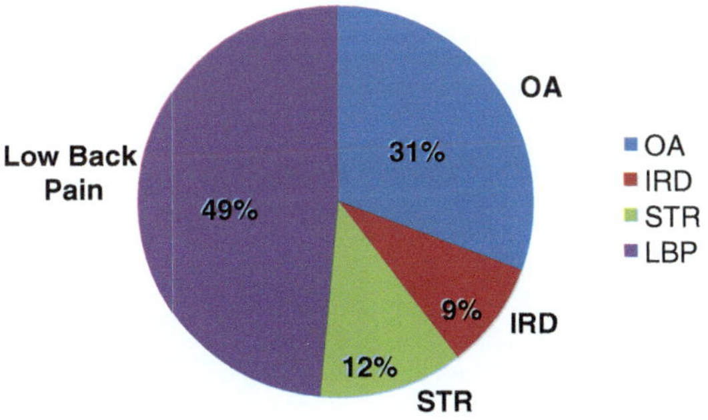

Fig. 3.1 "Big 4" of rheumatology (approximate percentages). *LBP* low back pain, *OA* osteoarthritis, *STR* soft tissue rheumatism, *IRD* inflammatory rheumatic diseases

Table 3.1 Natural history of acute low back pain

• 40% of cases recover within 1 week
• 80% of cases recover within 3 weeks
• 90% of cases recover within 6 weeks
• Less than 10% experience symptoms for >6 months
• Less than 1% require surgical intervention

3.2 Causes and Natural History

Back pain can be divided into acute, subacute, and chronic LBP based upon duration (acute <1 month, subacute from 1 to 3 months, and chronic >3 months or if pain occurs episodically within a 6-month period). The notable thing about acute LBP is its favorable natural history, with most episodes resolving in a few weeks (Table 3.1).

Table 3.2 lists the various causes of LBP. Mechanical causes of low back pain account for the majority (≥90%) of cases, while systemic diseases account for only ≤10% of cases. Nonspecific back pain is perhaps the commonest cause of LBP. It is defined as back pain that cannot be attributed or assigned to a recognizable or specific pathology such as cancer, infection, spinal stenosis, cauda equina syndrome, fracture, spondyloarthritis, etc. Degenerative changes on lumbar spine imaging are deemed nonspecific, as they correlate poorly with symptoms.

R. Handa, *Clinical Rheumatology*, https://doi.org/10.1007/978-981-33-4885-1_3

Table 3.2 Causes of low back pain

Mechanical ≥ 90%	Systemic/inflammatory/infectious diseases ≤10%
1. Nonspecific 2. Back sprain 3. Herniated disc 4. Osteoarthritis (lumbar spondylosis) 5. Spinal canal stenosis 6. Spondylolisthesis/spondylolysis 7. Scoliosis 8. Trauma	**1. Rheumatologic** – Spondyloarthitis (SpA) **2. Neoplastic diseases** – Multiple myeloma – Metastasis (breast, lung, prostate) – Benign tumors **3. Infections** – Pott's spine – Vertebral osteomyelitis – Epidural abscess **4. Metabolic** – Osteoporotic fracture – Osteomalacia – Fluorosis – Paget's disease **5. Hematologic.** – Myelofibrosis – Hemoglobinopathies. **6. Referred pain** – Pelvic inflammatory disease – Cystitis, prostatitis, endometriosis – Pancreatic disease 7. **Miscellaneous** – Rupture of an abdominal aneurysm – Postural – Aortic dissection – Psychosomatic/malingering

Common Risk Factors for LBP include heavy physical labor, lifting of heavyweights/objects, improper posture, prolonged sitting/driving, pregnancy, somatization, etc.

3.3 Clinical Approach to a Patient with Low Back Pain

The clinician should elicit a detailed history and perform a thorough general physical, systemic, and local examination with particular reference to musculoskeletal and nervous systems. The issues to the addressed are:

1. Is a serious/systemic disease responsible for LBP?
2. In acute LBP, are any "red flag" signs present?
3. Are psychological factors contributing to the LBP?

The various clues, which point toward a serious/systemic disease, are enumerated in Table 3.3. Inflammatory LBP (Table 3.4) is typical of spondarthritides. These conditions are characterized by male preponderance; HLA B27 positivity; asymmetric, oligoarthritis involving large joints of lower limbs; and sacroiliitis. Clinical evaluation helps one to arrive at a diagnosis in most cases. In acute low back pain, the clinician should rule out or rule in medical emergencies (the so-called red flag signs) like cauda equina syndrome, epidural abscess, rupture of aortic aneurysm, dissection of the aorta, etc. (Fig. 3.2). Features, which are suggestive of these serious causes, include saddle anesthesia, bladder/bowel involvement, asymmetric loss of deep tendon reflexes, pulse inequality, hypotension, circulatory instability, etc. Neurologic deficits warrant magnetic resonance imaging (MRI) and neurosurgical intervention if appropriate. Cardiovascular catastrophes warrant angiography and surgery. Malignancy as a cause of LBP is uncommon in primary care.

Sciatica, by definition, is LBP with radiation below the knee. It suggests nerve root compromise due to mechanical pressure or inflammation. A straight leg raise (SLR) is commonly performed in patients with sciatica. A positive SLR is a reproduction of the patient's sciatica between 30 and

Table 3.3 When to suspect systemic/serious disease as a cause of LBP?

- Fever
- Weight loss
- Pain with recumbency
- Nocturnal pain
- Morning stiffness ≥1 h
- Localized bone pain
- Visceral pain, abdominal mass, rectal mass
- Age >50 years
- Previous history of cancer
- Sphincter incontinence
- Neurological deficit.

Table 3.4 Differentiating inflammatory from mechanical low back pain

	Mechanical	Inflammatory
Example	Herniated disc	Spondyloarthritis (SpA)
Onset	May be acute	Insidious
Age	Any age	Usually <40 years
Morning stiffness	±	+++
Exercise	Aggravates	Relieves
Rest	Improves	Worsens
Precipitating factors	Strenuous task, e.g., weight lifting	Usually none
Acute phase reactants (ESR, CRP)	Normal	May be increased
Other features like buttock pain, rib pain, uveitis, peripheral arthritis, etc.	Absent	May be present

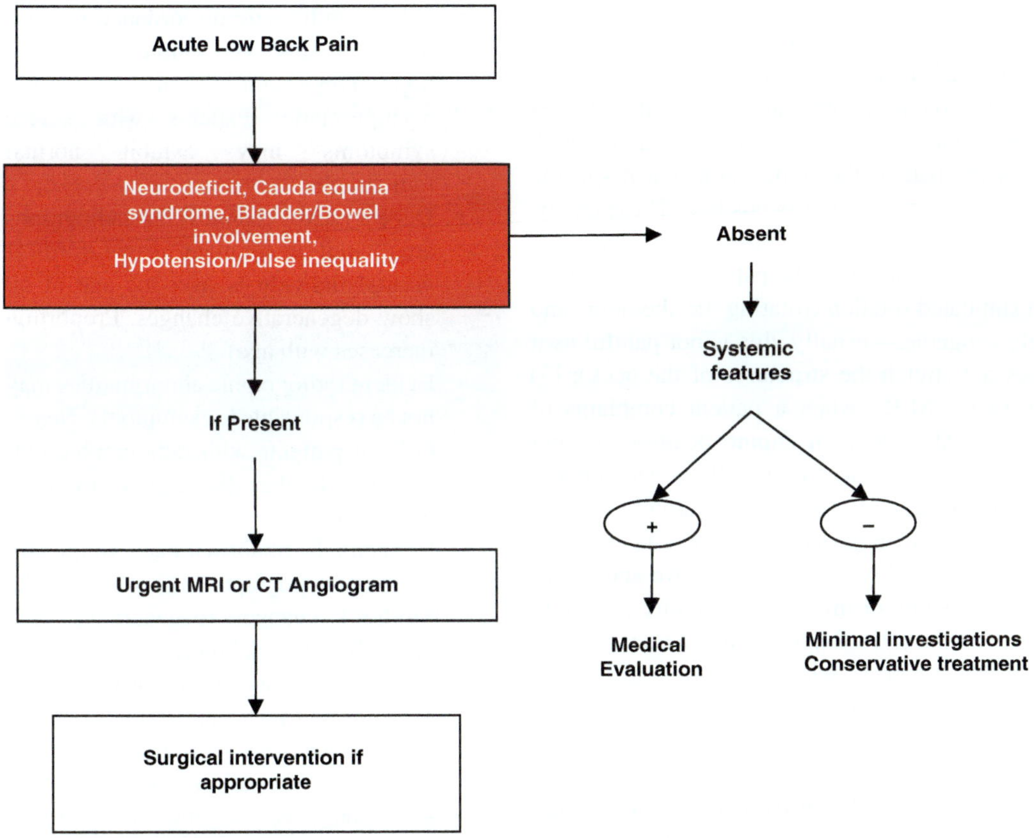

Fig. 3.2 Approach to acute low back pain (Red flag signs—highlighted in red—merit urgent attention)

70° of leg elevation and has a relatively high sensitivity (91%) but modest specificity (26%) for diagnosing a herniated disc. The crossed SLR test (when the unaffected leg is lifted) is more specific (88%) but less sensitive (29%).

Lumbar spinal stenosis may present with back pain and sciatica. The characteristic feature, however, is neurogenic (pseudo) claudication. In contrast to vascular claudication, the claudication distance is not fixed in lumbar spinal stenosis. Also, with lumbar spinal stenosis, the pain is relieved on leaning forward/sitting as these actions flex the body at the hip. Vascular claudication becomes worse while walking uphill in contrast to pseudo-claudication that is usually worse when going downhill. Causes of lumbar spinal stenosis include osteoarthritis, degenerative disc disease, etc.

Chronic LBP may be due to psychological reasons or malingering, a diagnosis of exclusion to be entertained only if physical causes have been carefully excluded. Waddell's signs are signs that indicate the nonorganic cause of chronic LBP. Waddell's signs include: (1) Superficial tenderness—generalized tenderness over the entire lumbar area when the skin is lightly pinched or rolled; (2) Simulation, which gives the patient the impression that a specific test is being carried out is positive. These can be done by axial loading (eliciting pain when pressing down on the top of the patient's head) or pain on simulated rotation (rotating the shoulders and pelvis together—usually, this is not painful as it does not stretch the structures of the back); (3) Distracted SLR—when a patient complains of pain on SLR done in supine position but not when it is done seated; (4) Regionalization—motor and sensory loss is nonanatomic or nonphysiological. Regional sensory change is a nondermatomal sensory loss in glove and stocking distribution or involving the entire extremity or side of the body. Regional weakness is a weakness that is jerky, with intermittent resistance (such as cogwheeling or catching) in contrast to organic weakness and can be overpowered smoothly; and (5) Overreaction—disproportionate verbalization, facial expression, etc. A high Waddell score (>3) may be indicative of symptom magnification or possible illness behavior.

3.4 Pain Assessment

Pain can be assessed by different scales: visual analog scales, verbal rating scales, and numerical rating scales. Pain drawings are commonly employed in pain clinics.

3.5 Investigations

Investigations in LBP should be kept to a minimum except in patients with neurologic deficits or where serious/systemic disease is suspected. Overreliance on radiographs/imaging should be avoided because of reasons enunciated in Box 3.1. In general, imaging studies should

Box 3.1 Pitfalls of Indiscriminate Radiographic Imaging in Low Back Pain

- The majority of patients with nonspecific back pain have normal X-rays
- Clinico-radiologic discordance is common: Patients with impressive radiologic abnormalities may be totally asymptomatic. Patients with severe symptoms may exhibit normal radiographs
- Degenerative changes on radiographs are ubiquitous (as many as two-thirds of normal individuals over the age of 50 show degenerative changes. Proportion increases with age)
- Evident radiographic abnormalities may not be responsible for symptoms. Nearly 60% of patients with radiographic evidence of lumbar disc degeneration are asymptomatic
- Congenital abnormalities frequently seen on radiographs like spina bifida, Modics's changes (degenerative endplate changes), Schmorl's nodes (herniation of the nucleus pulposus into the adjacent end plate) are unlikely causes of back pain
- Frequent X-rays add to radiation exposure but very little to clinical management

only be obtained if results are likely to influence surgical or medical treatment. However, patients with a history of trauma or pointers toward systemic/serious disease need appropriate laboratory investigations and radiological work. The imaging modality of choice in most circumstances is MRI.

3.6 Treatment

Patients with nonspecific low back pain should be advised to remain active. Bed rest is counterproductive in both acute and chronic LBP. Even patients with severe symptoms should be encouraged to return to normal activities as soon as possible. Patients with LBP are offered a plethora of nonpharmacologic treatments with varying degrees of evidence base to support these therapies. It is essential to realize that recommendations change with time as new data becomes available. Also, modalities of use in acute LBP may not help in subacute/chronic LBP.

3.6.1 Acute Low Back Pain

For acute low back pain, superficial heat and massage may help. Some studies report benefits from spinal manipulation. Bed rest, cold application, back exercises, lumbar belts, TENS, laser, epidural steroids, particular mattress type, and traction are not believed to be of much utility in acute LBP. Short-term NSAIDs for 2–4 weeks are used in acute LBP unless there are contraindications. Paracetamol (acetaminophen) can be employed as the first-line drug for pain relief in patients with contraindication to NSAIDs. In case of inadequate relief, a nonbenzodiazepine muscle relaxant can be added. Opioid analgesics or tramadol should be used only if the above measures do not yield benefits. Opioids should not be prescribed for long periods because of the potential for addiction. Failure to respond to a finite course of opioids should prompt reassessment and alternative treatments. There is no rationale for using steroids or antidepressants in acute LBP.

3.6.2 Subacute and Chronic Low Back Pain

Patients are encouraged to maintain activity as tolerated. Heat therapy is more beneficial than cold, although individual preference may vary. Nonpharmacologic treatments with evidence of efficacy for chronic or subacute low back pain are psychological interventions (cognitive-behavioral therapy and progressive relaxation), exercise, spinal manipulation, and interdisciplinary rehabilitation. Results with acupuncture are variable. Other noninvasive therapies (back schools, interferential therapy, low-level laser therapy, lumbar supports, TENS, traction, and ultrasonography) are not supported by robust evidence. NSAIDs, paracetamol, and muscle relaxants are used. The major adverse effect of muscle relaxants is sedation. Tricyclic antidepressants, duloxetine, and tramadol have been employed for pain relief in chronic LBP. Duloxetine seems to have a lesser potential for abuse or misuse as compared to tramadol. The duration of therapy has to be individualized. Risk factors or psychological factors, if identified, should also be addressed. The current evidence does not support the routine use of gabapentin or pregabalin.

Surgical intervention is needed in a small proportion of patients. The possible indications include fractures/dislocations, epidural abscess, Pott's spine, tumors, and aortic dissection/aneurysm rupture. Discectomy or epidural corticosteroid injections may be considered in patients with herniated lumbar disc and persistent radicular symptoms. Given the fact that as many as one-third of asymptomatic adults have a disc protrusion on MRI scans, surgical intervention based only on radiologic findings is often unsuccessful and should be avoided.

3.7 Conclusions

Low Back Pain can be acute, subacute, or chronic based upon duration. The natural history of acute LBP is favorable. Chronic LBP may be due to psychological reasons or malingering. Imaging plays a limited role in the workup of these patients. Early mobilization is preferred in most patients.

Suggested Reading

1. Hartvigsen J, Hancock MJ, Kongsted A, Louw Q, Ferreira ML, Genevay S, et al. What low back pain is and why we need to pay attention. Lancet. 2018;391(10137):2356–67.
2. Maher C, Underwood M, Buchbinder R. Non-specific low back pain. Lancet. 2017;389(10070):736–47.
3. Oliveira CB, Maher CG, Pinto RZ, Traeger AC, Lin CC, Chenot JF, et al. Clinical practice guidelines for the management of non-specific low back pain in primary care: an updated overview. Eur Spine J. 2018;27:2791–803.
4. Qaseem A, Wilt TJ, McLean RM, Forciea MA; Clinical Guidelines Committee of the American College of Physicians. Noninvasive treatments for acute, subacute, and chronic low back pain: a clinical practice guideline from the American College of Physicians. Ann Intern Med 2017;166:514–530.

4 Osteoarthritis

4.1 Introduction

Osteoarthritis (OA) is the most frequent joint disease encountered in clinical practice. It is also the commonest cause of locomotor disability in the elderly. The usual presentation is with joint pain and functional limitation. Typically the morning stiffness is mild, the pain is more on using the joints than at rest, and acute phase reactants are generally not elevated. Although aging is a significant risk factor for OA, aging alone does not cause OA. The present concept is that OA is not a single disease process. It is instead a heterogeneous group of illnesses with several risk factors (Fig. 4.1), the end result of which is joint failure

The brunt of the disease in OA is borne by the cartilage. However, it has become increasingly apparent that OA disease processes are panarticular and affect the subchondral bone, ligaments, capsule, synovial membrane, and periarticular muscles. Signs and symptoms like joint swelling and effusion reflect ongoing synovitis. OA was earlier thought to be a degenerative disease due to the lack of florid signs of inflammation. It is now believed that this watertight distinction is perhaps an oversimplification of a complex process. OA articular cartilage, in contrast to normal cartilage, is characterized by the superinduction of pro-inflammatory genes (like iNOS, COX-2, IL-1β, IL-6, and IL-8) and corresponding gene products. Since the chondrocytes are sequestered within the lacunae of articular cartilage, which is avascular and aneural, the localized *"molecular inflammation"* is sans the typical clinical signs of inflammation.

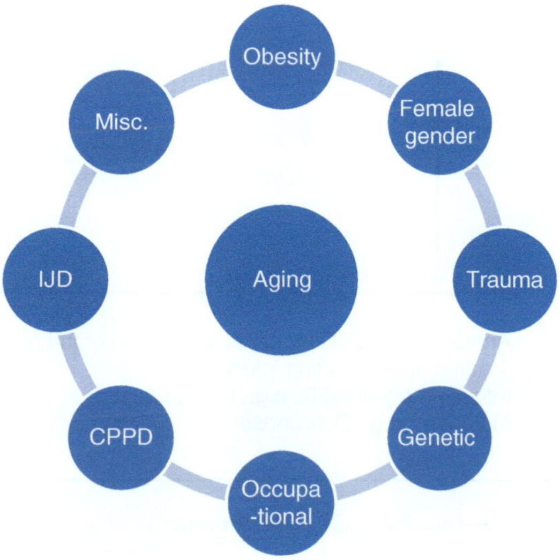

Fig. 4.1 Risk factors for osteoarthritis. *CPPD* calcium pyrophosphate deposition disease, *IJD* inflammatory joint diseases like rheumatoid arthritis, *Misc* miscellaneous conditions like hypermobility, neuropathic joints, Perthes disease, etc

R. Handa, *Clinical Rheumatology*, https://doi.org/10.1007/978-981-33-4885-1_4

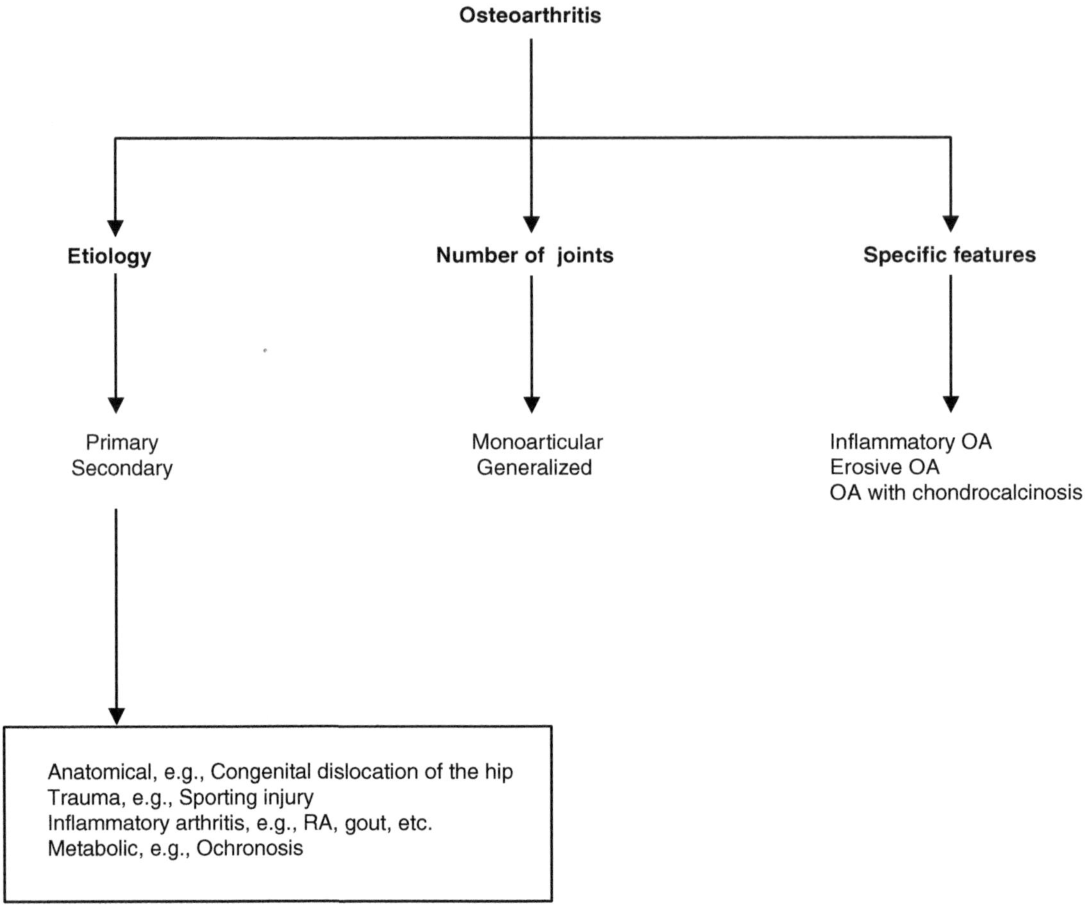

Fig. 4.2 Classification of osteoarthritis

4.2 Classification of OA

Osteoarthritis may be classified as primary (idiopathic) or secondary. Secondary OA has an identifiable underlying cause like rheumatoid arthritis, Perthes disease, trauma, etc. Secondary OA accounts for less than 20% of OA, and patients are approximately 10 years younger than patients with primary OA. The other methods of classifying OA are set out in Fig. 4.2. Erosive OA is a subset of OA characterized by the involvement of interphalangeal joints of the hand with florid inflammation and erosive changes (Fig. 4.3).

4.3 Clinical Features, Investigations, and Diagnosis

The commonest joint affected in Indian patients is the knee joint, possibly due to squatting. Other joints affected include the hips, distal and proximal interphalangeal joints, first carpometacarpal joint, first metacarpophalangeal (MCP) joint, first metatarsophalangeal joint, and the spinal apophyseal joints (mostly lower cervical and lower lumbar segments—cervical and lumbar spondylosis). The involvement of the other MCP joints, wrist, elbow, shoulder, or ankle is uncommon but may be seen occasionally. Nodular OA—

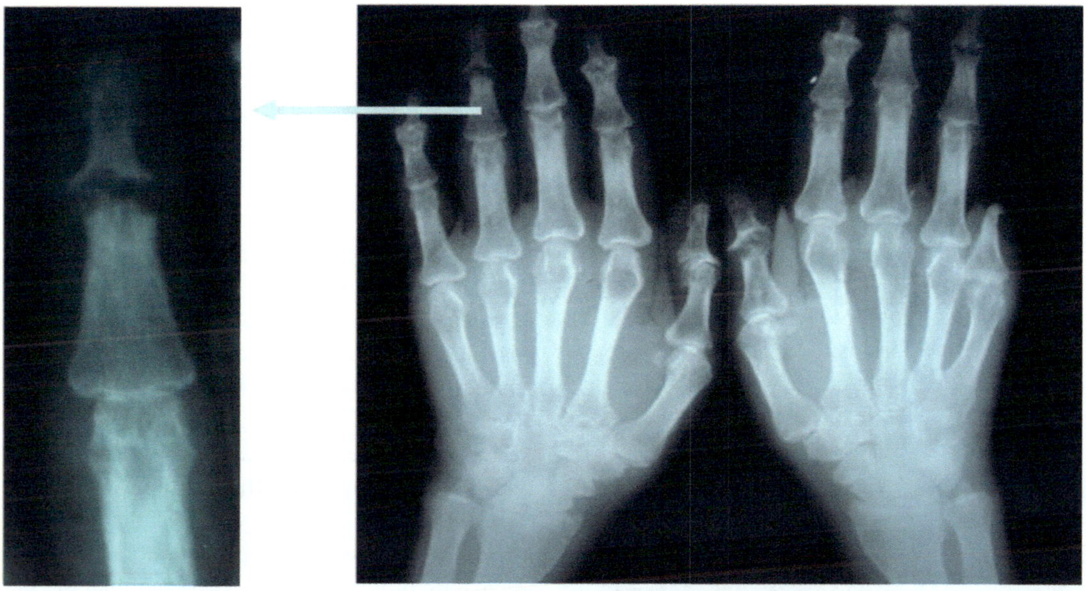

Fig. 4.3 Erosive OA. Note the presence of subchondral erosive changes. The amputation of right 5th finger is incidental

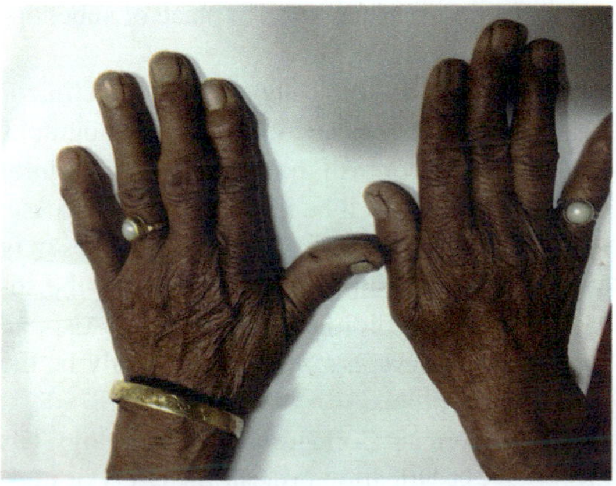

Fig. 4.4 Heberden and Bouchard nodes

Heberden and Bouchard's nodes—seem to be less common in Indians (Fig. 4.4).

The main symptom of OA is "use-related" pain seen in nearly 100% of symptomatic patients. Rest pain and nocturnal pain are seen in almost 50% and 30% patients, respectively. The exact cause of pain in OA is not known since cartilage lacks blood and nerve supply. The possible factors include raised intraosseous pressure in the subchondral bone as a result of venous outflow obstruction, periosteal elevation by osteophytes, inflammatory synovitis, secondary periarticular syndromes like bursitis, tenosynovitis, and muscle pain, central pain amplification mechanisms, etc. The patients also complain of stiffness—"gelling" after a period of inactivity. The morning stiffness is typically mild. Knee joint involvement is associated with pain on descending or ascending stairs, climbing into rickshaws, buses, etc. Patients have difficulty in squatting, using Indian toilets, and sitting cross-legged. The knee joint may "lock" or "give way"—buckling. In a patient with knee OA who has aggravation of pain, it is worthwhile to bear in mind that causes other than OA may be responsible (Box 4.1). Systemic involvement is not a feature of OA. Occasionally, OA and rheumatoid arthritis (RA) may coexist.

Examination reveals crepitus on joint movement (sensation of bone rubbing against bone),

Box 4.1 Possible Causes of Aggravation of Pain in Knee OA

- OA flare
- Septic arthritis
- Pseudogout (CPDD crystals)
- Rupture of Baker's cyst
- Osteonecrosis of the medial femoral condyle
- Ligament rupture/meniscal tear
- Anserine bursitis

CPDD calcium pyrophosphate dihydrate

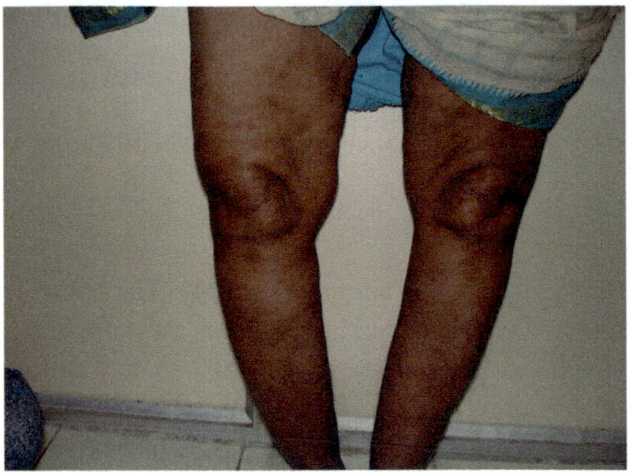

Fig. 4.5 Varus deformity in knee OA (medial compartment disease)

bony swelling, joint deformity, and muscle weakness and wasting. The knee joint may exhibit effusion. Medial compartment disease of the knee can give rise to varus (bow leg) deformity (Fig. 4.5).

Being predominantly noninflammatory, an acute phase response is not typical in OA. However, ESR may show an age-related increase. It is important to remember that 5% of healthy elderly individuals may show rheumatoid factor (RF) positivity without having RA. Careful attention to clinical profile is crucial to prevent an erroneous label of RA in these individuals with hand OA and RF positivity. Prominent wrist and MCP involvement (except first MCP joint) is unusual in OA. Also, the swelling in OA is bony in contrast to the boggy synovitis of RA. The cell count in synovial fluid is usually <2000/mm^3. Synovial fluid may show the presence of calcium pyrophosphate dehydrate (CPPD) crystals. Hydroxyapatite and Basic Calcium Phosphate crystals may also be detectable.

The radiographic features of OA include joint space (inter bone distance) narrowing (reflecting cartilage loss), osteophytes, subchondral sclerosis, and subchondral cysts. Loose bodies and chondrocalcinosis due to CPPD crystals may be seen. For knee OA, a weight-bearing anteroposterior view is recommended. Lateral or skyline views are employed to delineate the patellofemoral joint better. In primary OA of the knee, the medial tibiofemoral and patellofemoral compartments are more commonly involved than the lateral tibiofemoral compartment (Fig. 4.6). Features that suggest RA leading to secondary OA of the knee are involvement of both medial and lateral tibiofemoral compartments, erosions, and periarticular osteopenia in place of subchondral sclerosis (Fig. 4.7).

The diagnosis of osteoarthritis is clinico-radiologic with some caveats. Radiographs merely help to confirm the presence of structural changes but may well be normal in early disease. Patients with impressive radiologic changes may be totally asymptomatic and vice versa—the so-called "clinico-radiologic discordance." Also, an abnormal radiograph may not necessarily be the cause of symptoms.

The American College of Rheumatology has proposed classification criteria for OA. For idiopathic OA of the knee, the presence of knee pain is required plus 1 of the following three features—age >50 years, stiffness <30 min, and crepitus in addition to osteophytes (Sensitivity 91%, specificity 86%). Similarly, Hip OA requires the presence of hip pain and two of the following three features—ESR Westergren <20 mm/h, radiographic femoral or acetabular osteophytes, and radiographic joint space narrowing (superior, axial, and/or medial) [Sensitivity 89%, Specificity 91%].

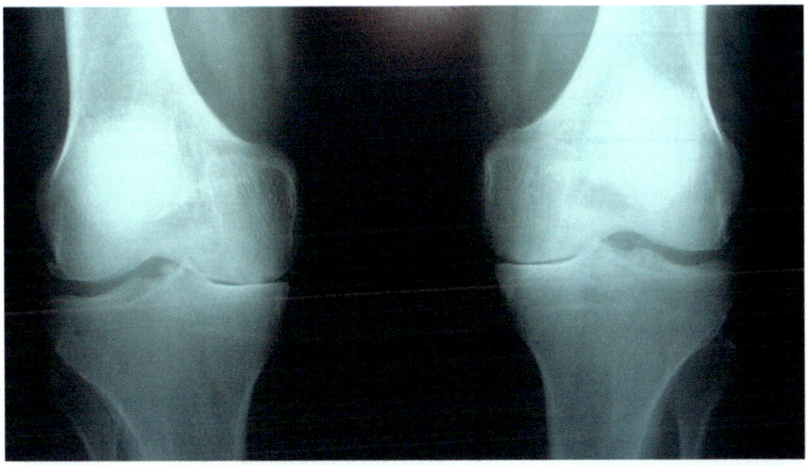

Fig. 4.6 Radiographic changes in knee OA

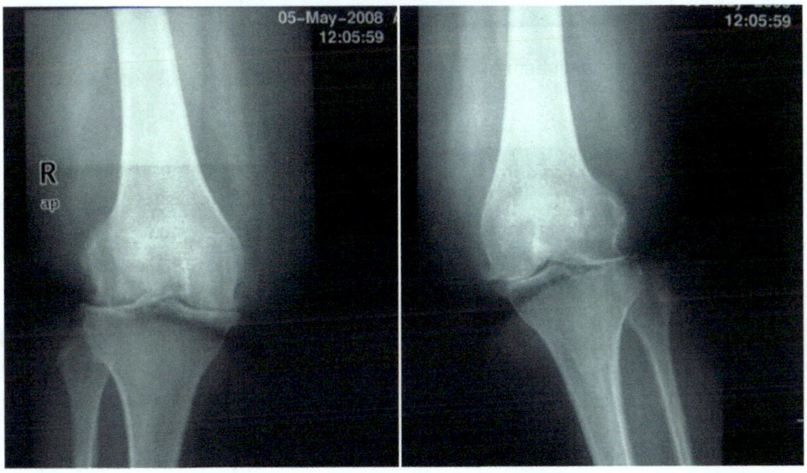

Fig. 4.7 Secondary OA of knees in a patient with rheumatoid arthritis. Note the absence of subchondral sclerosis and involvement of both medial and lateral tibiofemoral compartments

4.4 Treatment

There has been a remarkable change in the treatment paradigm of OA as the therapeutic options continue to expand (Fig. 4.8). The goals of treatment in OA are pain relief, optimization of function, and limitation of disability. The two critical components are pharmacologic and nonpharmacologic. The elderly patient with OA often has several comorbidities like hypertension, diabetes, chronic obstructive airways disease, coronary artery disease, benign prostate hypertrophy, etc. which require multiple drugs. The treatment plan needs to factor these in (Table 4.1). Physicians also need to be reminded about the ever-present danger of "prescription cascade" in the elderly wherein a medicine prescribed for one condition may lead to another condition that evokes prescription of another drug, giving rise to a vicious loop.

4.4.1 Nonpharmacologic Treatment Modalities in OA

Nonpharmacologic measures are an essential part of every OA treatment program. Patients should be educated about joint protection like avoidance

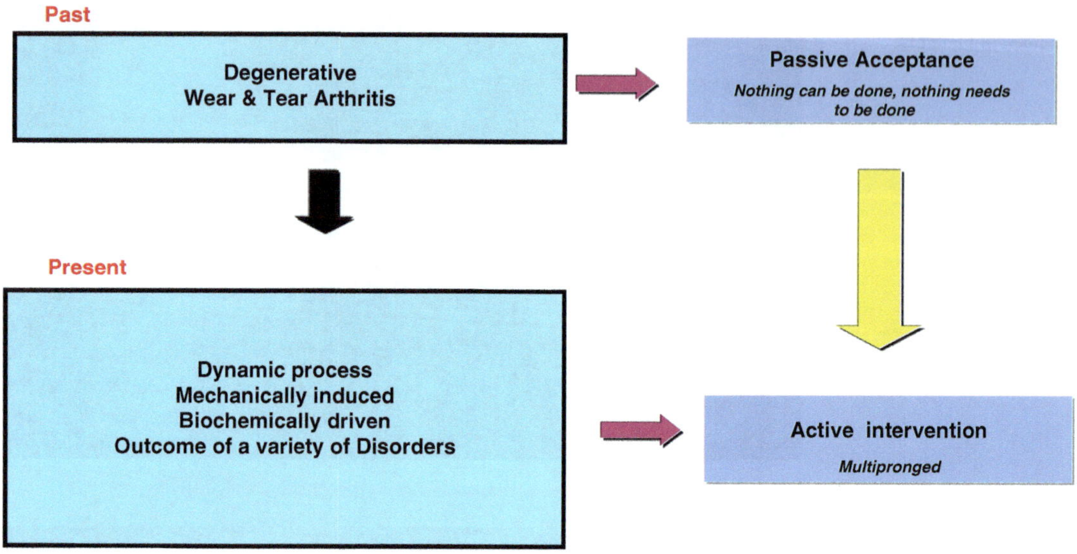

Fig. 4.8 The changed paradigm in OA

Table 4.1 OA with comorbidities

Condition	Comments
Diabetes mellitus	• Avoid oral NSAIDs • Glucosamine does not usually affect blood sugar levels or insulin sensitivity • Intra-articular steroids do not affect glycemic control in the majority of patients
Hypertension	• NSAIDs have a propensity to increase blood pressure • Intra-articular steroids safe
Coronary artery disease	• Avoid both selective and nonselective NSAIDs, if possible • Regular NSAID use should also be avoided in patients taking low-dose aspirin. Aspirin to be taken at least 2 h before the NSAID • Naproxen preferred NSAID • Some question marks have been raised about the safety of paracetamol also
Kidney disease	• NSAIDs best avoided
Peptic ulcer disease	• Use selective COX-2 inhibitors unless contraindicated • Use proton pump inhibitors (PPIs) with nonselective NSAIDs
Very old patients	• Avoid opioids • Limit paracetamol dose • Look out for drug interactions and multi-morbidities

of poor posture and excessive joint loading. Patients with knee OA are advised to avoid squatting, sitting cross-legged, low sofas, stair climbing, and Indian lavatory. Weight loss is very beneficial for patients who are obese. General muscle training improves joint function. Quadriceps exercises are recommended for knee OA. Exercise programs should be instituted only when the disease is relatively quiescent. During the active phase of the illness with significant pain, vigorous exercise should be avoided. High impact exercises such as running or jumping are usually discouraged in severe knee OA to prevent further joint damage. Muscle relaxation exercises are useful when there is muscle spasm, e.g., cervical spine OA. Thermal modalities like the application of superficial heat by hot packs and wax baths or deep heat by ultrasound alleviate pain and joint stiffness. In general, ice packs are used in acute inflammatory conditions, while hot fomentation is employed in chronic cases. Hydrotherapy also helps relieve pain and increase the range of joint movement. These modalities are useful adjuncts. Devices like walking sticks (contralateral cane) of appropriate length may help. The benefits of knee braces, orthotic shoes, shock-absorbing heel pads, and insoles are quite variable, and no firm recommendations can be made based on the available evidence. However, a team approach with the inclusion of a physiatrist, physiotherapist, and occupational therapist, among others, is helpful in the management of all patients with OA.

4.4.2 Pharmacologic Therapy

The drugs used for OA can be divided into four broad categories:

(a) Symptom relieving.
(b) Symptomatic slow acting drugs for OA (SYSADOA).
(c) Structure/disease-modifying drugs for OA (SMOADS/DMOADS).
(d) Intra-articular treatments.

4.4.2.1 Symptom Relieving Drugs in OA

Symptom relieving drugs include analgesics like paracetamol and nonsteroidal anti-inflammatory drugs (NSAIDs). Paracetamol has lost its sheen as the preferred first-line pain-relieving agent in OA because of a relative lack of efficacy. Pari passu with the questions about effectiveness, questions have been raised about the safety of long-term paracetamol, especially an increased risk of gastrointestinal bleeding, a small (~4 mmHg) increase in systolic blood pressure, liver and renal toxicity.

There are no firm guidelines or recommendations regarding which NSAID should be preferred. The decision has to be individualized and has to factor in comorbidities (Table 4.1). The European Society for Clinical and Economic Aspects of Osteoporosis, Osteoarthritis, and Musculoskeletal Diseases (ESCEO) task force recommends that oral NSAIDs may be used intermittently or continuously in longer cycles rather than chronic use, at the lowest effective dose, and for the shortest time necessary to control symptoms. NSAID combinations are not recommended. While switching NSAIDs may provide some benefit, the ESCEO task force does not recommend multiple successive rounds of NSAIDs before considering other treatment options.

Symptomatic patients where NSAIDs are contraindicated may be offered weak opioids like tramadol. Tramadol does not cause gastrointestinal and cardiovascular adverse events seen with NSAIDs. Respiratory depression is also very rare with tramadol. The other advantage is that the potential for abuse and addiction is notably low, unlike physical dependence commonly seen with conventional opioid drugs. Nausea and headache are the everyday adverse events that may be prevented by sustained-release (SR) formulations. SR formulations prevent the high plasma peaks associated with the immediate-release formulations. The daily dose ranges from 50 to 100 mg twice or thrice daily. Tramadol should not be co-administered with monoamine oxidase inhibitors or tricyclic antidepressants. Duloxetine is another agent that has been used in OA and other chronic pain syndromes because it acts centrally to alter pain neurotransmitters (serotonin and norepinephrine).

Topical treatments include NSAID gels and capsaicin. NSAID gels like diclofenac gel are useful for short periods during flare-ups in disease. Capsaicin is applied as a thin layer 3–4 times per day over the target joint. It depletes substance P, responsible for transmitting nociceptive stimuli from the periphery to the central nervous system.

4.4.2.2 Symptomatic Slow Acting Drugs for OA (SYSADOA)

These include agents like glucosamine, chondroitin, diacerein, avocado–soybean unsaponifiable (ASU), collagen fragments, methylsulfonylmethane, and herbal treatments like Boswellia serrata rosehip extract and turmeric (curcuminoid formulations). These nutraceutical agents are said to be chondroprotective and have attracted considerable attention and heated debate in recent times. The available trials mainly focus on knee OA. It has to be noted that numerous formulations of glucosamine as sulfate and hydrochloride salts are available. These are either patented (Rottapharm) or prescription-only generics or

OTC products and dietary supplements. The best trial evidence is for the patented crystalline glucosamine sulfate (pCGS) formulation (Rottapharm). Most studies show that prescription-grade glucosamine and chondroitin have modest efficacy and are safe, although structure modification/disease modification needs further verification. Whether it is advantageous to combine both agents is not known in the absence of high-quality trials. Diacerein or diacetylrhein is a cytokine modulator with IL-1ß inhibitory activity that has been used in knee and hip OA. It inhibits metalloproteases (collagenase, stromelysin) but does not inhibit prostaglandins. The usual starting dose is 50 mg daily that is gradually stepped up to 50 mg twice daily. The onset of action is in 4 weeks; the most typical side effect is diarrhea seen in nearly 40% of patients.

The earlier recommendations from professional bodies were ambivalent. The recent recommendations from Osteoarthritis Research Society International (OARSI) and the American College of Rheumatology (ACR) do not endorse these products for knee or hip OA. The ACR conditionally recommends chondroitin sulfate for hand OA (Table 4.2).

4.4.2.3 Structure/Disease-Modifying Osteoarthritis Drugs (SMOADS/DMOADS)

The drugs aim at slowing, stopping, or even reversing the structural changes of osteoarthritis. These are akin to disease-modifying antirheumatic drugs (DMARDs) in RA. As of now, no real disease-modifying drugs are available for OA.

4.4.2.4 Intra-articular Treatments for OA

These include corticosteroids, hyaluronic acid, and platelet-rich plasma.

1. **Intra-articular corticosteroids:** Almost all guidelines endorse the use of IAS for their short-term benefit. Triamcinolone and methyl prednisolone injections are commonly utilized. It is mandatory to rule out sepsis before injecting corticosteroids into the joint. Most authorities now believe that there is no real evidence that intra-articular steroids hasten joint destruction or cartilage degeneration. However, it is common practice not to inject the same joint more than three times a year. Strict aseptic technique is mandatory

Table 4.2 Recommendations/guidelines for knee osteoarthritis

	OARSI 2019	ACR 2019	EULAR 2003	NICE 2014[a]	AAOS 2013	Indian 2017
Glucosamine, chondroitin	Conditional recommendation AGAINST	No	May help	No	No	No
Hyaluronic acid intra-articular	Conditional recommendation FOR	Conditional recommendation AGAINST	May help	No	No	No
Intra-articular steroids	Conditional recommendation FOR	Yes	Yes	Yes	Inconclusive	Yes
PRP (platelet-rich plasma)	Strong recommendation AGAINST	Strong recommendation AGAINST	No mention	No major safety concerns. However, the evidence on efficacy is limited in quality.	Inconclusive	No mention

[a]National Institute for Health and Clinical Excellence guidance for OA was published in 2014 while the guidance on platelet-rich plasma injections for knee osteoarthritis was published in 2019

2. **Viscosupplementation with hyaluronic acid (HA):** Knee injection with HA may provide pain relief for up to 6 months. The evidence to date on the use of HA has been conflicting, and recommendations remain inconclusive (Table 4.2). It is uncertain if high-molecular-weight and cross-linked preparations of HA have superior efficacy compared with other HA preparations.

   Intra-articular hyaluronan is currently used in the following situations:
   (a) Patients who have not responded to a regimen of nonpharmacologic therapy and NSAIDs.
   (b) Patients in whom NSAIDs are contraindicated.
   (c) In patients who are otherwise candidates for surgery but surgery is contraindicated due to medical reasons, e.g., advanced cardiac disease or patients who refuse surgery.
3. **Platelet-rich plasma (PRP):** The evidence base for this modality is not robust. The use of PRP, especially a lower leukocyte concentration known as leukocyte-poor PRP, may relieve pain and improve function for about 2 months after application and lasting up to a year. The current ACR and OARSI guidelines recommend against PRP injections.

4.4.3 Surgery

Patients whose symptoms are not adequately controlled with medical therapy and who have moderate to severe pain and functional impairment are candidates for orthopedic intervention. The primary aim of surgery is to relieve pain. Options available include partial and total joint arthroplasty.

4.5 Conclusions

Osteoarthritis ranks among the top 10 causes of disability worldwide. The recent advances in understanding the pathogenesis of OA have firmly dispelled the myth that OA is an inevitable consequence of aging for which no treatment exists. The existing guidelines incorporate research-based evidence, expert opinion, and patient perspective in varying measure.

Suggested Reading

1. Bannuru RR, Osani MC, Vaysbrot EE, Arden NK, Bennell K, Bierma-Zeinstra SMA, et al. OARSI guidelines for the non-surgical management of knee, hip, and polyarticular osteoarthritis. Osteoarthritis Cartilage. 2019;27:1578–89.
2. Kolasinski SL, Neogi T, Hochberg MC, Oatis C, Guyatt G, Block J. 2019 American College of Rheumatology/Arthritis Foundation guideline for the management of osteoarthritis of the hand, hip, and knee. Arthritis Care Res (Hoboken). 2020;72:149–62.
3. Jordan KM, Arden NK, Doherty M, Bannwarth B, Bijlsma JW, Dieppe P, et al. EULAR Recommendations 2003: an evidence-based approach to the management of knee osteoarthritis: Report of a Task Force of the Standing Committee for International Clinical Studies Including Therapeutic Trials (ESCISIT). Ann Rheum Dis. 2003;62:1145–55.
4. National Institute for Health and Clinical Excellence. NICE guideline on osteoarthritis: The care and management of osteoarthritis in adults, NICE clinical guideline 177, 2014. Available at: http://guidance.nice.org.uk/CG177. Accessed 2 July 2020.
5. Jevsevar DS. Treatment of osteoarthritis of the knee: evidence-based guideline, second edition. J Am Acad Orthop Surg. 2013;21:571–6.
6. Management of Osteoarthritis Knee. Clinical Guidelines January 2017. Ministry of Health & Family Welfare. Government of India. Available at: http://clinicalestablishments.gov.in/WriteReadData/31911.pdf. Accessed 2 July 2020.
7. Liu X, Eyles J, McLachlan AJ, Mobasheri A. Which supplements can I recommend to my osteoarthritis patients? Rheumatology (Oxford). 2018;57(suppl_4):iv75–87.
8. Hunter DJ, Bierma-Zeinstra S. Osteoarthritis. Lancet. 2019;393(10182):1745–59. https://doi.org/10.1016/S0140-6736(19)30417-9.
9. National Institute for Health and Clinical Excellence. Platelet-rich plasma injections for knee osteoarthritis. Interventional procedures guidance IPG637, 2019. Available at: https://www.nice.org.uk/guidance/ipg637/evidence. Accessed 2 July 2020

5 Gout and Other Crystal Arthritides

5.1 Introduction

The spectrum of crystal arthritides includes gout, calcium pyrophosphate dihydrate deposition disease (CPPD), basic calcium phosphate (BCP) crystal arthritis, and calcium oxalate arthritis. Gout is the commonest crystal arthropathy seen in clinical practice followed by CPPD. BCP and calcium oxalate arthropathies are less common. The aging population and lifestyle changes, especially the epidemic of metabolic syndrome in Indians, have contributed to making gout ubiquitous. Gout primarily afflicts the joints and kidneys. Crystal identification is the gold standard of diagnosis. Treatment adherence is a significant issue.

5.2 Gout

Gout is the prototypic crystal arthritis characterized by hyperuricemia and urate crystal formation. Urate exists in the body in two forms: monosodium urate (MSU) at neutral and alkaline pH and uric acid at acidic pH, as in urine. Uric acid concentrations are influenced by age and gender. The mean SUA (serum uric acid) is around 3.5 mg/dl in prepubertal boys with a steep rise at puberty. In females, the surge is appreciated only after menopause since estrogens are uricosuric. Hyperuricemia is defined as SUA concentration greater than 7.0 mg/dl in males and 6.0 mg/dl in females. Concentrations greater than ~6.8 mg/dl, in conjunction with other tissue factors, favor crystal deposition in and around joints. The peak age of onset in males is between 30 and 50 years. Gout is rare in children and premenopausal females. The risk factors for primary gout (no cause identifiable) include male gender, age >40, renal insufficiency, hypertension, obesity, positive family history, and alcohol use. The onset of gout in early childhood with a positive family history should arouse suspicion of rare enzyme defects like hypoxanthine-guanine phosphoribosyl transferase (HPRT) deficiency, 5-phosphoribosyl-1-pyrophosphate (PRPP) synthetase superactivity, and glucose 6-phosphatase (G6P) deficiency. Secondary gout may be seen with tumor lysis syndrome, myeloproliferative disorders, hemolytic anemia, and psoriasis. Drugs known to cause hyperuricemia include low-dose aspirin (<2 Gm/day), cyclosporine A, diuretics, laxatives, ethambutol, pyrazinamide, etc. In most (80–90%) patients with gout, excretion of uric acid is impaired (under secretors). Increased production of uric acid (>800 mg/day) is seen in only 10–15% of subjects (over producers). Combined overproduction and underexcretion may be seen with alcohol intake.

5.2.1 Gouty Arthritis

Articular gout is divided into four clinical stages: asymptomatic hyperuricemia, acute gouty arthritis, intercritical gout, and chronic tophaceous

R. Handa, *Clinical Rheumatology*, https://doi.org/10.1007/978-981-33-4885-1_5

gout. Hyperuricemia is a common biochemical problem, and the vast majority of patients with hyperuricemia do not develop clinical problems like gout or renal disease. The development of gout depends on many factors, including age and degree of hyperuricemia. Acute gouty arthritis generally follows long-standing hyperuricemia. Urate solubility decreases with cooler temperatures accounting for the predilection of gout for distal joints. Repetitive minor trauma of the foot is invoked as an explanation for the frequent involvement of toes/lower limbs. The big toe (first metatarsophalangeal joint) is the classic site for gout (podagra). Nearly a third of patients may get their first attack at other areas such as the instep of the foot, ankle, knee, or hand joints. The afflicted joint and surrounding tissues are red, hot, and swollen (Figs. 5.1 and 5.2). The pain can be excruciating, and the patient may show fever with shaking chills. The intensity of the acute attack wanes over a few days. The skin over the joint may subsequently show desquamation. Factors known to precipitate acute attack include alcohol, red meat, surgical stress, trauma, starvation, dehydration, and drugs like diuretics, pyrazinamide, and low-dose aspirin. These factors lead to perturbations in serum uric acid levels. While gout typically causes monoarticular or pauciarticular (2, 3, or 4 joints) involvement, polyarthritis (>5 joints) can also be rarely seen, especially in the elderly and in postmenopausal women on diuretics. Other less common manifestations include tenosynovitis and bursitis. Intercritical gout refers to the symptom-free period in between attacks. The second attack may never occur or occur after a variable period. Chronic tophaceous gout is seen in individuals with uncontrolled, prolonged hyperuricemia (Fig. 5.3). Tophi represent the deposition of urates in soft tissues. Rarely, tophi may be seen in bones or other organs. They appear as firm, nodular swellings on the toes, small joints of hands, elbows, Achilles tendon, knees, and the pinna of the ear. Ulcerated tophi may exude a white chalky material. The tophi may be difficult to distinguish from rheumatoid nodules. The differential diagnosis of arthritis with nodules includes conditions like gout, rheumatoid arthritis (RA), rheumatic fever, erythema nodosum, methotrexate-induced nodulosis, vasculitis, sarcoidosis, and multicentric reticulohistiocy-

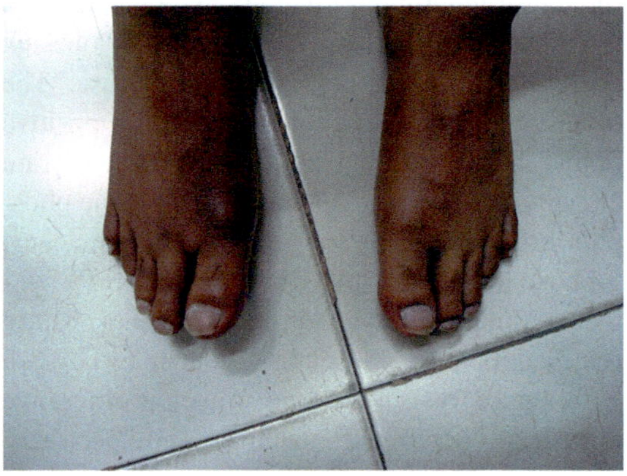

Fig. 5.1 Classical presentation of Gout affecting big toe

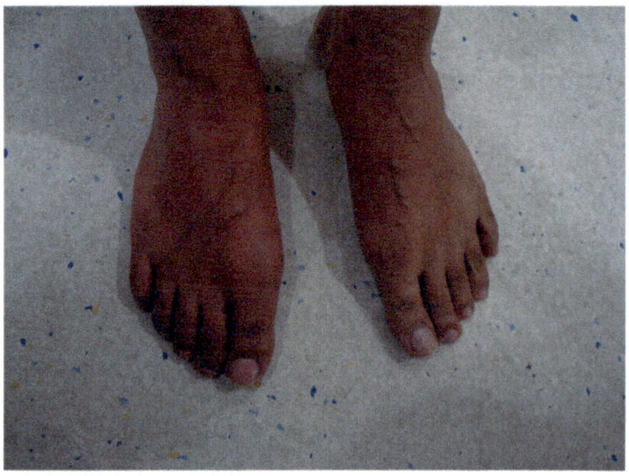

Fig. 5.2 Gout affecting fore and mid foot

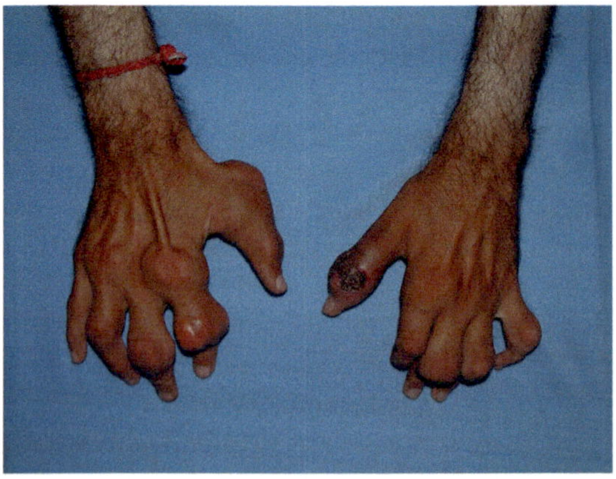

Fig. 5.3 Tophaceous Gout

Table 5.1 Gout in the elderly

• More equal sex distribution.
• Acute polyarticular presentation is not uncommon.
• Fewer bouts of classic monoarticular gout.
• More indolent chronic clinical course.
• Increased tophi in upper limbs.
• Greater propensity for colchicine/NSAID adverse events.

tosis. Gout in the elderly is being increasingly seen. Risk factors include diuretic use and renal insufficiency. Gout in the elderly, unlike classical gout, does not exhibit male preponderance, articular involvement may be polyarticular, and tophi may come up relatively early (Table 5.1).

Apart from gout, other conditions that come in the differential diagnosis of a red, hot joint include septic arthritis, reactive arthritis, and CPPD disease. Sometimes, cellulitis and trauma may mimic gout.

5.2.2 Renal Disease in Gout

Renal disease can assume three forms: urate nephropathy due to deposition of urate crystals in the renal interstitium; acute uric acid nephropathy due to precipitation of uric acid in the collecting tubules (usually in the setting of chemotherapy instituted for a lymphoproliferative disorder), and uric acid stones. It is interesting to note that not all patients with uric acid stones have hyperuricemia. Also, patients with gout have an increased tendency to develop stones other than uric acid. Other important contributory factors to renal dysfunction in gout include hypertension and nonsteroidal anti-inflammatory (NSAID) use.

5.2.3 Investigations in Gout

A definitive diagnosis of gout is based on the demonstration of MSU crystals in the synovial fluid or tophi. The synovial fluid is inflammatory with white counts >20,000/mm^3, mainly neutrophils. Though MSU crystals may be picked up on ordinary light microscopy, polarized light microscopy is ideal as it permits the detection of birefringence characteristics. Crystal identification relies on shape and birefringence. MSU crystals may be intracellular or extracellular, are needle-shaped, and exhibit strongly negative birefringence (Box 5.1). In contrast, CPPD crystals demonstrate positive birefringence (blue when parallel to the slow axis of the red compensator). A change in the orientation of the red compensator from parallel to perpendicular leads to a change in the color of the crystals. MSU crystals can often be demonstrated during the intercritical

Box 5.1 Characteristics of Gout Crystals

- Gout crystals are composed of monosodium urate (MSU).
- MSU crystals can precipitate within joints or soft tissues.
- MSU crystals may be intracellular or extracellular.
- MSU crystals are needle-shaped.
- Centrifugation may improve the pickup rate.
- MSU crystals may be detected on light microscopy.
- Polarized light microscopy is required to determine birefringence characteristics.
- MSU crystals exhibit *strong negative* birefringence.
- "Strong" birefringence means that the crystal is bright and easily seen whereas "weakly" birefringent crystal is subdued and difficult to see.
- "Positive" and "negative" birefringence refer to colors in reference to the red compensator's alignment. MSU crystals are yellow when parallel to the slow axis of the red compensator (negative birefringence).
- Polarized light microscopy is operator dependent.
- A negative report does not rule out crystal arthritis. The sensitivity of crystal analysis in synovial fluid is 63–78% depending on the experience of the lab. The specificity is 93–100%.

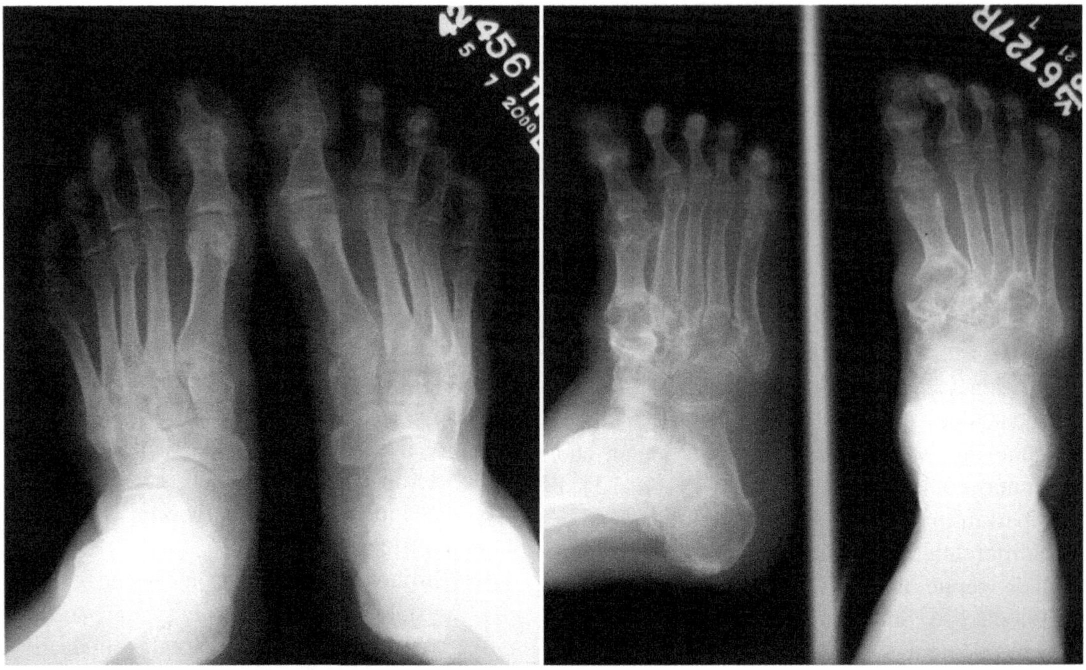

Fig. 5.4 Radiographic changes in Gout

period from quiescent joints that have been the sites of previous attacks.

Serum uric acid has limited utility in the diagnosis of gout, and a diagnosis of gout should never be based only on SUA levels. The levels of uric acid may be normal during an acute attack since the adrenocorticotrophic hormone (ACTH) released in response to stress is uricosuric. Conversely, not all patients with joint pains and a raised SUA have gout. Therefore, save in classical attacks or typical situations, attempts should be made to obtain synovial fluid for crystal studies. The primary utility of SUA is in following response to treatment in patients on urate-lowering drugs. Estimation of 24-h urinary uric acid (usually less than 800 mg) is sometimes required to differentiate overproducers from under excretors. Alcohol, radiographic contrast, and drugs like aspirin may interfere with urinary uric acid excretion.

Radiographs are normal in early gout except for soft tissue swelling, which may be seen in some patients. Patients with chronic gout show punched-out erosions with overhanging edges (Fig. 5.4). The erosions may be in the joint or away from the joint. The joint space is preserved till late, and periarticular osteopenia is absent or minimal. Table 5.2 lists the radiographic differences between gout and RA.

Table 5.2 Radiographic differences between gout and rheumatoid arthritis

	Gout	Rheumatoid arthritis
Erosions	May be located within the joint (punched-out appearance) or away from the joint (overhanging margins).	Within the joint
Joint space	Preserved till late in the disease	Reduced
Periarticular osteopenia	Absent or minimal	Characteristic feature

Ultrasound is being increasingly adopted in rheumatology, and gout is no exception. Nonspecific findings in gout include erosions, joint effusion, and synovitis. More characteristic of gout is the "snowstorm appearance" due to hyperechoic floating crystal aggregates and the "double contour sign"—an irregular hyperechoic line because of crystal deposition on the hyaline cartilage which is anechoic. This hyperechoic line and the underlying anechoic line give rise to this characteristic sonographic feature.

Dual-energy CT (DECT) is another new modality employed to assess the distribution and quantity of MSU crystals. Dual-energy X-ray tubes at 80 kv and 140 kv are placed at 90 degrees to each other and the two detectors. After simultaneous image acquisition, the materials are color-coded and overlaid on multi-planar reformatted cross-sectional and volumetric-rendered images. DECT can help assess the volume of urate crystals in tophaceous gout. It has limited sensitivity in patients with acute gout without prior episodes of gouty arthritis because patients with early disease may not demonstrate evidence of MSU deposition on DECT images. The specificity of DECT is reduced in knee osteoarthritis (OA), which may show false-positive pixilation suggestive of crystals. Nail bed artifacts may be seen in more than three-fourths of imaged feet due to the overlap of DECT values of crystals and the keratin in nails. Calluses on feet may also produce artifacts for a similar reason.

5.2.4 Treatment of Gout

Diet and lifestyle changes are crucial adjuncts. Blanket dietary prescriptions and proscriptions, and overly strict restrictions are most often unsuccessful. Diets tailored to insulin resistance and weight reduction are preferred. Purines in the diet should be restricted to <200 mg/day. Items rich in purine include red meat, liver, kidney, sardines, shellfish, and some other seafood. The total amount of purine in the diet is more important than the item consumed. Spinach, pulses (lentils), peas, mushrooms, cauliflower, soya beans, etc. are rich in purines but cause a much lower rise in SUA than red meat. Most patients do not need to restrict these vegetables or pulses in their diet. Dietary purine restriction has only a modest effect on SUA lowering (no more than 1–2 mg/dL). It is not enough to avoid ULT in most patients. Tomatoes, while not being purine-rich, can precipitate gout in some patients and may be avoided should such a history be available in a given patient. It needs emphasis that a low purine diet is not the same as a low protein diet. Protein intake needs to be restricted only to those consuming very high amounts of proteins, which is not common in Indians. Patients with gout should be encouraged to abstain from alcohol. Amongst alcoholic drinks, beer is the biggest offender, while wine (especially red wine) is the least. Skimmed milk and curd (yogurt) are beneficial. Comorbidities like hyperlipidemia and hypertension need adequate treatment. Precipitating factors, if identifiable, need appropriate attention.

Physical modalities to treat acute gout include rest, elevation, and ice. The drug treatment of gout has three facets: treatment of acute attack, prevention of further attacks, and treatment of hyperuricemia. NSAIDs are the treatment of choice for acute attacks of gout. No one agent is superior to another. Preference should be given to fast-acting NSAIDs with a short half-life. The use of NSAIDs has replaced the use of colchicine to treat acute attacks because of gastrointestinal (GI) toxicity associated with the latter and the slower onset of action. Intravenous colchicine is no longer recommended. NSAIDs are continued till the acute attack subsides over a few days. Patients at GI risk should be offered coxibs if no contraindications exist or prophylaxis with proton pump inhibitors like omeprazole, pantoprazole, etc. Corticosteroids may be used in patients with contraindications for NSAIDs, e.g., renal failure or congestive cardiac failure. Oral (prednisolone 20–40 mg daily tapered over 2 weeks) or intramuscular methylprednisolone 40–120 mg may be used. There is no consensus on agent, dose, or route of administration. Intra-articular corticosteroids are also very effective in acute gout. Urate-lowering treatments (ULT) like allopurinol should not be started during an acute attack of gout as they may precipitate another attack or prolong the duration. Patients already on ULT should continue the drugs. Patients with recurrent attacks (>3 per year) may be advised colchicine prophylaxis (0.5 mg twice daily) for 6–12 months in addition to ULT. Table 5.3 outlines the various myths and facts about gout.

Table 5.3 Prevalent myths and scientific facts

Myth	Fact
Hyperuricemia and gout are synonymous.	Hyperuricemia is a biochemical abnormality that may or may not culminate in gout. Gout is a clinical syndrome where hyperuricemia is but one of the risk factors. Environmental factors play a significant role in determining which patient with hyperuricemia will get gout.
Serum urate is the most important test for the diagnosis of gout.	Crystal identification is the gold standard.
The primary utility of serum urate is for the diagnosis of gout.	The paramount importance of serum urate lies in monitoring response to treatment.
Joint pains with elevated serum urate translate into a diagnosis of gout.	Clinical correlation is most important. Psoriasis, drugs like pyrazinamide, hematologic malignancies, hemolytic anemia, and sarcoidosis may have arthralgias/arthritis with concomitant hyperuricemia but not gout.
The gouty attack is invariably associated with elevated serum urate levels.	During an acute attack, the levels are sometimes normal because of increased urinary uric acid excretion (ACTH released in response to stress promotes this along with other inflammatory factors). Levels rise subsequently. Normouricemic gout is rare but not unknown.
Crystal detection cannot be done without polarized light microscopy.	MSU crystals can be detected on ordinary light microscopy, while polarized light microscopy, which permits detection of birefringence characteristics, is ideal.
Gout always causes monoarthritis.	The typical presentation is monoarthritis. Oligoarthritis (2, 3, 4 joints) is uncommon, and polyarthritis (5 or more joints) is rare in gout. However, these are not unknown. Polyarticular presentation is common in the elderly.
Gout is a disease of young persons only.	Elderly onset gout is increasingly being recognized. The presentation in the elderly may be more indolent, involve upper limbs, and be polyarticular.
Gout only involves the big toe.	While podagra is the characteristic presentation, midfoot, hindfoot, ankles, knees too can be affected. Upper limb involvement is well described, although rare.
Gout means goodbye to proteins.	Moderation of portion size rather than total removal from the diet is advocated. Diet of most Indians has suboptimal quantities of proteins. A blanket ban on milk or pulses not required in most instances.
Gout patients should be asked to stop milk, curd, and cheese.	Low-fat dairy should be encouraged.
Since most patients with gout are under excretors, uricosurics are the preferred agents to treat gout.	In clinical practice, xanthine oxidase inhibitors are preferred.
Low-dose aspirin should not be used in gout.	Aspirin doses in the range of 600–2400 mg/day cause uric acid retention, while doses above 4000 mg/day are uricosuric. Low-dose aspirin for cardioprotection does not have meaningful untoward effects and may be continued or instituted if so warranted by the cardiac condition.
The maximum daily dose of allopurinol is 300 mg.	The dose of allopurinol ranges from 100–800 mg daily. Dosing is determined by the target serum urate, which should be kept below 5.5–6 mg/dl.
Allopurinol should be given in divided doses.	Does up to 300 mg daily can easily be given as a single daily dose. Higher doses and gastrointestinal intolerance may require divided doses
Combination of allopurinol and febuxostat is superior to either agent alone.	Current guidelines do not recommend a combination of these agents. Uricosurics, however, can be combined with allopurinol or febuxostat.
Febuxostat is superior to allopurinol since it is a newer drug.	Both drugs are equally effective. Cardiovascular safety is a concern with febuxostat.
Colchicine is the drug of choice for acute gout.	NSAIDs, corticosteroids, and colchicine are equally effective in the treatment of acute gout. The choice is governed by patient characteristics.
Urate-lowering therapy (ULT) should be immediately started in acute gout.	ULT should not be started during an attack of acute gouty arthritis till there is adequate control of the gouty inflammation.
ULT should be discontinued after the acute attack subsides.	ULT often needs to be continued indefinitely in most patients. The dose can be titrated up or down according to serum urate levels.

In the past, most authorities did not recommend long-term pharmacologic treatment to reduce SUA after the first attack in patients with uncomplicated gout because several patients never developed another attack. Drugs to reduce SUA were instituted only if a second attack occurred within a year. There were exceptions to this thumb rule, and hyperuricemia was treated even after a single attack in the following settings: tophaceous gout, renal insufficiency, uric acid stones, and patients on diuretics. However, the current guidelines favor a stricter approach with ULT initiation close to the time of the first diagnosis in all patients presenting at a young age (<40 years), setting of very high SUA level (>8 mg/dL), and comorbidities (renal impairment, uric acid stones, hypertension, ischemic heart disease, heart failure, patient on diuretics).

Asymptomatic hyperuricemia does not warrant knee jerk treatment with ULT. It should provoke a search for other comorbidities associated with metabolic syndrome like obesity, hypertriglyceridemia, insulin resistance, etc. and correction thereof. Prophylactic use of allopurinol is recommended in situations like tumor lysis syndrome or very high SUA levels. There is no cut-off limit above which asymptomatic hyperuricemia should be treated. The 5-year cumulative risk of developing gout is nearly 30% in those with SUA >10 mg/dl, and such patients may be candidates for allopurinol despite being asymptomatic. All attempts should be made to identify risk factors and institute lifestyle changes in such patients before initiating allopurinol.

Drugs to treat hyperuricemia include xanthine oxidase (XO) inhibitors like allopurinol and febuxostat (uricostatics) or uricosuric agents like probenecid, benzbromarone, and sulfinpyrazone, which inhibit urate transporter 1 (URAT1). Despite the majority of the patients being under-excretors of uric acid, allopurinol is used as the first-line drug for lowering urate in all patients because of its efficacy, safety, and excellent benefit to risk ratio in both over producers and under-excretors of urate. The institution of allopurinol is deferred until 1–2 weeks after the acute attack. The dose varies from 100 to 800 mg p.o. given once daily—usual dose being 300 mg daily. The dose is governed by the SUA levels. The ideal SUA to aim for is below 5 mg/dl. The duration of antihyperuricemic therapy is indefinite. Side effects of allopurinol include skin rash, dyspepsia, diarrhea, and headache. Uncommon side effects include fever, bone marrow suppression, interstitial nephritis, hepatitis, and toxic epidermal necrolysis. The dose of allopurinol needs to be reduced in renal insufficiency. Notable drug interactions are with warfarin and azathioprine. The decreased metabolism of the latter with the potential for bone marrow toxicity is important in renal transplant patients.

Febuxostat in doses ranging from 40 to 120 mg daily as a single dose is another agent widely used to lower serum urate. Dose adjustment of febuxostat may not be necessary for patients with mild to moderate renal insufficiency. Common adverse reactions are abnormal liver function tests, headaches, and gastrointestinal symptoms, usually mild and transient. Concerns have been raised about the cardiovascular safety of febuxostat. In 2019, the FDA added a boxed warning for increased risk of death with febuxostat advising that it be reserved for use only in patients who were failing or having intolerance to allopurinol.

Uricosuric agents are rarely used in practice. These are ineffective in renal insufficiency and carry a small risk of uric acid stone formation. Benzbromarone (50–200 mg daily), a potent uricosuric drug used in patients who do not tolerate allopurinol or in the setting of renal insufficiency, carries a risk of hepatotoxicity. Losartan and fenofibrate also lower SUA.

Lesinurad is a recently approved selective uric acid reabsorption inhibitor. The approved dose is 200 mg once daily in combination with XO inhibitors. It acts by inhibiting the urate transporter, URAT1, which accounts for the bulk of the renal reabsorption of uric acid. It also inhibits OAT-4 (organic anion transporter 4), a uric acid transporter associated with diuretic-induced hyperuricemia.

Pegloticase, a recombinant pegylated uricase, is approved for the treatment of refractory gout. The adult dose is 8 mg given as an intravenous infusion over no less than 2 h every 2 weeks. Patients need to be premedicated with antihistamines and corticosteroids. It should never be given as an intravenous push or bolus. Oral urate-lowering agents are discontinued before starting pegloticase. Infusion reactions due to the development of antipegloticase antibodies are common.

Biologics targeting interleukin-1 (IL-1) are being tried. These include the IL-1 receptor antagonist anakinra and rilonacept (also called IL1 Trap). An exciting new drug on the horizon is arhalofenate, an anti-inflammatory uricosuric drug that reduces the risk of gout flares while also lowering SUA. It is the only drug that does not increase the risk of flares when lowering SUA. Its dual benefit action decreases the incidence, duration, and severity of flares while lowering SUA. Other benefits of arhalofenate include improvements in insulin sensitivity, as well as reductions in serum glucose and triglycerides.

A practical question often asked is regarding the continuation or start of low-dose aspirin (75–150 mg/day) for cardiovascular prophylaxis in patients with gout. Such a dose does not have clinically meaningful untoward effects and may be continued or instituted if so warranted by the cardiac condition. Aspirin doses in the range of 600–2400 mg/day cause uric acid retention, while doses above 4000 mg/day are uricosuric. Thiazide diuretics also cause a rise in SUA. In patients with hypertension, these may be substituted by other antihypertensives as far as possible. In contrast, in patients with gout and congestive cardiac failure as a comorbidity, it might be necessary to continue thiazides.

5.3 Calcium Pyrophosphate Dihydrate (CPPD) Crystal Deposition Disease

CPPD disease may be idiopathic or associated with metabolic disorders like hyperparathyroidism, hemochromatosis, hypothyroidism, etc. The prevalence increases with age. CPPD may coexist with osteoarthritis. The clinical presentation can be varied. Some of the recognized clinical patterns of CPPD deposition disease are:

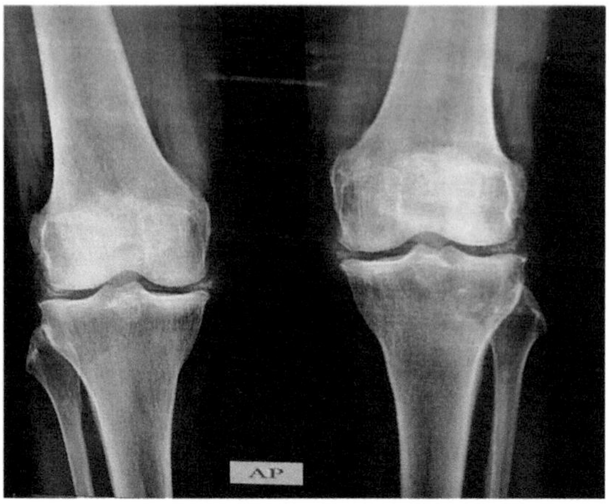

Fig. 5.5 Chondrocalcinosis

Pseudo-osteoarthritis This accounts for about 50% of all CPPD patients. Degenerative arthritis of knees and other joints like wrists, elbows, shoulders, metacarpophalangeal joints, and ankles is seen. The disease is usually symmetric. The involvement of joints like wrists, elbows, and ankles is unusual in primary OA and should arouse suspicion of CPPD. Unlike primary OA, the knee shows valgus deformity, and the finding of a valgus deformity in an elderly individual is suggestive of CPPD disease. X-rays of the knees may reveal typical calcification of the articular cartilage termed chondrocalcinosis (Fig. 5.5).

Pseudo-gout This is seen in nearly one-fourth of the patients. It presents as an acute inflammation of one or more joints. The knee joint is most commonly affected though any joint can be involved. The clinical picture mimics gout or septic arthritis.

Pseudo-rheumatoid Arthritis This presentation may mimic RA and is seen in ~5% of CPPD patients. Serologic markers of RA like rheumatoid factor and anti-CCP (cyclic citrullinated peptide) antibodies and radiographic evidence of RA in the form of erosions on radiographs of hands and feet are absent. Marked degenerative changes in joints and the presence of chondrocalcinosis point toward CPPD disease.

Pseudo-neuropathic Deposition of CPPD crystals in ligamentum flavum and spinal canal may give rise to neck pain, cervical myelopathy, radiculopathy, and spinal canal stenosis. The lumbar spine, too, may be affected. CPPD deposits can occasionally cause problems at other sites like median nerve compression at the wrist.

The diagnosis of CPPD disease can only be confirmed by the demonstration of typical crystals of CPPD in the synovial fluid of an affected joint. CPPD crystals are short, rhomboid, and demonstrate weakly positive birefringence on polarizing light microscopy. Radiologic survey for chondrocalcinosis involves three X-rays: AP views of the knees (preferably not standing), AP view of pelvis (for symphysis pubis and acetabular labrum of hips), and PA views of both hands including wrists.

The treatment of CPPD disease is symptomatic. NSAIDs are the mainstay of therapy. In pseudo-gout, aspiration of the joint followed by an intra-articular steroid injection helps. Colchicine is used though it is less effective as compared to gout. Unfortunately, treatment of associated conditions like hyperparathyroidism or hypothyroidism does not help in the resorption of CPPD crystals.

5.4 Basic Calcium Phosphate and Calcium Oxalate Crystal Disease

Basic calcium phosphate crystals comprise hydroxyapatite, octacalcium phosphate, and tricalcium phosphate. Deposition in joints and periarticular tissues causes musculoskeletal symptoms. BCP crystals are common in OA. Destructive arthritis of shoulders with a rotator cuff tear, periarticular calcification, and large effusion may occur in older women due to apatite crystal deposition (Milwaukee shoulder). The detection of BCP crystals is difficult. The small size makes identification by light microscopy difficult. Since hydroxyapatite crystals do not show birefringence, they cannot be picked up by polarized light microscopy. Synovial fluid staining with alizarin red is used to identify these crystals. Sophisticated methods like X-ray diffraction and electron microscopy may be needed in some cases.

Calcium oxalate crystals are seen in chronic renal failure. These are rod-shaped, positively birefringent crystals.

5.5 Conclusions

Crystal arthritides are common in day-to-day practice. The incidence and prevalence of gout are increasing worldwide. The diagnosis is based on a suggestive clinical picture supported by elevated serum uric acid. Crystal analysis constitutes the gold standard of diagnosis. Ultrasound and dual-energy CT have expanded the investigative armamentarium. NSAIDs, corticosteroids, or colchicine treat acute attacks of gout. ULT is the cornerstone of treatment for hyperuricemia underlying gout and often needs to be continued indefinitely.

Suggested Reading

1. Richette P, Doherty M, Pascual E, Barskova V, Becce F, Castaneda J, et al. 2018 updated European League Against Rheumatism evidence-based recommendations for the diagnosis of gout. Ann Rheum Dis. 2020;79:31–8.
2. FitzGerald JD, Dalbeth N, Mikuls T, Brignardello-Petersen R, Guyatt G, Abeles AM, et al. 2020 American College of Rheumatology guideline for the management of gout. Arthritis Care Res (Hoboken). 2020;72:744–60.

6 Rheumatoid Arthritis

Although early treatment produces better results, it is never too late to treat RA. There is nothing like burnt-out RA. The fire continues to smolder inside. Do not deny treatment to patients who present late. Tight control of disease activity is the goal of treatment. Disease-modifying antirheumatic drugs (DMARDs) should be offered to all patients with RA. Methotrexate (MTX) is the anchor drug for the treatment of RA. Folic acid should be given to all patients on MTX. DMARD combinations can be used in patients not responding to single-agent DMARD. Corticosteroids are beneficial adjuncts in the management of RA. These should not be used as the sole agents. Use minimum possible dose for the shortest possible time. Biologics and targeted synthetic DMARDs (JAK inhibitors) represent a major advance, especially in refractory, aggressive RA. Their efficacy is similar. Biologics should preferably be combined with MTX. The JAK inhibitors can be used as monotherapy. A switching of biologic agents may help in patients not responding to one agent.

Extra-articular problems in RA, like osteoporosis, premature coronary artery disease, need appropriate attention and treatment. Disease flares are a part of the disease course. During quiescence, drug dosages can be reduced. During flares, the doses are hiked up. In general, dose escalation for disease flare should be rapid. Once remission or low disease state is achieved, de-escalation is very gradual. "Top-down" rather than the "Bottom-up" approach is preferred. Seronegative RA is treated no differently from seropositive RA.

6.1 Introduction

Rheumatoid Arthritis (RA) is the commonest inflammatory polyarthritis seen in clinical practice. It is an autoimmune disease of insidious onset and unknown etiology afflicting 1% of the adult population, women more than men. RA can affect any joint, but it is common to find involvement of the metacarpophalangeal (MCP), proximal interphalangeal (PIP) joints of the fingers, the interphalangeal joints of the thumbs, the wrists, the knees, and the metatarsophalangeal (MTP) joints of the toes. The affected joints are swollen and tender. The axial skeleton is usually spared except for the cervical spine. Malaise, morning stiffness, and fatigue are common.

Investigations reveal elevated acute phase reactants. The serologic abnormalities include rheumatoid factor (RF) and anti-citrullinated peptide antibodies (ACPA). Radiographs of hands and feet show joint space narrowing and bony erosions. Ultrasound imaging and magnetic resonance imaging (MRI) are useful in the detection of early changes with many rheumatologists considering the former as an extension of physical examination.

Current treatment strategies employ disease-modifying antirheumatic drugs (DMARDs), often in combination, to achieve tight disease control. A

R. Handa, *Clinical Rheumatology*, https://doi.org/10.1007/978-981-33-4885-1_6

better understanding of the disease pathobiology has led to the development of several targeted treatments. Extra-articular complications of RA, notably osteoporosis and accelerated atherosclerosis, need to be sought and addressed.

6.2 Clinical Recognition

RA is an entity diagnosed on clinical grounds when a patient presents with bilateral, symmetrical, inflammatory polyarthritis of the small joints of hands and feet with a duration in excess of 6 weeks (Fig. 6.1). Of note, rheumatoid factor (RF) is not essential to diagnose RA, since as many as 20% of patients with RA do not exhibit RF (seronegative RA). Careful attention to the clinical description helps the clinician to avoid mistakes. Duration exceeding 6 weeks enables the exclusion of viral arthritides, which are self-limited. The insistence on a cutoff of 6 weeks has been dropped in the current classification criteria (vide infra). In the absence of clinical involvement of small joints of hands, one should be extremely reluctant to make a diagnosis of RA.

Extra-articular involvement may take the form of anemia, pleuropericarditis, interstitial lung disease, episcleritis, scleritis, sicca syndrome, vasculitis, neuropathy, splenomegaly, and osteoporosis (Figs. 6.2 and 6.3). Almost any organ may be affected. Accelerated atherosclerosis is a major contributor to mortality.

The usual age of RA is 30–50 years. Late-Onset Rheumatoid Arthritis (LORA) is a subset where the age of onset is more than 60 years. It is characterized by a more equal sex distribution, a higher frequency of abrupt disease onset, greater involvement of large joints, and a lower frequency of rheumatoid factor positivity. It is worth reiterating that low titers of RF are seen in ~5% of healthy older people without any disease. Also, ESR elevation is normal in older people

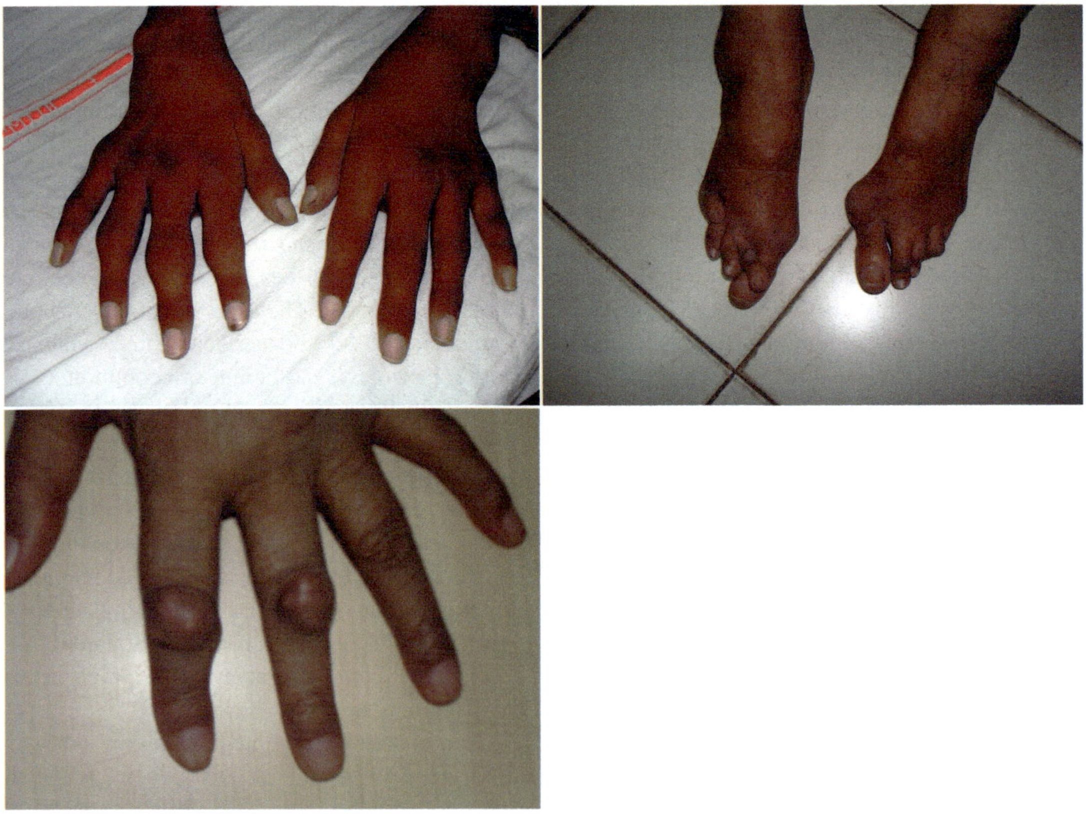

Fig. 6.1 Clinical phenotype of rheumatoid arthritis

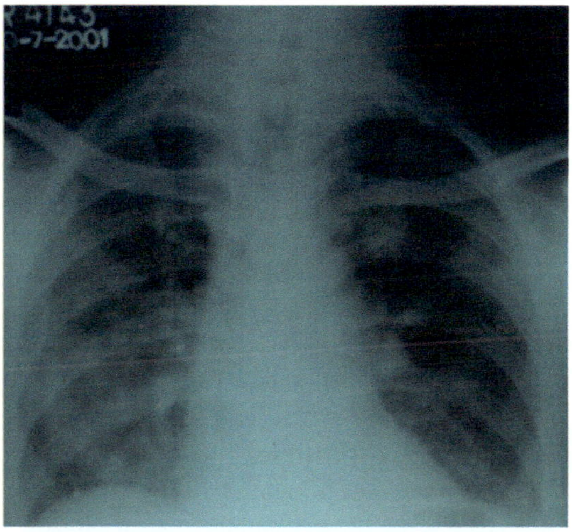

Fig. 6.2 Interstitial lung disease in rheumatoid arthritis

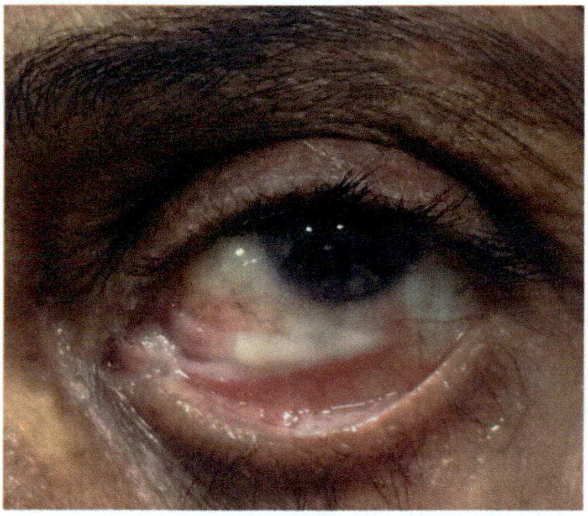

Fig. 6.3 Scleral melt in rheumatoid arthritis

(thumb rule: ESR = Age in years divided by 2, for males. For females, age+10 divided by 2. Equally important is the fact that nodular OA and RA may coexist in the same patient.

6.3 Classification Criteria for Rheumatoid Arthritis

Rheumatology as a specialty has an abundance of criteria of several different types: classification criteria, prognostic criteria, diagnostic criteria, remission criteria, etc. While being an unavoidable necessity in this era of evidence-based medicine, criteria can be quite daunting for the uninitiated. To add to the complexity, criteria do change as knowledge advances. Germane to this discussion is the need to understand that classification criterion evolved in response to the fact that most systemic rheumatic diseases lack a single pathognomonic or distinguishing feature. Features like arthritis, morning stiffness, fever, Raynaud's phenomenon, skin rash are common to several diseases. Also, many of the features do not occur concurrently but sequentially. These features present in a particular combination, along with certain laboratory investigations, help identify a specific disease. Despite being (mis) used as surrogate diagnostic criteria, classification criteria are not meant (and were never meant) to be used for diagnostic purposes. This difference is crucial. "Classification" criteria are applicable to groups and are more specific than "diagnostic" criteria, which are applied to individuals and are more sensitive. While using criteria, the clinician should never lose sight of the fact that therapeutic decisions in an individual patient should not be governed solely by fulfillment or lack of fulfillment of criteria.

The earlier 1987 criteria for RA were developed using cases with long-standing disease (mean disease duration of 7.7 years). These criteria incorporated the typical features of symmetric inflammatory polyarthritis and did away with definite, possible, and probable categories. These criteria were simple to use and required only one laboratory test, rheumatoid factor, and only one set of radiographs, posteroanterior view of hands and wrists. These criteria had a sensitivity of 91–94% and specificity of 89% when comparing RA with non-RA. These criteria served their purpose admirably well for several years. Over a period of time, a few shortcomings became apparent. The most important was the poor performance characteristics of the 1987 criteria in early RA (sensitivity 40–60%, specificity 80–90%). Two things fuelled interest in early RA: an explosion of targeted therapies, and the growing realization that the time to treat is a crucial driver of outcome. The cutoffs between "early" and "established" RA have progressively decreased. Currently, "early RA" is defined as a disease duration of less than 6 months. The 1987 criteria did not incorporate anti-citrullinated peptide antibodies (ACPA) because they were formulated prior to the advent of ACPA.

The 2010 ACR/EULAR criteria were born out of the need to pick up RA early. In the new criteria set, classification as "definite RA" is based on the confirmed presence of synovitis in at least one joint, absence of an alternative diagnosis better explaining the synovitis, and achievement of a total score of 6 or greater (of a possible 10) from the individual scores in four domains: number and size of involved joints (range 0–5), serological abnormality (range 0–3), elevated acute phase response (range 0–1), and symptom duration (two levels; range 0–1). (Table 6.1). These criteria have done away with features that are typical of late disease, namely symmetry, rheumatoid nodules, and radiographic changes. There is no longer insistence on a disease duration of 6 weeks. The criterion of morning stiffness has been dispensed with, and the serologic marker of ACPA included. This practically means that a patient with one small joint involvement (2 points), high levels of RF/ACPA (3 points), and high ESR/CRP (1 point) can be classified as RA even on day 1 of symptoms. Overdiagnosis, therefore, remains an area of concern. Clearly, the quest for ideal criteria is far from over. We need to strike a balance between sensitivity and specificity. Finally, when in doubt, the reasoned judgment of an experienced clinician prevails.

Table 6.1 ACR/EULAR 2010 classification criteria for RA

Domain: Joint involvement • 1 large joint (0 points) • 2–10 large joints (1 point) • 1–3 small joints (2 points) • 4–10 small joints (3 points) • >10 small joints (5 points)	*Domain: Duration of synovitis* • Less than 6 weeks (0 points) • 6 weeks or longer (1 point)
Domain: Serology • RF/CCP negative (0 points) • RF or CCP positive at low titer, <3 times ULN (2 points) • RF or CCP positive at high titer, defined as >3 times ULN (3 points)	*Domain: Acute phase reactants* • Normal ESR/CRP (0 points) • Abnormal ESR/CRP (1 point)

Aletaha et al. Arthritis Rheum 2010; 62:2569–81

6.4 Current Treatment Paradigm of RA

The current treatment paradigm hinges around three basic tenets (Fig. 6.4):

1. Time to Treat
2. Treat to Target
3. Targeted Treatments

RA is now deemed a time-critical illness. The philosophy of laid back "go slow, go low" approach has been discarded. Intervention, irrespective of the drug chosen, should be early since irrefutable evidence shows that irreversible damage occurs within the first 2 years of the disease when the rate of progression is significantly higher than in later years. Apart from the clinical and radiological benefits, early DMARD therapy

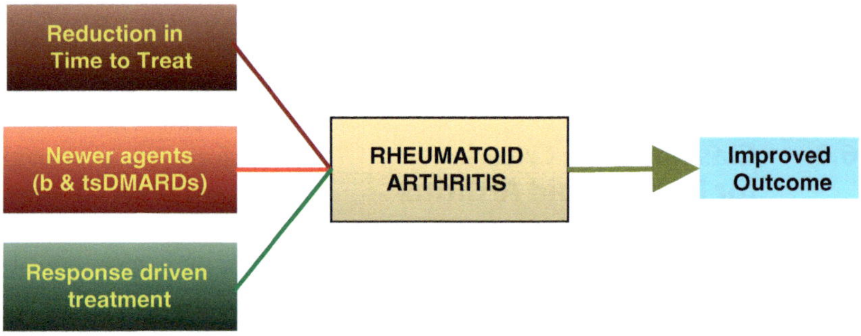

Fig. 6.4 Current treatment paradigm of rheumatoid arthritis. *bDMARDs* biologic DMARDs, *ts DMARDs* targeted synthetic DMARDs

also favorably influences mortality, which is lower in patients who present early than those who present late.

The other significant conceptual change in RA management has been the adoption of quantitative measures in the routine clinical care of patients. There is a unanimity of opinion on the need for objective measurements rather than subjective impressions. The modern-day treatment is "response-driven" rather than "routine care" whereby one sets up a predefined threshold of disease activity (target) for a patient and escalates treatment until the target is achieved. The target of treatment is clinical remission. Failing this, the next best goal is low disease activity. These targets should ideally be reached within 6 months of treatment. Of this, nearly 80% improvement in disease activity should take place within 3 months.

The third important change is the advent, and now, widespread adoption of targeted treatments comprising biologics and drugs targeting intracellular pathways—the targeted synthetic DMARDs. These are discussed in greater detail below.

6.5 How to Monitor Treatment in RA (Aligning Treatment to Targets)

RA is a multidimensional disease. The different domains include disease activity, disability, damage, and quality of life (Fig. 6.5). Validated tools to measure the different domains are available. The disease activity reflects the underlying inflammatory burden and helps decide the quantum of treatment. It is assessed by several parameters which include duration of morning stiffness, tender joint count (TJC), swollen joint count (SJC), observer global assessment, patient global assessment, visual analog scale (VAS) for pain, health assessment questionnaire for activities of daily living, erythrocyte sedimentation rate (ESR), nonsteroidal anti-inflammatory drug (NSAID) pill count, etc. The 28 joints assessed for swelling and tenderness include the 10 PIP joints, 10 MCP joints, 2 wrists, 2 elbows, 2 shoulders, and the 2 knees. Scores that integrate several parameters are now frequently employed, e.g., Disease Activity Score (DAS) 28 score, Simplified Disease Activity Index (SDAI), and Clinical Disease Activity Index (CDAI). The latter two are replacing the first one in clinical practice. Patient-reported outcome measures (PROMs) are also being increasingly employed.

The DAS 28 requires four simple inputs: 28 tender joint count, 28 swollen joint count, ESR, and general health assessment by the patient on a VAS from 0 to 100. The formula used is: DAS-28 $= 0.56\sqrt{\text{TJC}} + 0.28\sqrt{\text{SJC}} + 0.7\ln \text{ESR} + 0.014$ GH. The SDAI is a simple numerical summation of 28 SJC, 28 TJC, CRP in mg/dL (range 0.1–10), patient's global disease activity on a 10-cm VAS and physician's global assessment on a 10-cm VAS. The CDAI excludes CRP. Online

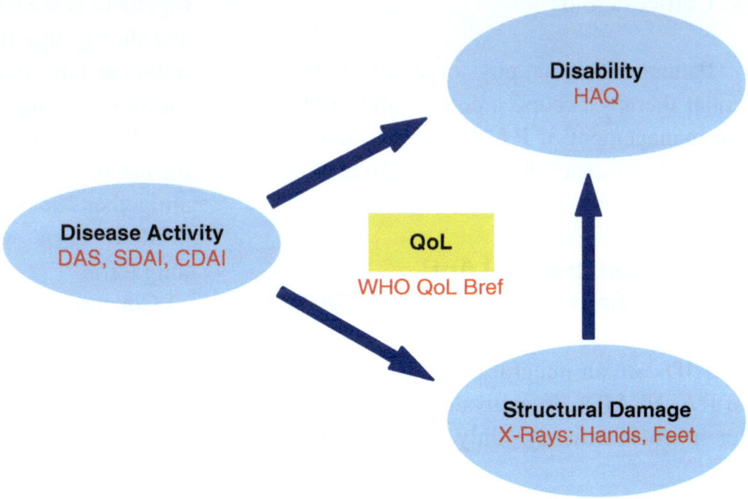

Fig. 6.5 Different domains of rheumatoid arthritis and some common measurement tools. *DAS* disease activity score, *SDAI* simplified disease activity index, *CDAI* clinical disease activity index, *HAQ* health assessment questionnaire, *QoL* quality of life, *WHO QoL Bref* World Health Organization quality of life abbreviated

Table 6.2 Disease activity measurement in rheumatoid arthritis

	Score range	Remission	Low	Moderate	High
DAS28	0–9.4	<2.6	<3.2	>3.2 and <5.1	>5.1
SDAI	0.1–86	<3.3	<11	>11 and <26	>26
CDAI	0–76	<2.8	<10	>10 and <22	>22

DAS disease activity score, *SDAI* simplified disease activity index, *CDAI* clinical disease activity index

calculators and apps are available for calculation. The cutoffs are mentioned in Table 6.2. A detailed exposition of HAQs, radiographic scoring methods, and QoL instruments is beyond the scope of this chapter.

Frequent monitoring is advocated in active disease (every 1–3 months). The aim is clinical remission or at least low disease activity within 6 months, of which about 80% improvement should occur within 3 months of starting treatment. Lack of substantial improvement at 3 months calls for a strategy change.

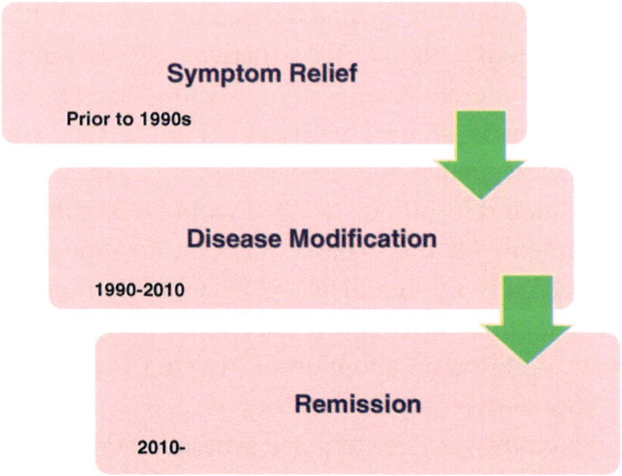

Fig. 6.6 Evolution of treatment goals of rheumatoid arthritis

6.6 Treatment Modalities for RA

The goals of treatment today have become more ambitious. The mantra today is durable remission as quickly as possible (Fig. 6.6). The various drugs used for the treatment of RA include:

1. NSAIDs
2. DMARDs
3. Corticosteroids

Patient education, physiotherapy, and occupational therapy occupy a central and vital role in the management of RA. Surgical considerations are beyond the purview of this chapter.

6.6.1 Nonsteroidal Anti-inflammatory Drugs (NSAIDs)

NSAIDs are an integral part of the management of RA. NSAIDs, in equivalent doses, do not differ much in efficacy. Only the side effects may differ. Combining two or more NSAIDs should be avoided since it does not increase efficacy but increases the incidence of side effects. The use of a particular NSAID is more a matter of choice and patient tolerance than anything else. NSAIDs are adjuncts to and not substitutes for DMARDs in the treatment of RA. Both agents are started together. DMARDs take several weeks to act, and during this time, NSAIDs are invaluable in reducing pain and inflammation. They are also useful in treating rheumatoid flares. Once the disease has been brought into clinical quiescence by the use of DMARDs, the NSAIDs can be stopped altogether or used intermittently on an "as needed" basis while DMARDs are continued long term.

Concerns about the cardiovascular (CV) safety of coxibs have led to revised recommendations taking into account gastrointestinal (GI) safety and CV effects. Nonselective NSAIDs are appropriate for patients at low risk for GI complications (i.e., under age 65 years, with no other risk factors for upper GI complications). In the elderly, in the absence of cardiovascular risk factors, coxibs are preferred to nonselective NSAIDs because they are less frequently associated with either upper/lower GI bleeding. Coxibs should generally be avoided in patients at risk of cardiovascular disease.

6.6.2 Disease-Modifying Antirheumatic Drugs (DMARDs)

The early and universal use of DMARDs is the cornerstone of current treatment strategies for RA. Since patients with active disease develop erosions within the first few months of disease onset, DMARD therapy should be initiated as soon as the diagnosis of RA is firmly established. This is analogous to the concept of "window period" for the administration of thrombolytic therapy in acute myocardial infarction. The only caveat is a situation where the diagnosis of RA is not on firm grounds, as might happen in some cases of early arthritis or situations of protracted viral arthritis like chikungunya arthritis. In such a scenario, careful observation and close follow-up are essential with the institution of DMARDs deferred until the diagnosis of RA is either ruled in or ruled out. The current nomenclature of DMARDs is spelled out in Table 6.3.

Table 6.3 The current nomenclature for disease-modifying antirheumatic drugs (DMARDs)

Synthetic DMARDs	
Conventional csDMARDS	Methotrexate, Leflunomide, Hydroxychloroquine, Sulfasalazine
Targeted tsDMARDS	Tofacitinib, Baricitinib, Upadacitinib, Peficitinib
Biological DMARDs	
Bio-originator DMARDs	Infliximab, Etanercept, Adalimumab, Golimumab, Certolizumab, Rituximab, Tocilizumab, Abatacept, Anakinra, Sarilumab
Biosimilar DMARDS	Infliximab, Etanercept, Adalimumab, Rituximab

6.6.2.1 Conventional Synthetic (cs) DMARDs

The commonly used csDMARDs include methotrexate (MTX), sulfasalazine (SSZ), hydroxychloroquine (HCQ), and leflunomide (LEF). Other agents like gold, D-penicillamine, bucillamine, iguratimod, levamisole, chloroquine, cyclosporine, cyclophosphamide, azathioprine, chlorambucil, etc. are seldom used these days.

Methotrexate is the most widely prescribed csDMARD in the world. Once weekly administration, a wide dose range from 7.5 to 25 mg, choice of oral or parenteral route, low cost, high retention rate, compatibility with other csDMARDs, targeted synthetic DMARDs or biologics, and decades of experience have contributed to MTX attaining this status. MTX should be used with caution in patients with preexisting liver disease or alcoholics. The liver function needs to be monitored regularly. A rise in aminotransferase levels necessitates a dose reduction or even temporary cessation of the drug. The transaminitis could also be a result of NSAIDs or nonalcoholic steatohepatitis that is common in Asian Indians. The concomitant administration of folic acid can mitigate the mucositis and hair loss seen in some patients on MTX. Nausea may require the use of antiemetics like ondansetron or granisetron. It is now customary to start MTX at a dose of 15 mg/week and escalate to 25 mg/week over 3–6 months, depending on tolerance and requirement. The rapidity of dose escalation and the selection of maintenance dose is governed by clinical status, patient tolerance, and the absence or presence of adverse effects. Once durable remission is achieved, the dose can be gradually reduced to the minimum, which keeps the disease activity in control, which is then continued indefinitely. Some people in remission may need as little as 2.5 mg per week. The practical points about MTX are described in Box 6.1.

In the case of MTX intolerance, adverse effects, or occasionally, patient concerns, alternative DMARDs include HCQ, LEF, or SSZ. There are no guidelines about which DMARD to choose first. The bottom line is tight disease control, no matter how it is achieved. Patients with

Box 6.1 Methotrexate: Fact File for the Clinician

- Methotrexate is the anchor DMARD for RA.
- Dose ranges from 7.5 to 25 mg weekly depending on disease activity and patient tolerance.
- Folic acid is given along with methotrexate. There is no fixed regimen. Some rheumatologists use it daily, some on alternate days, and some weekly. It is by convention administered either before or after the weekly dose of methotrexate. Even simultaneous administration does not reduce the efficacy of methotrexate significantly.
- Adherence drops with complex dosing schedules.
- Nausea may require the use of antiemetics like ondansetron or granisetron before methotrexate.
- In patients with suboptimal relief to oral MTX, subcutaneous MTX may be used as it offers better bioavailability.
- It is also recommended that doses of more than 15 mg be administered by the parenteral route.
- Oral doses higher than 15 mg per week can be split into two doses on the same day, spaced out 12 h to improve absorption. For example, a patient on 25 mg methotrexate on Sundays can split the dose to 15 mg morning and 10 mg evening to improve bioavailability.
- Methotrexate needs to be stopped 3 months before planning a pregnancy.
- Methotrexate does not compromise fertility.
- Methotrexate is not compatible with breastfeeding.
- Males wishing to father a child can continue methotrexate.
- Methotrexate can be combined with other DMARDs like hydroxychloroquine, sulfasalazine, leflunomide.
- Methotrexate can be combined with JAK inhibitors and biologics.
- Blood counts and liver function should be monitored in all patients.
- Methotrexate dose needs to be reduced in renal insufficiency.
- Methotrexate-induced interstitial lung disease (ILD) is extremely rare. The mere presence of mild-moderate ILD due to RA does not warrant a stoppage of methotrexate if needed for joints.
- There is no cumulative dose beyond which methotrexate cannot be continued. If clinically needed and if LFT is normal, the drug is continued indefinitely. Routine surveillance liver biopsies are not recommended.
- Some patients cannot continue methotrexate despite its efficacy because of adverse effects like hair loss, oral ulcers, and nausea. Anticipatory emesis may require drug cessation. Dose reduction, temporary cessation, or drug withdrawal may be needed and requires patient participation in decision-making.
- General recommendations, as mentioned above, cannot replace physician judgment in an individual patient.

mild disease can be treated with HCQ alone. DMARDs compatible with pregnancy and lactation include SSZ and HCQ. The effects of MTX, SSZ, and LEF become apparent within 2–3 months of treatment, while antimalarials take 3–6 months to produce results. Table 6.4 gives practical information about the commonly employed csDMARDs.

Patients may discontinue DMARDs because of the emergence of side effects or loss of efficacy with time (secondary failure). The former requires a change of DMARD while the latter is tackled by dose escalation, combining DMARDs or switching to alternate drugs. Disease flares punctuate the course of RA and are managed by

Table 6.4 Clinical information about common csDMARDs

Name	Usual adult dose	Side effects	Routine monitoring
Hydroxychloroquine (HCQ)	200 mg twice daily × 3 months, then once daily orally. Dose may be further reduced in quiescent disease.	Skin pigmentation, retinopathy, nausea, psychosis, myopathy	Baseline eye check-up. Then yearly screening after 5 years of use. Amsler grid is not recommended. Fundoscopy is insensitive. Baseline fundoscopy obtained to rule out preexisting maculopathy. The primary screening tests currently are automated visual fields and spectral-domain optical coherence tomography.
Methotrexate (MTX)	7.5–25 mg once a week orally, subcutaneous or intramuscular	Bone marrow suppression, hepatotoxicity, pulmonary fibrosis, mucositis, nausea, hair loss. Females should stop at least 3 months before pregnancy.	Blood counts, liver function tests (LFT), serum creatinine every 3 months. Chest X-ray at baseline.
Sulphasalazine (SSZ)	2–3 g daily orally	Rash, myelosuppression, may cause reversible reduction in sperm counts	Blood counts, LFT 3 monthly
Leflunomide (LEF)	10–20 mg daily orally	Nausea, diarrhea, alopecia, hepatotoxicity, teratogenic (females should stop at least 2 years before pregnancy)	Blood counts, LFT 3 monthly

SSZ and HCQ are compatible with pregnancy and lactation. MTX and LEF need to be discontinued before pregnancy in women. MTX and LEF are not permitted in breastfeeding mothers.

an escalation of DMARD dose with short periods of corticosteroids. Regular follow-up of patients to detect DMARD toxicity is mandatory.

6.6.2.2 Combination Therapy with csDMARDs

The advent and increasing use of biologics and tsDMARDs has diminished the importance of combination therapy with csDMARDs. Beginning 2016, the EULAR recommendations do not advocate the use of csDMARD combination therapy because the data available does not conclusively prove that combinations of csDMARDs are superior to MTX monotherapy, especially if MTX is combined with corticosteroids. Notwithstanding this, csDMARDs combinations continue to be used in large parts of the world where the penetration of biologics and tsDMARDs is not high due to resource constraints. Combination therapy with csDMARDs is employed in patients exhibiting suboptimal response to a single csDMARD. Combinations should preferably include methotrexate as an anchor drug. Combinations of methotrexate with leflunomide may be synergistic since the mode of action of these drugs is different. Leflunomide acts on the pyrimidine pathway, while methotrexate acts on the purine pathway. Liver toxicity requires careful monitoring when using this combination. The other combination frequently used is the classical triple-drug combination of MTX, SSZ, and HCQ. MTX is also commonly combined with biologics or tsDMARDs. For a clinician, perhaps more important than the drugs used in combination is the fact that "tight control" of disease activity is the goal, no matter how it is achieved.

6.6.2.3 Biologics

The conventional DMARDs have several shortcomings: onset of action takes several months, remission induced in many cases is partial, and drugs used tend to lose effectiveness with time—"slip out." These drawbacks have made researchers look for alternative treatment strategies for RA. The targeted treatments comprise biologics and the tsDMARDs. They target particular cytokines, cells, or specific pathways. Biologic therapies refer to genetically engineered treatments such as monoclonal antibodies (mAbs) or receptor-immunoglobulin fusion proteins (cepts). Examples of mAbs are infliximab, adalimumab, golimumab, certolizumab, rituximab, etc. while etanercept and abatacept are the prototypes of a receptor construct fusion protein where the naturally occurring receptor is linked to the immunoglobulin frame. The lineage can be ascertained by the name where "mo" refers to murine, "xi" to chimeric, "zu" to humanized, and "mu" to fully human mAbs. For example, infli***xi***mab is a chimeric mAb (75% human and 25% murine), tocili***zu***mab is humanized while adali***mu***mab is fully human.

The biologics may target cytokines (both ligands and receptors) or cells. Table 6.5 lists the targets of various FDA-approved biologics and their usual doses in RA.

When to Initiate Biologics in RA?
Biologics, in general, are initiated in patients who have:

- Inadequate response to csDMARDs in adequate doses (refractory disease)
- Aggressive disease with poor prognostic factors (high titer autoantibodies, high disease activity, early erosions)
- Intolerance to or adverse effects with csDMARDs
- Special situations like RA with corneal melt, rheumatoid vasculitis, some patients with RA-ILD (interstitial lung disease)

Table 6.5 Biologicals for rheumatoid arthritis

Biologic	Target	Route of administration	Usual adult dose
Infliximab	TNF	Intravenous	In conjunction with methotrexate, 3 mg/kg at 0, 2, and 6 weeks, then every 8 weeks.
Etanercept	TNF	Subcutaneous	50 mg weekly.
Adalimumab	TNF	Subcutaneous	40 mg every other week.
Golimumab	TNF	Subcutaneous	50 mg once a month.
Certolizumab	TNF	Subcutaneous	400 mg initially and at weeks 2 and 4, followed by 200 mg every other week; For maintenance dosing—400 mg every 4 weeks can be considered.
Tocilizumab	IL-6R	Intravenous and subcutaneous	Intravenous: Recommended starting dose is 4 mg per kg every 4 weeks, followed by an increase to 8 mg per kg every 4 weeks based on clinical response. Subcutaneous: 162 mg administered subcutaneously every other week, followed by an increase to every week based on clinical response.
Sarilumab	IL-6 R	Subcutaneous	200 mg once every 2 weeks.
Anakinra	IL-1R	Subcutaneous	100 mg daily.
Rituximab	CD 20 on B cells	Intravenous	The dose for RA in combination with methotrexate is two—1000 mg intravenous infusions separated by 2 weeks (one course) every 24 weeks or based on clinical evaluation, but no sooner than every 16 weeks.
Abatacept	Selective T cell costimulation modulator	Intravenous and subcutaneous	500–1000 mg intravenous injection (depending on body weight) given initially and at 2 and 4 weeks, then every 4 weeks. Subcutaneous dose is 125 mg once a week.

TNF tumor necrosis factor, *IL-6R* interleukin 6 receptor, *IL-1R* interleukin 1 receptor. Table 6.5 lists only those biologics that have FDA approval for RA. The doses mentioned are usual adult doses and may need modification in renal disease/liver disease/intercurrent infection. Please refer to the full prescribing information of each drug before use. Subcutaneous rituximab is approved only for hematologic conditions

How to Initiate Biologics in RA?

Biologics are initiated only after screening for infections. The investigations employed include Hepatitis B surface antigen (HBsAg), Hepatitis B total core antibody (HBcAb), Hepatitis C antibody, HIV screening, and tests for latent tuberculosis (TB). Screening for latent TB includes the Mantoux test, IGRA (interferon-gamma release assays), and chest radiograph. Infections, including latent TB, if present, should be appropriately treated before commencing biologics. It is also recommended that all patients initiating biologic therapy should complete vaccinations for influenza and pneumococcal pneumonia. Herpes zoster vaccination is offered to patients >50 years, depending on availability. Inactivated, adjuvanted, subunit vaccine (Shingrix) is preferred over the earlier live, attenuated vaccine (Zostavax), and immunization entails two 0.5 ml doses intramuscularly given 2–6 months apart. These recommendations may vary according to geographic location, national guidelines, and resource availability. Live vaccines such as yellow fever should be avoided.

What Do Biologics Achieve in RA?

Biologics help control disease activity in RA in a multitude of ways. They:

- Reduce signs and symptoms
- Improve physical function
- Enhance the quality of life
- Inhibit the progression of structural damage

Biologics are superior to MTX in inhibiting radiographic progression. Trial evidence reveals that the combination of a biologic and MTX inhibits radiographic progression more than either agent alone, reducing both the proportion of patients progressing and the degree of progression of those who do progress.

Place of Biologics in the Treatment Matrix of RA

Despite trial data reaffirming the utility of biologics both in early and established RA, cost and various other practicalities mean that biologic DMARDs are used primarily after csDMARD failure. It is recommended that biologics and tsDMARDs should be combined with a csDMARD, ideally MTX. When MTX is a component of such combination therapy, high doses may not be necessary. Modest MTX doses of 10 mg/week may suffice. In patients unable to tolerate MTX, IL-6R antagonists like tocilizumab or sarilumab are preferred. Nearly 40% of patients in registry data are on biologic monotherapy for various reasons, primarily csDMARD intolerance. Once sustained remission has been achieved (usually 6 months or even longer), an attempt can be made to reduce the frequency of administration or dose of biologics.

Efficacy of Biologics

Biologics may not work for all patients. In general, the efficacy of biologics in patients failing MTX is given by the broad thumb rule of American College of Rheumatology-ACR-20/−50/−70 response of 60%/40%/20%. That is, ACR 20 response is seen in 60% of such patients, ACR 50 response in 40% patients while ACR 70 response is seen in 20% of patients. Besides primary nonresponse, some patients may exhibit partial response or even exhibit worsening disease control over time (secondary nonresponse). Such situations necessitate a change of drug or increase in dose or frequency of administration.

Switching of Biologics

This is required in patients failing a biologic or for reasons of intolerance/adverse effects. If a bDMARD has failed, treatment with another bDMARD or a tsDMARD should be considered. In patients failing one TNFi therapy, biologics with another mechanism of action or another TNFi or tsDMARD may be considered.

Which Biologic for Whom?

All biologics have roughly the same efficacy and no one agent can be recommended over others for reasons of efficacy. In absence of biomarkers that predict response, the choice of a biologic is more or less empiric. Patient preference, physician familiarity, drug availability, cost sensibility, and insurer requirements play a role. For patients preferring to avoid daycare visits/hospitalization, self-administered subcutaneous injections via pen devices/auto-injectors are preferred. Some drugs like golimumab offer ease of once-a-month administration, unlike weekly etanercept or fortnightly adalimumab, sarilumab, or certolizumab. Rituximab needs to be administered intravenously once in 6 months. For patients with a past history of tuberculosis/latent TB, non-TNF agents like rituximab, tocilizumab, abatacept may be preferred over TNF inhibitors with respect to TB risk. Biosimilars may provide a cost advantage, whereas tsDMARDs may provide equal efficacy with the oral route of administration. Notwithstanding the fact that methotrexate combined with biologics is preferred over biologic monotherapy, some patients cannot tolerate methotrexate and continue only with biologic monotherapy in RA. In such instances, IL-6R antagonists are more efficacious than adalimumab monotherapy.

Biologics and Safety Issues

Injection site or infusion reactions, opportunistic infections, and reactivation of TB can be seen with almost all biologics. Drug-induced lupus, psoriasis, demyelinating syndromes may occasionally be encountered with TNFi. Rituximab can rarely be associated with hypogammaglobulinemia or progressive multifocal leukoencephalopathy. GI perforation, hypercholesterolemia, and neutropenia have been reported with tocilizumab. Readers are advised to check the full prescribing information provided by various manufacturers for a detailed understanding of adverse effects associated with these agents.

Biologics in Pregnancy and Breastfeeding

TNF inhibitors like certolizumab, infliximab, etanercept, adalimumab, golimumab can be continued throughout pregnancy if required. Certolizumab has reduced placental transfer compared with other TNFi. To ensure low/no levels of TNFα inhibitors (TNFi) in cord blood at delivery and if the disease activity permits, etanercept and adalimumab should be avoided in the third trimester and infliximab stopped at 16 weeks because of theoretical increased infection risk in newborns. If these drugs are continued later in pregnancy to treat active disease, the live vaccines should be avoided in the infant until 7 months of age. Rituximab, anakinra, abatacept, and tocilizumab should be stopped when pregnancy is confirmed.

Biologics compatible with breastfeeding include the TNFi infliximab, etanercept, adalimumab, golimumab, and certolizumab. The ACR conditionally recommends the use of rituximab, abatacept, tocilizumab during lactation, if required.

6.6.2.4 Biosimilars

The spiraling costs of bDMARDs in developed countries, limited access in resource-constrained countries, and expiry of patent periods have stimulated interest in Biosimilars. A biosimilar is a bio-therapeutic product similar in terms of quality, safety, and efficacy to an already licensed reference bio-therapeutic product. Unlike bio-originator DMARDs that require demonstration of clinical efficacy and safety for each indication, extrapolation to other indications is permitted in the case of biosimilars.

Recommendations regarding switching from bio-originator DMARDs to biosimilars or vice versa and substitution/interchangeability are continuously evolving.

6.6.2.5 Targeted Synthetic (ts) DMARDS

The advent of biologics heralded the transition from serendipity to specificity in the therapeutics of RA. Drugs like MTX were used in RA more by accident than by design. A better understanding of the pathobiology of RA led to targeted treatments, of which TNF inhibitors were the first to be put to routine clinical use. Several other agents followed this. These biologic DMARDs have a high molecular weight, are difficult to manufacture, and require parenteral administration. To overcome these drawbacks, drug development subsequently focused on small molecules with low molecular weight that are orally bioavailable and easier to manufacture. Janus kinases (JAKs) are phosphotransferases that bind to the intracellular domains of various cytokine receptors and trigger intracellular signaling.

There are four JAKs (JAK1, JAK2, JAK3, and TYK2). First-generation JAK inhibitors (jakinibs) include tofacitinib and baricitinib. These are pan-JAK inhibitors. JAK selectivity is relative rather than absolute and is dose-dependent. Selective JAK inhibitors limit the activity of a lesser number of cytokines and may have lesser adverse effects. Tofacitinib and baricitinib are available in India. These drugs have been investigated in robust global trials in various situations: methotrexate-naïve patients, patients with an inadequate response to csDMARDs, and patients with inadequate response to biologics. Trials have used adalimumab as a comparator. JAK inhibitors are initiated very much like biologics. The screening protocols are similar to those employed for bDMARDs (vide supra). The efficacy matches that of bDMARDs. JAK inhibitors can be used as monotherapy. The major impediment to widespread use is cost. The available JAK inhibitors are listed in Table 6.6.

6.6.3 Corticosteroids

Corticosteroids are invaluable in the treatment of RA. The drugs are good; their indiscriminate use is bad. It is essential to differentiate low-dose from high-dose steroids because the side effect profile of "low-dose" corticosteroids as used in RA is very different from "high-dose" steroids as used in some other conditions. Low dose refers to a daily prednisolone dose of 7.5 mg or less. A medium dose refers to a prednisolone dose between 7.5 and 30 mg daily, while a high dose is >30 mg per day. The dose advocated in RA is usually <7.5 mg/day. It could be as low as 2.5 mg daily or even on alternate days and needs to be individualized. In general, the lowest dose should be used for the shortest possible time.

The rationale for use in early RA differs from established RA. In newly diagnosed, early RA (<6 months), steroids are used as "bridge therapy" and to inhibit radiographic progression. The csDMARDs start showing effects after 2–3 months, and corticosteroids used for 8–12 weeks bridge the gap between the institution of csDMARDs and their onset of action. Also, the addition of low-dose prednisolone to DMARDs like methotrexate leads to a reduction in radiographic progression. Such use to harness the disease-modifying potential of steroids is advocated only in early RA with the caveat that steroids should never be used as monotherapeutic agents but always combined with DMARDs like methotrexate. The retardation of radiographic damage is over and above that achieved by DMARDs alone. While earlier Cochrane review discussed such use for 1–2 years, the optimum duration to capitalize on the radiographic inhibition is unknown.

In established RA, corticosteroids are used in:

(a) As "bridge therapy" for 8–12 weeks when initiating or switching csDMARDs.
(b) For the treatment of rheumatoid flares.
(c) For extra-articular RA like rheumatoid vasculitis, mononeuritis multiplex, interstitial lung disease, etc.
(d) Low doses of 7.5 mg or less of prednisolone daily in patients with refractory RA to maintain quality of life.
(e) Pregnancy and lactation if the disease is active despite the permitted DMARDs.

Table 6.6 Targeted synthetic (ts) DMARDs

Agent	JAKs targeted	Usual oral dose	Comments
Tofacitinib	JAK1, JAK2, JAK3	5 mg BD or 11 mg ER OD	Increased incidence of reactivation of herpes zoster is likely a class effect of JAK1 inhibitors. Deep vein thrombosis and pulmonary embolism have been reported. Pefcitinib is approved in Japan only.
Baricitinib	JAK1, JAK2	2–4 mg OD	
Upadacitinib	JAK1	15 mg OD	
Peficitinib	JAK1, JAK2, JAK3 and Tyk 2	150 mg OD	

JAK Janus kinase, *OD* once daily, *BD* twice daily, *ER* extended release

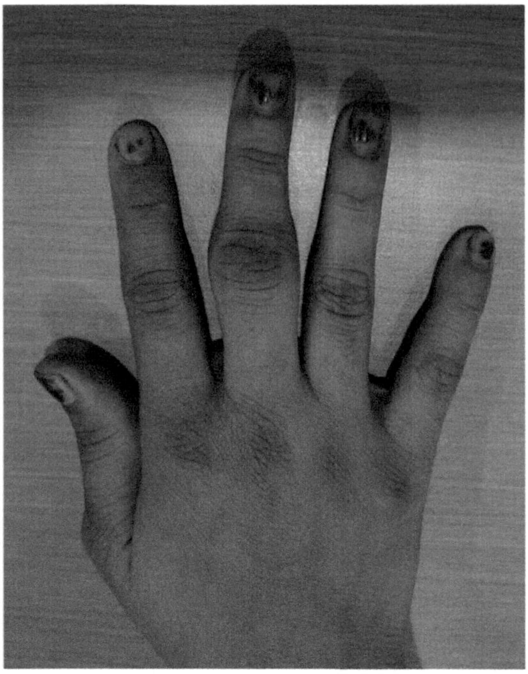

Fig. 6.7 Intraarticular steroids in rheumatoid arthritis (The third PIP joint is active while other joints are quiescent. This can be injected)

Most of the aforementioned conditions require low-dose corticosteroids. Some conditions like vasculitis may require higher dosages for initial disease control. Eye inflammation may require topical corticosteroids. The odd, recalcitrant joint that is active in the face of the globally quiescent disease can be injected with intra-articular steroids rather than hiking systemic treatment (Fig. 6.7). Joint infection should always be ruled out before local steroid injections.

Low dose does not confer exemption from steroid side effects. No dose is absolutely safe. Due diligence must be exercised as with any other drugs. Thus, strategies to minimize complications like bone protective agents should be instituted concurrently with the steroids. Prolonged use, even of low doses, carries with it the risk of all the well-known side effects of steroids. There is no robust evidence to suggest that methylprednisolone and deflazacort confer any advantage over simple prednisolone.

How Long Should Treatment Be Continued
Once remission is achieved, drug doses can be reduced. Treatment with maintenance doses for long periods is recommended. Relapse, within weeks to months, is the norm on drug discontinuation. In a patient on corticosteroids, biologics, and csDMARDs, it is recommended that corticosteroids be withdrawn first, followed by biologic DMARDs, and lastly, if remission persists, csDMARDs. While several patients can sustain remission with dose reduction of biologic DMARDs, total cessation of bDMARDs may be associated with flares (increasing with time since discontinuation). In such a scenario, biologics are reinstituted, and satisfactory control of disease activity can usually be regained. It is to be reiterated that csDMARDs are continued virtually indefinitely, albeit at reduced dosages appropriate to maintain remission.

6.7 Conclusions

RA is a chronic polyarthritis associated with substantial disability. The common pitfalls in diagnosis and treatment are summarized in Box 6.2. Current treatment protocols advocate the early use of DMARDs or a combination of therapies to achieve tight disease control. The need of the hour is to strike a balance between efficacy, toxicity, and cost. Intense efforts are underway to identify which drug would work best in what patient. This precision medicine is likely to incorporate a multiomic approach using information from the genome, epigenome, transcriptome, proteome, metabolome, and microbiome of the RA patient. Stratification and better delineation of RA's clinical, immunological, and molecular phenotype hold the key to the inevitable shift from "protocol-driven" treatments of *today* to "individualized protocols" of *tomorrow*!

Box 6.2 Common Pitfalls in Diagnosis and Treatment of RA

- Failing to consider a diagnosis of RA when RF is absent.
- Basing the diagnosis of RA on serology without clinical correlation.
- Attributing a lot of importance to borderline serologic abnormalities.
- Frequently repeating RF.
- Ordering ACPA without RF.
- Treating subjectively without measuring disease activity objectively.
- Underplaying the pivotal role of patient (*and family*) education.
- Suboptimally utilizing physiotherapy and occupational therapy services.
- Combining NSAIDs.
- Underdosing of methotrexate.
- Injudicious use of corticosteroids.
- Projecting biologics as a potential cure without factoring socioeconomic realities.
- Being oblivious to pill burden, and patient's beliefs and desires.
- Delaying treatment escalation in face of a flare. Premature de-escalation of treatment when the disease is quiescent. Escalations should be rapid. De-escalations should be gradual.
- Drug continuation without adequate monitoring.
- Labeling the disease as refractory without checking adherence.
- Paying inadequate attention to comorbidities and extra-articular manifestations.

Suggested Reading

1. Smolen JS, Landewé RBM, Bijlsma JWJ, Burmester GR, Dougados M, Kerschbaumer A, et al. EULAR recommendations for the management of rheumatoid arthritis with synthetic and biological disease-modifying antirheumatic drugs: 2019 update. Ann Rheum Dis. 2020;79:685–99.
2. Singh JA, Saag KG, Bridges SL Jr, Akl EA, Bannuru RR, Sullivan MC, et al. 2015 American College of Rheumatology Guideline for the treatment of rheumatoid arthritis. Arthritis Care Res. 2016;68:1–25.
3. Lau CS, Chia F, Dans L, Harrison A, Hsieh TY, Jain R, et al. 2018 update of the APLAR recommendations for treatment of rheumatoid arthritis. Int J Rheum Dis. 2019;22:357–75.

Spondyloarthritides

7

7.1 Introduction

Spondyloarthritides or Spondarthritides (SpA) is a big group of inflammatory rheumatic diseases that primarily involve the axial skeleton and the sacroiliac (SI) joints. The prototype disease is Ankylosing Spondylitis (AS). The absence of rheumatoid factor led to the prefix "seronegative," and the earlier nomenclature of seronegative spondyloarthropathies or SSA syndrome. The SpA primarily involves the entheses (sites where tendons and ligaments attach to bone) in contrast to rheumatoid arthritis, where synovium is the major pathologic site. Osteoproliferation rather than osteodestruction is typical. The term SpA is actually a misnomer because it is the SI joint involvement that characterizes SpA rather than spinal involvement. SpA includes several overlapping conditions: ankylosing spondylitis (AS), reactive arthritis (ReA), non-radiographic SpA (nRSpA), psoriatic arthritis (PsA), inflammatory bowel disease (IBD) associated arthritis (enteropathic arthritis), and juvenile-onset SpA (Fig. 7.1). This chapter deals primarily with AS. Reactive arthritis and PsA are discussed separately.

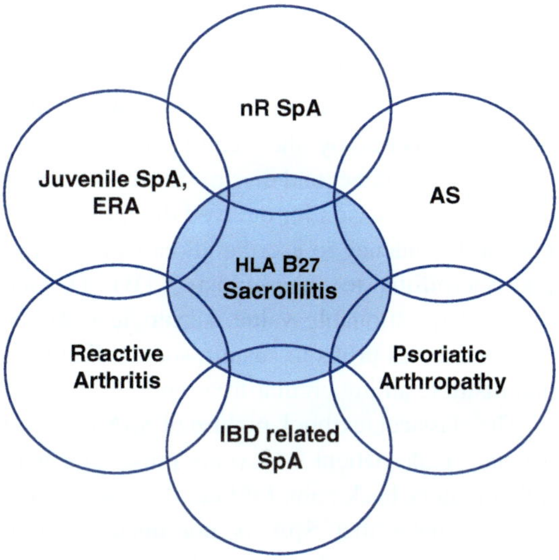

Fig. 7.1 Spectrum of spondyloarthritis (SpA)

7.2 Clinical Recognition and Investigations

The characteristic features of SpA are listed in Box 7.1. The diagnosis is suspected on clinical grounds in patients presenting with inflammatory low back pain (LBP). In routine practice, mechanical causes of LBP outnumber inflammatory causes (90% vs. 10%). Mechanical causes include conditions like herniated disc, osteoarthritis, spondylolisthesis, back sprain, nonspecific LBP, etc. The differences between mechanical and inflammatory LBP are outlined in Chap. 3.

Diagnostic delays of several years are common with SpA. Indiscriminate ordering of magnetic resonance imaging (MRI) scans in patients with LBP, and the subsequent attribution of symptoms to the "disc prolapse" that is apparent on the MRI, contributes to this in no small

R. Handa, *Clinical Rheumatology*, https://doi.org/10.1007/978-981-33-4885-1_7

Box 7.1 Characteristic Features of SpA

- Age of onset <45 years
- Males > Females
- Inflammatory low back pain
- Sacroiliitis
- Peripheral arthritis (asymmetrical, oligoarticular, large joints of lower limbs predominantly)
- Enthesitis
- Tendency to familial aggregation
- Association with HLA-B27

measure. The pernicious belief of the lay public that "disc prolapse" is the cause of all back symptoms, coupled with the perpetuation of this unfounded belief by the health care providers who fail to think beyond disc prolapse, is a major bane. Another reason for delayed diagnosis is the knee jerk tendency to ascribe all cases of unilateral sacroiliitis to tuberculosis (TB). Despite being of questionable value, serologic tests for TB are used as props to sustain such a diagnosis and institute antitubercular treatment.

The classical textbook picture of SpA is that of a young male patient <45 years presenting with inflammatory back pain. Of late, there is a growing awareness that SpA is not uncommon in women. Current studies put male-to-female ratio of 2:1 for radiographic axial spondyloarthritis and a ratio of 1:1 for non-radiographic axial spondyloarthritis. The diagnostic delay in women exceeds diagnostic delay in men because of the failure of the treating doctor to consider this possibility in women. Women exhibit less spinal and more peripheral involvement as compared to men.

Typical features of SpA are alternating buttock pain, chest pain that aggravates on coughing/sneezing, difficulty in turning side while in bed, and pain which awakens the patient during the second half of night. Enthesitis, pain along tendinous insertion sites, is another classical clinical feature of SpA. Thus, the patient can have Achilles tendinitis, plantar fasciitis (heel pain), or tenderness at patellar tendon insertion into the tibial tubercle. Other enthesopathy sites are the insertion of intercostal muscles on ribs (anterior chest pain), superior and inferior aspects of the patella, metatarsal heads, base of the fifth metatarsal, and spinal ligament insertions on the vertebral bodies. Extra-articular structures involved are the gut, skin, mucous membranes, eye, and aortic valve. Apical fibrosis may be seen in the lungs.

The ESR and CRP may be elevated, and patients may exhibit anemia of chronic inflammation. HLA B27 is a useful adjunctive test but is by no means confirmatory. Routine HLA B27 testing in all patients of back pain is not clinically helpful because SpA can occur in B27 negative individuals. Also, the presence of HLA B27 should not be taken to imply a diagnosis of SpA because it is present in a variable proportion of healthy individuals. For example, nearly 6% of healthy north Indians exhibit the presence of HLA B27, of whom only 10% develop SpA, while about 90% never develop this disease. Some of the clinical conundrums are listed and answered in Table 7.1. The presence of the HLA B27 gene varies with the type of SpA and according to ethnicity. In general, it may be as high as 90–95% in AS and 40–50% in psoriatic arthritis and reactive arthritis.

The radiologic hallmark of SpA is sacroiliitis, which may be unilateral or bilateral. AP radiographs of the pelvis are used to assess SI joints. Oblique views are no longer recommended. The changes in radiographs include narrowing of SI joints, irregularity of joint margins, and eventually bony fusion (ankylosis). Apart from the X-ray pelvis AP view, the radiologic workup of patients with suspected AS should include radiographs of the lumbar spine and thoracic junction. The changes of spondylitis include squaring of vertebra, shiny corner sign, syndesmophytes, apophyseal joint fusion, and in late stages, "bamboo spine." These changes are commonly seen at the dorsolumbar junction and may even antedate radiographic sacroiliitis in some patients. There may be subtle radiographic differences between various SpA entities. Symmetric sacroiliitis with marginal, delicate syndesmophytes is seen in AS and enteropathic SpA, while asymmetric sacroiliitis with non-marginal, chunky syndesmophytes are encountered in PsA and ReA. Symphysitis is

Table 7.1 Frequently asked questions

Question	Answer
Does HLA B27 mean AS?	HLA B27 is present in 5% healthy individuals, of whom >90% never develop the disease. The risk of developing AS in a healthy HLA B27+ person is <(10%). The risk is much higher for HLA B27+, first degree relatives of HLA B27+ AS patients (10–30%).
Can you have AS without HLA B27?	10–15% of patients with AS may be HLA B27 negative.
Should children of patients be tested?	In the absence of any preventative treatment, asymptomatic children should not be tested. HLA B27 is transmitted to 50% of offspring. Of children with the gene, only 1 in 4 get AS. Testing is recommended only in symptomatic children.
What is the difference between HLA B27 positive and HLA B27 negative patients	HLA-B27 positivity, in general, confers a greater risk of disease severity and also a concentration of disease in the spine and the eye. HLA-B27-negative patients are more likely to develop peripheral arthritis, skin, and nail disease, or IBD.
Is bamboo spine inevitable in AS?	Bamboo spine is seen in some patients only Not all AS patients develop syndesmophytes. With symptom duration <10 years, approximately 25% of patients show syndesmophytes. They may be seen in ~50% of patients with more advanced disease.
Is axSpA the only cause of Bone Marrow Edema (BME) of SI joints?	BME indistinguishable from that seen in axSpA may be seen in young athletes and postpartum women underscoring the need for clinical correlation.
What conditions can mimic SpA?	Osteitis condensans ilii (OCI) may mimic SpA. OCI may be an incidental finding on X-rays of the pelvis without any symptoms. It is common in multiparous women who present with low back pain. The classic picture is triangular sclerosis on the iliac side of SI joints (Fig. 7.11). It may be unilateral. Tuberculosis of SI joints is another mimic. Unlike SpA, TB may have a prominent soft tissue component, and the inflammation often crosses the anatomical borders (Fig. 7.12).

more commonly seen in AS. However, these features are not pathognomonic. In early disease, sacroiliitis may not be evident on plain radiographs.

MRI is the recommended imaging modality in early disease with equivocal or no changes on plain radiographs. Patients where plain X-rays reveal clear-cut sacroiliitis without any ambiguity in diagnosis do not need MRI. The greater sensitivity of MRI is because it visualizes not only the joint but also inflammatory changes like subchondral bone marrow edema (BME). A CT scan can image joint well but cannot detect bone edema. Tc^{99} bone scans to detect scintigraphic evidence of sacroiliitis have been abandoned.

7.3 Ankylosing Spondylitis (AS)

This is the flagship disease of the group termed SpA. Epidemiologic data about the prevalence of AS in Indians is not available. The prevalence of the HLA B27 gene in the Indian population is around 2–6% with 83–94% of patients with AS exhibiting the gene. Though the disease is more common in males, milder disease is being increasingly recognized in females. The usual age of disease onset is the early 20s. Onset after the age of 45 is rare. Late-onset SpA is uncommon but not unknown. Patients complain of inflammatory low back pain, which is often dull in character and poorly localized. Sometimes, enthesitis by way of plantar fasciitis, Achilles tendinitis, etc. may precede axial involvement. Peripheral arthritis may occur in one-third of cases. Typically, large joints of the lower limbs are involved in an asymmetric fashion.

Juvenile onset (<16 years of age) and hip joint involvement are suggestive of poor prognosis. In early disease, the physical examination may be unremarkable, leading to missed diagnosis. Physical findings may reveal the restriction of spinal movements and reduced chest expansion. In advanced disease, the patient assumes an abnormal hunched forward posture because of the loss of normal lumbar lordosis and the devel-

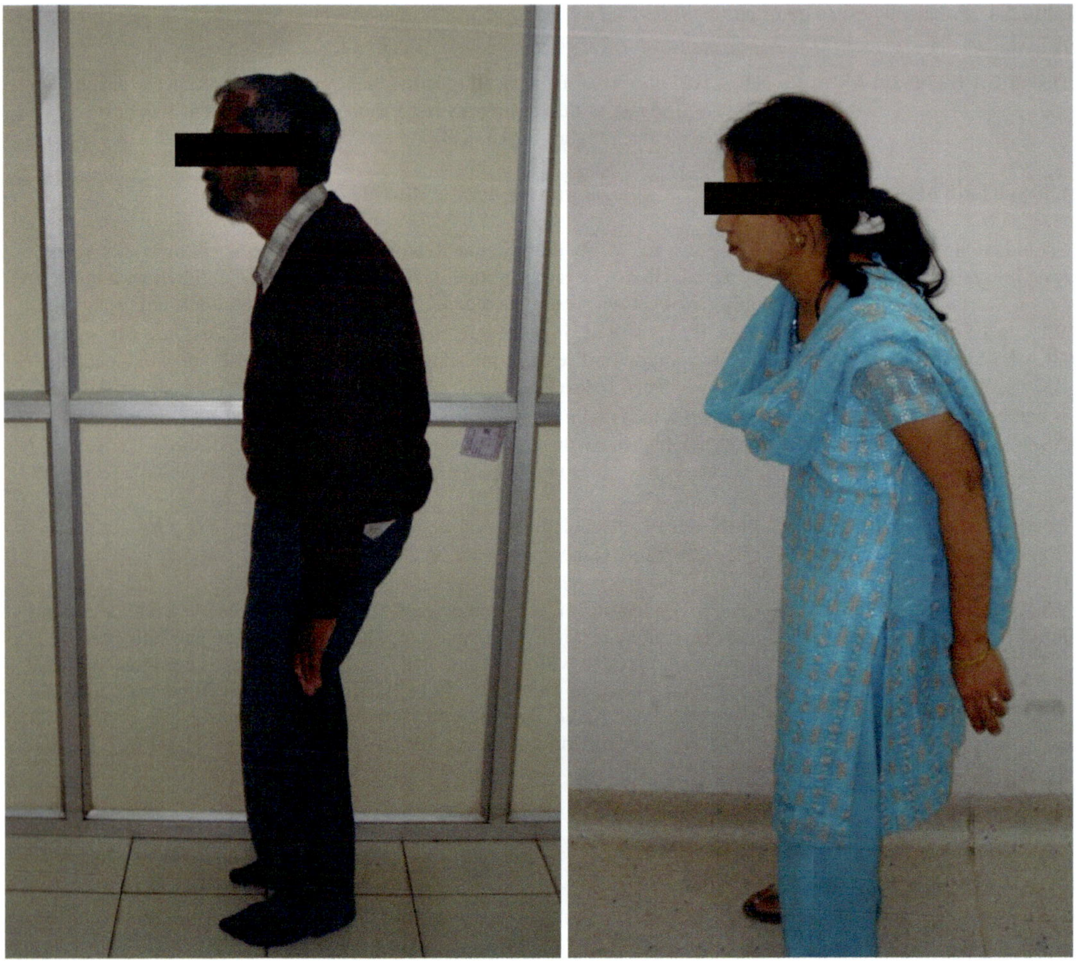

Fig. 7.2 Typical ankylosing spondylitis

opment of thoracic kyphosis (Fig. 7.2). The involvement of the cervical spine leads to a progressive limitation of neck motion. The patient may complain of difficulty in reversing a car due to the limitation of neck movements.

A variety of measurements have been described, like the modified Schober test, wall occiput distance, wall tragus distance, etc. The modified Schober test is the one most frequently employed at the bedside to assess lumbar flexion (Fig. 7.3). Clinical detection of sacroiliitis by maneuvers like pelvic compression test is unreliable.

Acute anterior uveitis, mostly unilateral, is seen in 25–30% of cases. Recurrent episodes may be seen. Occasionally, it may be the presenting symptom of AS. Other extra-articular features include apical lung fibrosis, aortic ring dilatation, aortic valve incompetence, conduction abnormalities, osteoporosis, and neurological involvement due to spinal fracture, atlantoaxial dislocation (AAD), or cauda equina syndrome. As many as 30–60% of patients may exhibit clinically silent (asymptomatic) mucosal lesions in the terminal ileum and colon on colonoscopy. Inflammatory bowel disease is seen in 5–10% of patients of AS with Crohn's being seen more often than ulcerative colitis. Psoriasis is seen in nearly 10% of patients with AS. Osteoporosis and accelerated atherosclerosis are important extra-spinal manifestations that should be sought and addressed.

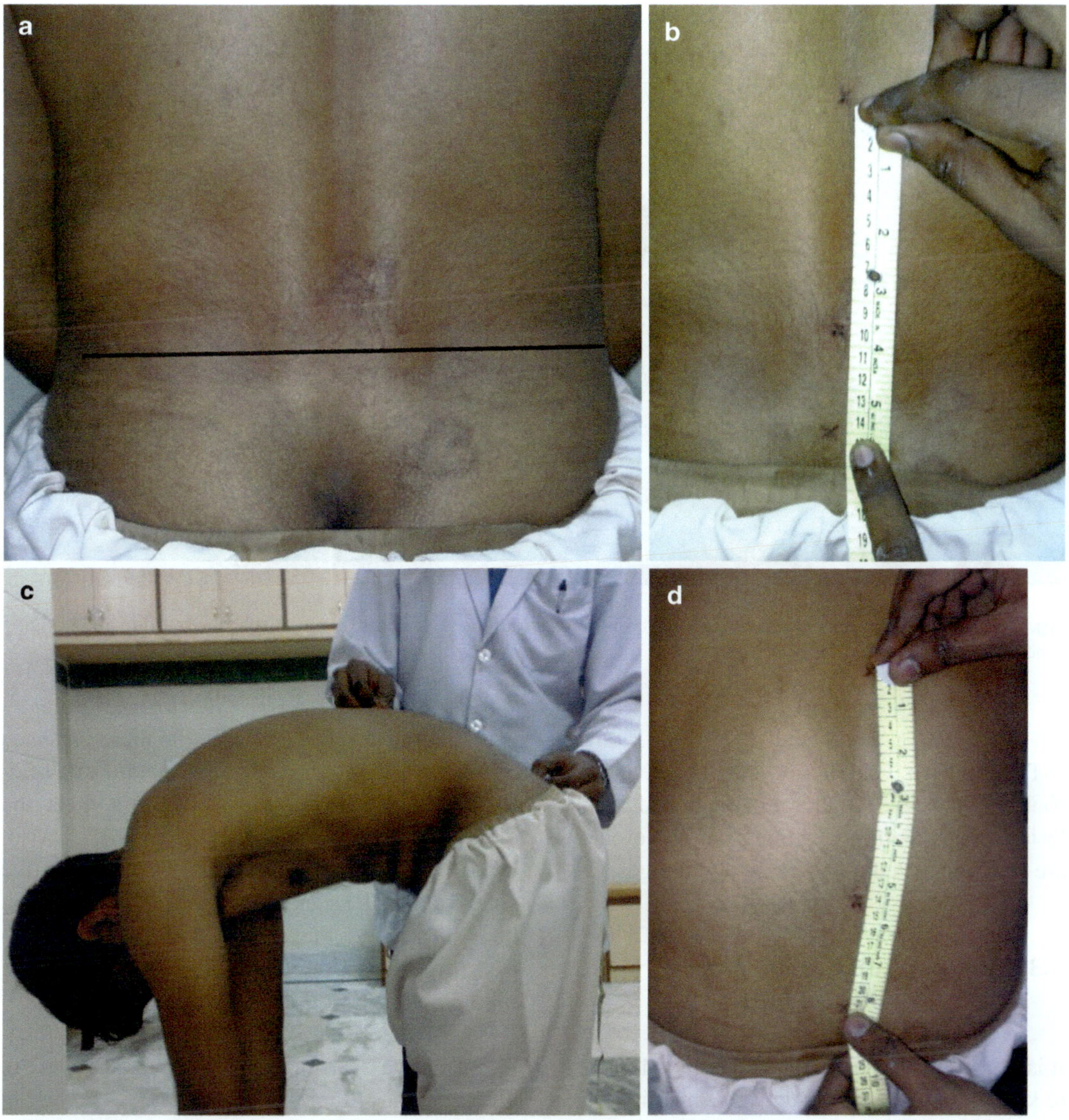

Fig. 7.3 Modified Schober's test (**a**) Draw a line joining the posterior superior iliac spines (Dimples of Venus), (**b**) Place a mark 10 cm above this point and another 5 cm below this point in the midline, (**c**) Ask the patient to bend forwards without bending the knees, (**d**) The distance between the two marks should increase by 5 cm or more in normal persons. A positive test is an increase of less than 5 cm suggesting reduced lumbar spine movement

The diagnosis of AS is clinico-radiologic. Sacroiliitis is considered the radiographic hallmark of AS. Anteroposterior radiographs of the pelvis allow visualization of both hips and symphysis pubis on the same plate in addition to the SI joints. Syndesmophytes can be picked up on radiographs of the dorsolumbar spine (Fig. 7.4). Peripheral joints may show erosions, periostitis, and fluffy periosteal reaction at the sites of enthesopathy.

In patients in whom clinical suspicion of disease is high, but X-rays of the SI joints are unremarkable, MRI is the imaging modality of choice. MRI is also invaluable in picking up sacroiliitis in children and adolescents. Active inflammatory lesions are best visualized on fat-suppressed

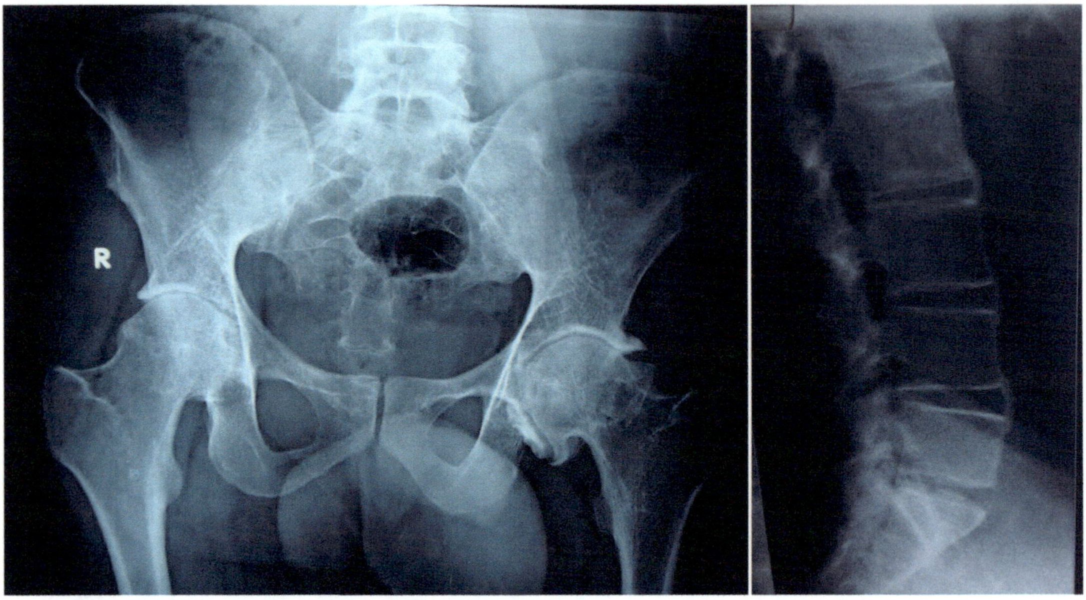

Fig. 7.4 Radiographic changes in ankylosing spondylitis. Note fused SI joints, hip joint space narrowing and bridging syndesmophytes in the spine

T2-weighted or short tau inversion recovery (STIR) images. Gadolinium enhancement is not routinely needed. Structural damage and chronic lesions, such as fatty degeneration and erosions, are best visualized on T1-weighted images.

7.3.1 What Constitutes Active Sacroiliitis on MRI

It is essential for clinicians who order MRI scans to know what constitutes active sacroiliitis on an MRI. Bone marrow edema (BME) is the radiologic hallmark of active sacroiliitis. The Assessment of Spondyloarthritis International Society (ASAS) has defined BME as a hyperintense signal on STIR images and a hypointense signal on T1-weighted images. The more intense the signal, the more likely that it reflects active inflammation. A strong hyperintense signal is similar to the signal of cerebrospinal fluid. The sacral interforaminal bone marrow signal forms the reference for the assignment of normal signal in the bone. The typical location is subchondral. BME may be accompanied by signs of structural damage such as sclerosis or erosion. The caveat is that in the absence of BME, the mere presence of structural lesions such as fat metaplasia, sclerosis, erosion, or ankylosis does not meet the definition of "active sacroiliitis on MRI." Also, BME has to be seen on at least two consecutive slices of an MRI scan. Detection of inflammation on a single slice may be sufficient for the criterion "highly suggestive of SpA" if more than one inflammatory lesion is present in the same slice. It is to be noted that BME, while being an indicator of active sacroiliitis, may also be found in other diseases (Table 7.1).

7.3.2 Classification Criteria for AS

Several classification criteria have been proposed for AS. Two, which need mention include the 1984 modified New York (mNY) criteria and the currently in vogue ASAS criteria (Figs. 7.5, 7.6, and 7.7). The mNY criteria are mentioned for historical reasons and to place in perspective the evolution of the concept of non-radiographic and peripheral SpA. The mNY criteria were specific but not sensitive and had three major shortcomings:

Clinical criteria

1. LBP & stiffness > 3 months that improves with exercise, but is not relieved by rest.
2. Limitation of lumbar spine movements in the sagittal (sideways) and frontal (forward and backward) planes.
3. Limitation of chest expansion.

Radiological criterion

- Sacroiliitis grade 2 bilaterally or grade 3–4 unilaterally or bilaterally.

grade 0: normal
grade 1: some blurring of the joint margins-suspicious
grade 2: minimal sclerosis with some erosions (mild sacroiliitis)
grade 3: severe erosions with widening of joint space +/-some ankylosis (moderate sacroiliitis)
grade 4: complete ankylosis

Fig. 7.5 Modified NY criteria for AS. [van der Linden et al. Arthritis Rheum 1984; 27:361]

Fig. 7.6 ASAS criteria for the classification of axial spondyloarthritis

Sacroiliitis on imaging plus one or more SpA features OR **HLA-B27 plus two or more other SpA features**

SpA Features
- Inflammatory back pain
- Arthritis
- Enthesitis(heel)
- Uveitis
- Dactylitis
- Psoriasis
- Crohn disease/Ulcerative colitis
- Good response to NSAIDs
- Family history of SpA
- HLA-B27
- Elevated C-reactive protein

Sacroiliitis on imaging
- Active (acute) inflammation on MRI, highly suggestive of sacroiliitis associated with SpA
  or
- Definite radiographic sacroiliitis according to the modified New York criteria.

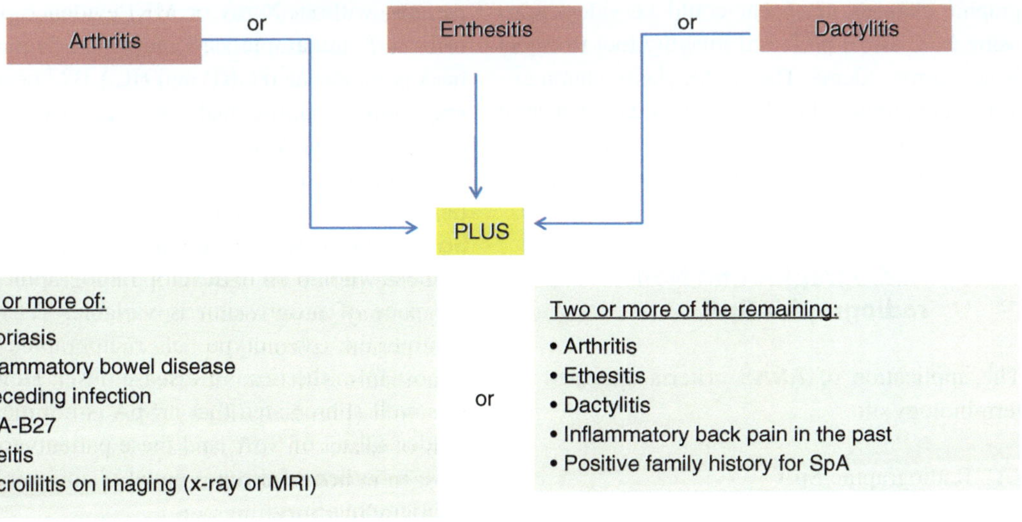

Fig. 7.7 ASAS criteria for the classification of peripheral spondyloarthritis

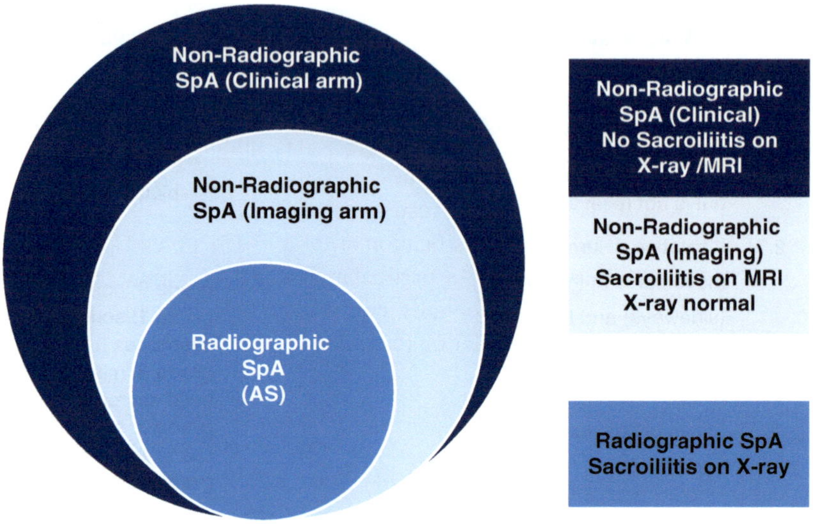

Fig. 7.8 SpA: radiographic and nonradiographic

(a) Insistence on X-ray changes of sacroiliitis, a late feature
(b) Focus on axial disease
(c) Noninclusion of HLA B27

Since LBP is ubiquitous, the thrust of mNY criteria was to identify which of these patients had AS. In the absence of treatment choices, early detection of AS did not matter much in 1984. Specificity was deemed more important than sensitivity. With the advent of biologics, there was a sea change in this paradigm. Early detection ensured timely intervention. The increasing availability of MRI meant that the interminable wait for radiographic changes to appear could be sidestepped using MRI as the preferred imaging tool to detect bone marrow edema. The ASAS classification criteria were published in 2009 to facilitate detection of early disease which could not be picked by the 1984 modified New York (mNY) criteria for AS.

7.3.3 Radiographic and Non-radiographic SpA

The application of ASAS criteria spawned the terminology of:

(A) Radiographic SpA
(B) Non-radiographic SpA (nrSpA)

Radiographic SpA includes patients with sacroiliitis evident on plain X-rays. This is virtually the same patient population as the classical AS of yore. Non-radiographic SpA includes two subsets of patients (Fig. 7.8):

(a) Those with MRI evidence of sacroiliitis but normal plain X-rays (imaging arm)
(b) Those with HLA B27 positivity plus ≥2 clinical criteria like inflammatory back pain, elevated CRP, uveitis, etc. (clinical arm)

Thus, the concept was expanded to include patients without X-ray or MRI evidence of sacroiliitis. For example, patients with inflammatory back pain, elevated CRP, and HLA B27 positivity and normal imaging could be categorized as non-radiographic SpA (clinical arm).

Opinion whether nrSpA is a forerunner of radiographic SpA or a different disease is divided. Some patients with nrSpA never progress. Even in those who go on to develop radiographic SpA, the pace of progression is variable. Yet others exhibit the phenotype of radiographic SpA almost from the time of disease onset. However, it is well appreciated that nrSpA is not merely a milder subset of SpA, and these patients too can have a burden of disease equal if not more than radiographic SpA.

7.3.4 The Concept of Peripheral SpA

Nearly 50% of patients with AS have arthritis in peripheral joints or enthesitis at some point in their disease course. Peripheral arthritis, dactylitis, or enthesitis may be the presenting, only, or predominant features in some patients with SpA. Axial symptoms may either be inconspicuous or absent. This group can now be classified as peripheral SpA using the ASAS criteria (Fig. 7.7). In addition to arthritis, enthesitis, or dactylitis, a patient can be classified as peripheral SpA if he/she demonstrates either: (1) presence of uveitis, psoriasis, or inflammatory bowel disease, preceding infection, HLA B27 positivity, or evidence of sacroiliitis on imaging, or (2) presence of at least two relevant items, which includes either arthritis (if the patient was not included on that basis), enthesitis (if the patient was not included on that basis), or dactylitis (if the patient was not included on that basis) together with inflammatory back pain (ever) or a family history of SpA.

7.3.5 Disease Assessment of AS

Validated tools like BASDAI and ASDAS are available as paper versions, on the internet, and as apps for smartphones. The Bath AS Disease Activity Index includes six questions related to five major symptoms of fatigue, spinal pain, joint pain/swelling, localized tenderness, morning stiffness over the past week. The score ranges from 0 to 10 with a higher score indicating greater disease activity.

The Ankylosing Spondylitis Disease Activity Score (ASDAS) is the more recent index that combines patient-reported symptoms and acute phase reactants. It offset the criticism that the assessment of disease activity in AS is dominated by patient-reported domains. It has two versions: ASDAS-CRP (preferred) and ASDAS-ESR (alternative) (Table 7.2). The cutoffs are shown in Fig. 7.9.

Other metrological indices include assessment of function by BASFI (Bath AS Functional Index) with ten items that ask respondents about their perception of their functional ability and how well they are able to function in their everyday life during the last 1 week. The first eight questions relate to functional anatomy, the last two to global assessment with a score range from

Table 7.2 Ankylosing spondylitis disease activity score (ASDAS)

ASDAS-CRP	0.12 × Back Pain + 0.06 × Duration of Morning Stiffness + 0.11 × Patient Global + 0.07 × Peripheral Pain/Swelling + 0.58 × Ln(CRP+1)
ASDAS-ESR	0.08 × Back Pain + 0.07 × Duration of Morning Stiffness + 0.11 × Patient Global + 0.09 × Peripheral Pain/Swelling + 0.29 × √(ESR)

√(ESR), square root of the erythrocyte sedimentation rate (mm/h); Ln (CRP+1), natural logarithm of the C-reactive protein (mg/L) + 1. Back pain, patient global, duration of morning stiffness, and peripheral pain/swelling are all assessed on a visual analog scale (from 0 to 10 cm) or a numerical rating scale (from 0 to 10). Back pain, BASDAI question 2: "How would you describe the overall level of AS neck, back, or hip pain you have had?". Duration of morning stiffness, BASDAI question 6: "How long does your morning stiffness last from the time you wake up?". Patient global: "How active was your spondylitis on average during the last week?" Peripheral pain/swelling, BASDAI question 3: "How would you describe the overall level of pain/swelling in joints other than the neck, back, or hips you have had?"

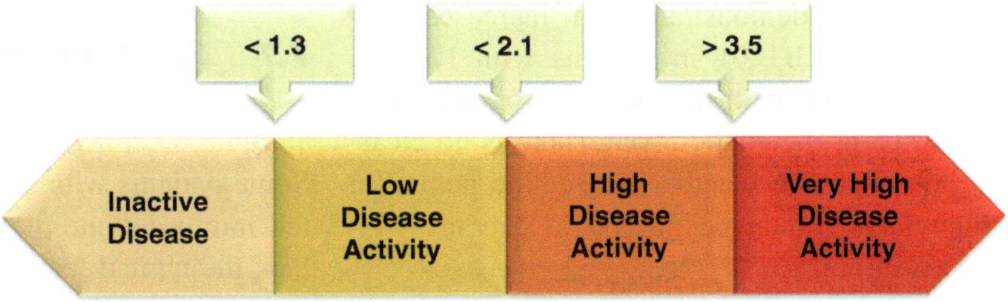

Fig. 7.9 ASDAS cut offs

0 (easy) to 10 (impossible). The Bath Ankylosing Spondylitis Metrology Index (BASMI) is a combined index to assess the spinal mobility in patients with AS. It includes Tragus-to-wall distance, Lumbar flexion (modified Schober test), Cervical rotation, Lumbar side flexion, and Intermalleolar distance. Indices employed to assess enthesitis include the SpA Research Consortium of Canada (SPARCC) Enthesitis Index, Maastricht Ankylosing Spondylitis Enthesitis Score (MASES), Leeds index, etc. A detailed discussion of these is beyond the scope of this chapter.

Radiographs of the SI joints are too insensitive to monitor the disease course. Similarly, disease monitoring by sequential spinal radiographs is of limited value because of the slow progression rate in most patients. MRI scoring systems are available for use in clinical trials.

7.4 PostStreptococcal Reactive Arthritis (PSReA)

An entity designated poststreptococcal reactive arthritis (PSReA) is mentioned in the literature. The syndrome has been considered part of the spectrum of acute rheumatic fever by some, whereas others have stressed the differences between the two diseases. As distinct from acute rheumatic fever, PSReA is characterized by a shorter latency period between the inciting streptococcal infection and the onset of arthritis, a higher frequency of involvement of the small joints and axial skeleton, poor response to aspirin and other nonsteroidal anti-inflammatory drugs (NSAIDs), a protracted course of arthritis, a low incidence of carditis, and absence of other major manifestations of acute rheumatic fever. Some studies have demonstrated an increased frequency of DRB1*01 in patients with PSReA, which contrasts with the increased frequency of DRB1*16 in rheumatic fever. There is no clear-cut consensus on whether benzathine penicillin prophylaxis should be offered to patients with PSReA or not.

7.5 Arthritis Associated with Inflammatory Bowel Disease (Enteropathic SpA)

The inflammatory bowel diseases (ulcerative colitis and Crohn's disease) may exhibit peripheral arthritis as well as axial involvement. Both forms are more common in Crohn's disease. Peripheral arthritis associated with IBD is seen in 15–20% of patients. It is asymmetric, pauciarticular, and involves the lower limbs predominantly. Both small and large joints may be affected. Arthritis may be migratory in some cases. The flare of peripheral arthritis may correspond with the flare of bowel disease in 60–70% of cases. Colectomy is said to cure arthritis in ulcerative colitis. Axial involvement similar to ankylosing spondylitis occurs in 15–20% of the patients. The sacroiliitis is usually symmetric. Enthesitis may be present. The course of the axial disease is independent of bowel inflammation. Another rheumatic problem encountered in patients with IBD is erythema nodosum.

7.6 Juvenile Spondyloarthritis

This term is used when SpA develops in a child below the age of 16 years. It is now termed Enthesitis related arthritis (ERA) and is a type of JIA (juvenile idiopathic arthritis). It mainly affects male children after the age of 6 and is characterized by enthesitis and arthritis involving joints of the lower extremities. Hip involvement is common. In some children, arthritis affects the SI joints and spine in a manner akin to AS. Most children with juvenile SpA are HLA-B27 positive.

7.7 Undifferentiated Spondyloarthritis (USpA)

Some patients with SpA features cannot be slotted into a definite disease entity. These patients lack the typical features of AS, and there are no recognizable bacterial triggers, psoriatic skin lesions, or associated inflammatory bowel disease. These patients were earlier classified as undifferentiated SpA. Some may go on to develop AS after several years. Using the ASAS criteria, some of these patients can now be reclassified as non-radiographic SpA.

7.8 Management

7.8.1 General Measures and Pain Relief

Patient education, like in other rheumatic diseases, is important. NSAIDs and spinal extension exercises form the cornerstone of therapy. Full therapeutic doses of agents like indomethacin, diclofenac, naproxen, celecoxib, etc. should be used for extended periods of time. There is no data to suggest that any one NSAID is superior to another. Whether continuous NSAIDs benefit radiologic progression is controversial with one study showing that patients with AS treated continuously over 2 years with daily NSAIDs had less radiologic progression than patients who took NSAIDs only irregularly on demand. However, this data needs validation in other studies. Physical therapy includes postural training and range of motion exercises. Swimming and hydrotherapy are very useful in SpA. Local heat or cold can be used for symptomatic relief. Splints, corsets, braces, radiotherapy to the spine do not help. Since osteoporosis is common in AS, these patients should be offered adequate calcium plus vitamin D, and if needed, bisphosphonates. Acute anterior uveitis requires mydriatics and corticosteroids—local or systemic.

7.8.2 DMARDs

DMARDs, in general, help the peripheral joints and are not effective for axial involvement. Patients with persistent peripheral synovitis like knee or ankle involvement may benefit from conventional synthetic DMARDs like sulfasalazine or methotrexate. Sulfasalazine is the most widely used agent. It has not been shown to be very effective in axial disease. The active ingredient is the sulfapyridine moiety. Methotrexate, too, may be used in the treatment of peripheral arthritis. The dosages are similar to those used for RA (methotrexate 7.5–25 mg/week; sulfasalazine 2–3 Gm/day). Gold, chloroquine, and D-penicillamine, unlike in rheumatoid arthritis, are not useful in SpA. Current guidelines do not recommend leflunomide, apremilast, thalidomide, azathioprine, and pamidronate. In resource-poor countries, many clinicians do try sulfasalazine even in axial disease. Tofacitinib, a targeted synthetic DMARD, has shown benefit in both clinical and imaging outcomes of axial disease over 12 weeks in a phase II study. It is not yet FDA approved for AS. The general principles of treatment are depicted in Fig. 7.10.

7.8.3 Biologic Agents

Two different types of biological have been approved for use in AS:

(A) TNF (tumor necrosis factor-α) inhibitors: infliximab, etanercept, adalimumab, golimumab, and certolizumab.
(B) IL-17 inhibitors: Secukinumab and ixekizumab

Anti-TNF monoclonal antibodies viz. infliximab, adalimumab, golimumab, and certolizumab are preferred for treating patients with axSpA who have recurrent uveitis or inflammatory bowel disease (IBD). Etanercept and IL-17 blockers are not recommended in the setting of uveitis and IBD. Unlike rheumatoid arthritis, routine co-administration of methotrexate with TNFi is not recommended in SpA. The usual doses are listed in Table 7.3. More details about biologics and biosimilars can also be obtained in the chapter on RA.

The biologics rapidly improve peripheral arthritis, enthesitis, and axial signs and symp-

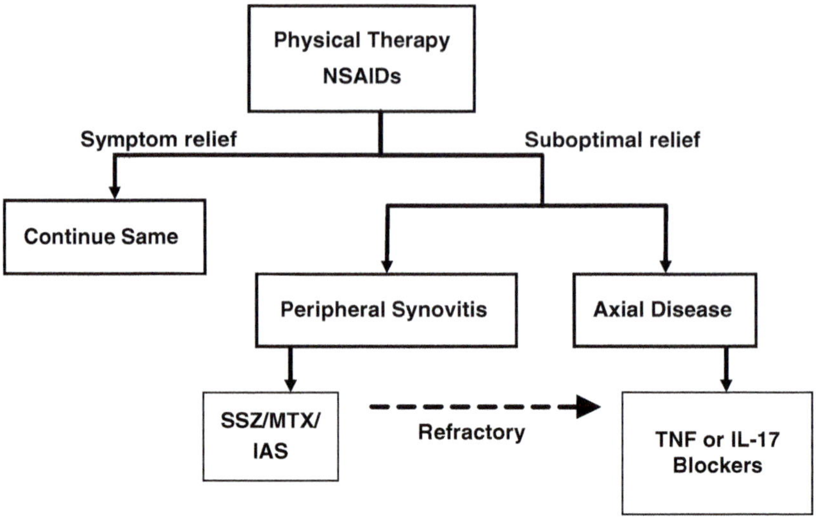

Fig. 7.10 Treatment algorithm for Ankylosing Spondylitis

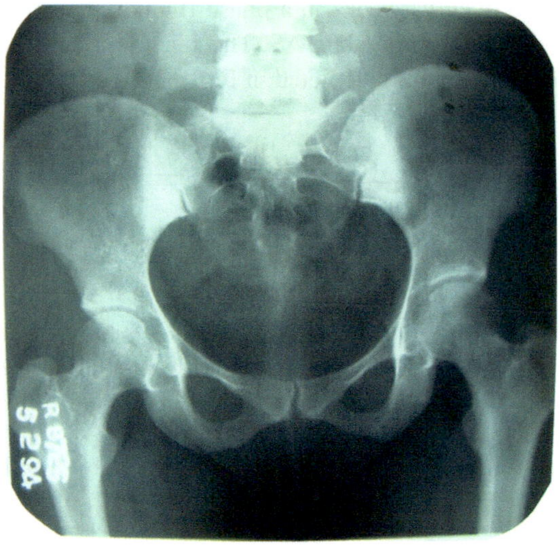

Fig. 7.11 Osteitis Condensans Ilii

toms. Improvement is also seen in imaging studies with a clearing of inflammatory lesions suggestive of disease activity on MRI. Nearly 80% of patients achieve >20% improvement in measures of disease activity. Adverse effects of biologics include predisposition to bacterial infections, reactivation of tuberculosis, and demyelination.

7.8.3.1 Indications for Biologics

Biologics are indicated for a disease that is active and refractory. Refractory axial disease is defined as one that has not responded to at least 2 NSAIDs tried in full doses over 4 weeks. Refractory peripheral disease is one that is unresponsive to intra-articular steroids (if indicated) and sulfasalazine (2–3 Gm/day) or methotrexate (up to 25 mg/week) given for 3 months after reaching the target dose. Active AS is defined by BASDAI score ≥4/10 or ASDAS ≥2.1. Like all other recommendations, these are meant as guidance. A positive rheumatologist opinion is needed before embarking on biologics. This is also embedded in the EULAR recommendations, thereby underscoring the importance of physician judgment like in other branches of medicine.

7.8.3.2 Sequence/Choice of Biologics

Most recommendations place the use of TNFi ahead of IL-17 inhibitors. This is primarily because of the earlier introduction and greater familiarity with these agents. This might change in the future. Approved biosimilars are being increasingly used for cost reasons. Nonresponders to TNFi are classified as primary or secondary. In primary nonresponders, to TNFi, secukinumab or ixekizumab are preferred over treatment with a different TNFi. In secondary nonresponders, a different TNFi can also be tried.

7.8.3.3 When to Stop Biologics

EULAR recommendations suggest the continuation of biologics if there is ASDAS improvement of ≥1.1 or BASDAI improvement of ≥2 at 12 weeks. Biologics need to be stopped/switched if

Table 7.3 Biologicals for SpA

Biologic (bio-originator)	Target	Route of administration	Usual adult dose	Biosimilar available
Infliximab (Remicade)	TNF	i.v.	5 mg/kg at 0, 2, and 6 weeks, then every 8 weeks	Yes
Etanercept (Enbrel)	TNF	s.c.	50 mg weekly	Yes
Adalimumab (Humira)	TNF	s.c.	40 mg every other week	Yes
Golimumab (Simponi)	TNF	s.c.	50 mg once a month	No
Certolizumab (Cimzia)	TNF	s.c.	400 mg initially and at weeks 2 and 4, followed by 200 mg every other week; For maintenance dosing, 400 mg every 4 weeks can be considered	No
Secukinumab (Cosentyx)	IL-17A	s.c.	Administer with or without a loading dosage. Loading dose is 150 mg at weeks 0, 1, 2, 3, and 4 and every 4 weeks after that. Without loading, the dosage is 150 mg every 4 weeks. In active disease with suboptimal response to 150 mg consider a dosage of 300 mg every 4 weeks	No
Ixekizumab (Taltz)	IL-17A	s.c.	160 mg at week 0, followed by 80 mg every 4 weeks.	No

TNF tumor necrosis factor, *s.c.* subcutaneous, *i.v.* intravenous
The doses mentioned are usual adult doses and may need modification in renal disease/liver disease/intercurrent infection. Please refer to the full prescribing information of each drug before use
Infliximab: Some clinicians in India start with 3 mg/kg and omit the loading dose for reasons of cost and risk of reactivation of Tuberculosis

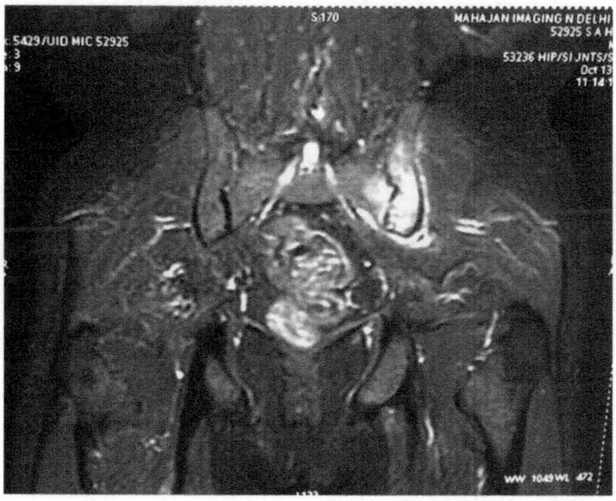

Fig. 7.12 Tuberculosis of left SI joint. Note the periarticular fluid collection. Patent had fever, and left buttock pain. CT chest revealed Miliary TB. Fever is not seen in SpA

there is no response or inadequate response, intolerance, or adverse effects. Many clinicians reduce dosages and reduce the dosing frequency once satisfactory disease control is achieved. Though recommendations call for indefinite continuation, in real-world practice, patients stop treatment for various reasons, one of which is cost. Interrupted treatment courses are common in India. Whether this promotes antidrug antibodies with loss of efficacy has not been systematically studied.

7.8.3.4 Does the Treatment of Radiographic SpA Differ from Non-radiographic SpA?

In practical terms, these entities are a spectrum of the same disease. The treatment principles remain the same. However, in some countries, regulatory requirements stipulate that TNFi can be used in radiographic axSpA (AS) without further limitations. However, in non-radiographic axSpA patients are eligible for biologicals only if there is an elevated CRP and/or inflammation on MRI. Thus, patients with axSpA need to have one or more of the three stipulations: (a) X-ray evidence of sacroiliitis; (b) MRI evidence of sacroiliitis; and (c) Elevated CRP. In some European countries, infliximab is not approved for nr-axSpA because formal trials are not available in this indication.

7.8.4 Corticosteroids

Unlike RA, the response to systemic corticosteroids is not as good in AS. Prolonged oral corticosteroid therapy does more harm than good and should be avoided. Intra-articular corticosteroids for the persistently active joint are helpful, provided septic arthritis has been ruled out. Painful enthesopathy or refractory plantar fascitis may also benefit from local corticosteroid injection. Direct injection into tendons is best avoided because of risk of tendon rupture.

7.8.5 Surgery

The commonest procedure is hip replacement. The results of surgical procedures on the spine are by and large disappointing.

7.9 Conclusions

The SpA is a cluster of overlapping chronic inflammatory diseases associated with HLA-B27. Patients present with inflammatory low back pain. The diagnosis is based on clinical pattern recognition. Sacroiliitis is the radiologic hallmark. Better elucidation of the underlying pathogenetic mechanisms and the availability of newer agents like TNF and IL-17 blockers are important advances in this field.

Suggested Reading

1. van der Heijde D, Ramiro S, Landewé R, Baraliakos X, Van den Bosch F, Sepriano A, et al. 2016 update of the ASAS-EULAR management recommendations for axial spondyloarthritis. Ann Rheum Dis. 2017;76:978–91.
2. Ward MM, Deodhar A, Gensler LS, Dubreuil M, Yu D, Khan MA, et al. 2019 Update of the American College of Rheumatology/Spondylitis Association of America/Spondyloarthritis Research and Treatment Network Recommendations for the Treatment of Ankylosing Spondylitis and Nonradiographic Axial Spondyloarthritis. Arthritis Rheumatol. 2019;71:1599–613.
3. Baeten D, Sieper J, Braun J, et al. Secukinumab, an interleukin-17A inhibitor, in ankylosing spondylitis. N Engl J Med. 2015;373:2534–48.
4. Sieper J, Listing J, Poddubnyy D, et al. Effect of continuous versus on-demand treatment of ankylosing spondylitis with diclofenac over 2 years on radiographic progression of the spine: results from a randomised multicentre trial (ENRADAS). Ann Rheum Dis. 2016;75:1438–43.

8 Psoriatic Arthritis

8.1 Introduction

Psoriasis is a common skin disorder. Psoriatic arthritis (PsA) occurs in 4–30% of patients with psoriasis. Unlike rheumatoid arthritis, there is no gender predilection. Usually, arthritis appears *after* at least 1 year of the onset of psoriasis (70% patients). However, in 15%, it appears *simultaneously* or *prior* to the development of psoriasis. The annual incidence of PsA is reported to be 2–3% in patients with psoriasis, with the skin manifestations preceding arthritis by 10 years on an average. PsA is considered a part of the spectrum of Spondyloarthritides or Spondarthritides (SpA). The similarities and differences between various entities are listed in Table 8.1. The severity of arthritis in psoriasis usually does not correlate with the extent of skin involvement. The activity of arthritis may or may not parallel the skin disease (Fig. 8.1).

The onset of joint pains in a patient with preexisting psoriasis should alert the clinician to the possibility of PsA. Sometimes, the primary caregiver in psoriasis, the dermatologist, may overlook joint symptoms, or the patient may fail to link the joint symptoms with skin disease and thus not volunteer history to the dermatologist. Physician and patient awareness play a vital role in bridging the gap. Not all joint pains in psoriasis should be reflexly attributed to PsA. Nodular osteoarthritis of hands can mimic PsA. Hyperuricemia is not uncommon in psoriasis, and gout is more common than in the general population. Clinical correlation and a careful joint examination can help avoid these pitfalls.

8.2 Clinical Recognition

PsA has multiple domains, as shown in Fig. 8.2. Moll and Wright's classification is widely employed for joints wherein there are five patterns: oligoarticular type (four or fewer joints affected); a polyarticular type (five or more joints affected); a pattern with predominant distal interphalangeal (DIP) joint involvement with nail changes; arthritis mutilans; and axial involvement with sacroiliitis and spondylitis. The oligoarticular asymmetric variety is most commonly seen in clinical practice and accounts for more than two-thirds of cases. The distinction among subtypes may not be clear cut. It is relevant to point out that the proportion has changed over the years, overlaps and crossovers are not infrequent, and oligoarthritis evolving into polyarthritis is not uncommon.

When arthritis antedates skin psoriasis, the diagnosis may be difficult. A careful search for psoriatic skin lesions in hidden sites such as umbilicus, scalp, natal cleft, behind ears, palms, and soles may be rewarding (Fig. 8.3). Dactylitis or sausage digit is a common feature of PsA occurring in 30–40% of cases. Nail changes are seen in 80–90% of patients and may take the form of pitting, ridging, onycholysis, or hyperkeratosis. These may be obscured by nail

R. Handa, *Clinical Rheumatology*, https://doi.org/10.1007/978-981-33-4885-1_8

Table 8.1 Spondarthritides

Clinical feature	PsA	AS (radiographic ax-SpA)	Reactive arthritis	Enteropathic (IBD-associated) SpA
Gender distribution	1:1	2:1	3:1	2:1
HLA-B27	45–50%	90–95%	70%	30%
Peripheral arthritis	95%	30%	90%	30%
Axial arthritis (%)	50%	100%	15–50%	30%
Dactylitis	+++	–	+	–
Enthesitis	++	+++	+	–
Skin psoriasis	All	10%	Rare	Rare

This data is pooled from several studies and reviews and is meant to enable a broad comparison among various entities

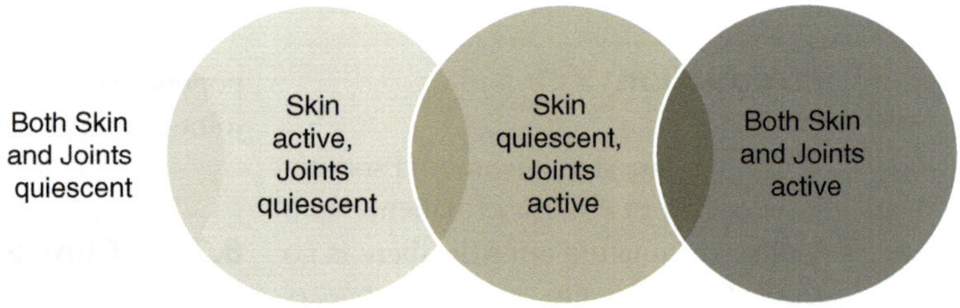

Fig. 8.1 Interrelationship between skin and joints in psoriatic arthritis

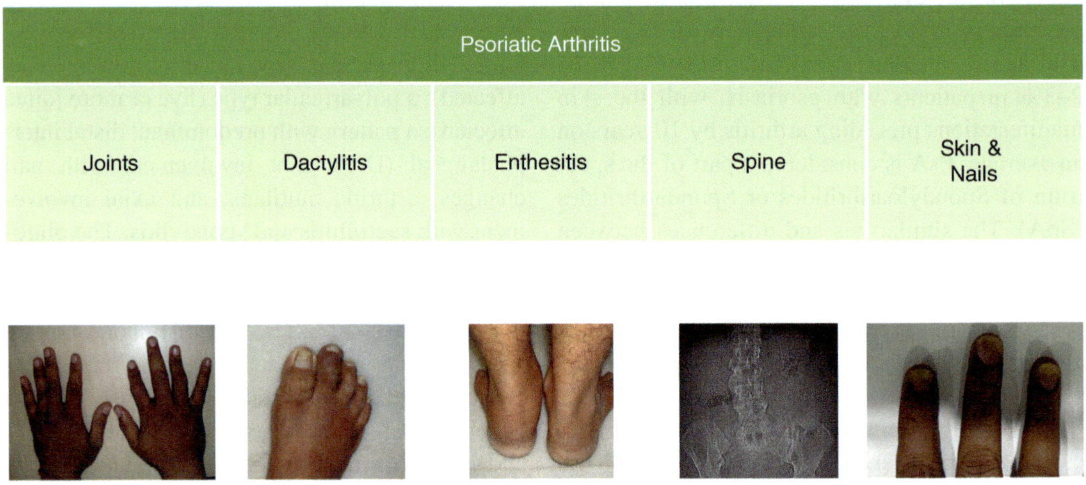

Fig. 8.2 Disease domains in PsA [Spine radiograph courtesy Dr Abhishek Patil]

paint in female patients and should be diligently sought.

The asymmetric, oligoarticular involvement with DIP joint affliction and nail changes serve to differentiate it from rheumatoid arthritis (RA), which is a bilaterally symmetrical polyarthritis sparing the DIP joints. The joint disease in symmetric variety is indistinguishable from RA and is often labeled as seronegative RA unless skin changes of psoriasis are evident.

It is now clear that PsA is not a mild disease. As many as 47% of patients develop erosive disease in 2 years. Nonalcoholic fatty liver disease, accelerated atherosclerosis, and osteoporosis are common extra-articular manifestations that need attention.

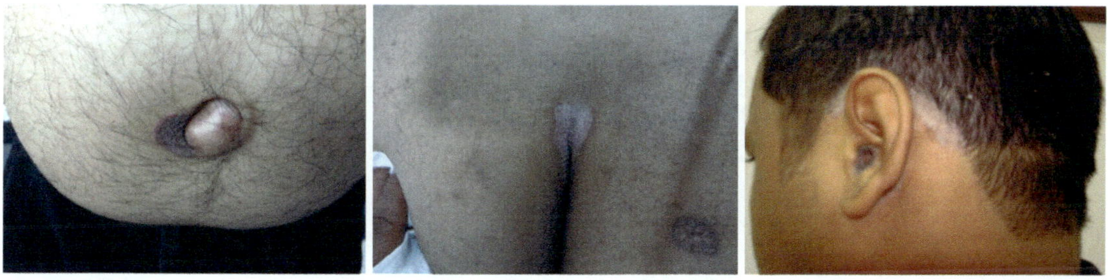

Fig. 8.3 Psoriasis in hidden areas

SAPHO syndrome (synovitis, acne, pustulosis, hyperostosis, and osteitis) is an uncommon variant of PsA. Palmo-plantar pustulosis is common in this variant. The osteoarticular associations include sternoclavicular hyperostosis, chronic sterile recurrent multifocal osteomyelitis, hyperostosis of the spine, and peripheral arthritis. Sternoclavicular hyperostosis, in India, frequently gets labeled as tuberculosis leading to a delay in diagnosis.

There are no pathognomic blood investigations. HLA B27 is present in nearly 50% of cases. Radiographs in PsA reveal erosive arthritis, with frequent DIP joint involvement and pencil-in-cup changes because of marked resorption of bone (Fig. 8.4). Other findings include enthesitis with periosteal reaction, sacroiliitis, and spondylitis. The sacroiliitis is frequently asymmetrical. In contrast to the symmetrical and marginal syndesmophytes seen in AS, the syndesmophytes in PsA are less frequent, asymmetrical, non-marginal, and chunky. These differences in syndesmophyte morphology may not be apparent in all patients.

8.3 Management

Validated instruments like DAPSA (disease activity in psoriatic arthritis), PASDAS (psoriatic arthritis disease activity score), CPDAI (composite psoriasis disease activity index) are available. The treatment approach has to be multidisciplinary and look at all five disease domains. Skin and nail disease require dermatology inputs. The current EULAR recommendations stipulate that the treatment target should be remission or low disease activity. Furthermore, if improvement does not exceed 50% of a composite measure for PsA within 3 months or the treatment target is not reached within 6 months, such conventional synthetic (cs) DMARD therapy should not be pursued longer and changed.

The American College of Rheumatology defines severe PsA as the presence of ≥1 of the following: a poor prognostic factor (erosive disease, elevated levels of CRP or ESR), joint deformities, active psoriatic inflammatory disease at many sites ([including dactylitis, enthesitis] or function-limiting inflammatory disease at few sites), and rapidly progressive disease. Moderate to severe skin disease is body surface area involvement of ≥5%.

NSAIDs are employed for pain relief. Corticosteroids should be used sparingly in PsA. Low doses for short periods or intra-articular injections are employed. Skin psoriasis may flare after withdrawal. The disease-modifying anti-rheumatic drugs (DMARDs) used in PsA are listed in Table 8.2. Initial treatment of peripheral arthritis comprises the cs DMARDs. Methotrexate is widely employed as the first agent. Despite little evidence on the efficacy of csDMARD combinations, these may be considered in resource-constrained countries. Cyclosporine is useful for skin psoriasis but not recommended for PsA in the current EULAR guidelines. In patients with severe disease or suboptimal response to csDMARDs, biologics are recommended. No particular sequence of biologics is mentioned for PsA. Both IL-12/23i and IL-17i have shown greater efficacy in skin than TNFi. This has led to recommendations that in

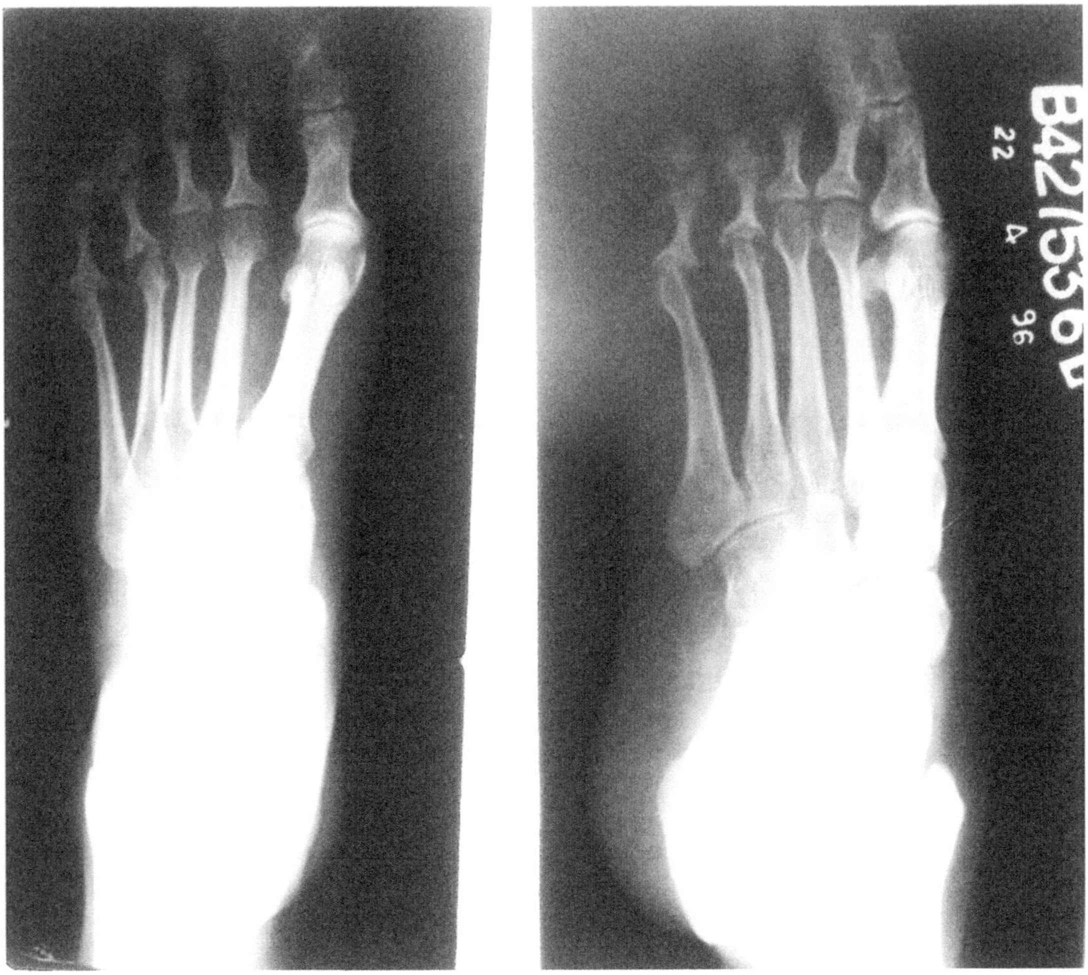

Fig. 8.4 Pencil in cup deformity

Table 8.2 DMARDs in PsA

Synthetic DMARDs	
Conventional csDMARDS	Methotrexate, Leflunomide, Sulfasalazine
Targeted tsDMARDS	Apremilast, Tofacitinib
Biological DMARDs	
TNFi	Monoclonal antibodies: Infliximab, Adalimumab, Golimumab, Certolizumab
	Receptor construct: Etanercept
IL-17i	Secukinumab, Ixekizumab
CTLA4 Ig	Abatacept
IL 12/23i	Ustekinumab

Note: Cyclosporine is not recommended for PsA

patients with relevant skin involvement, where "relevant" is defined as either extensive or as important to the patient, IL-12/23i and IL-17i are preferred over TNFi. The presence or absence of comorbidities also plays a role in the selection of biologics. IL-12/23 inhibition is not effective for axial involvement while IL-17 inhibition is not appropriate for patients with concomitant inflammatory bowel disease (Table 8.3). The various FDA-approved biologics for skin psoriasis and PsA are listed in Table 8.4.

Not all drugs work on all domains (Table 8.5). Axial disease and enthesitis do not respond to csDMARDs and need biologics in patients not

Table 8.3 Factors influencing choice of targeted treatments (Biologics/PDE4i/JAKi)

Condition	Comment
Psoriatic arthritis	TNFi, IL-17i, IL-12/23i, abatacept, tofacitinib, apremilast. No one biologic prioritized over another. Apremilast recommended for mild disease in absence of poor prognostic factors.
PsA with skin involvement that is extensive or of particular concern to the patient	IL-17i and IL-12/23i preferred to TNFi. Abatacept has no role in skin psoriasis. Tofacitinib has lower efficacy in skin psoriasis.
PsA with inflammatory bowel disease	TNFi monoclonal antibodies or IL-12/23i. Etanercept and IL-17i not recommended.
PsA with uveitis	TNFi monoclonal antibodies preferred. Etanercept is not recommended.
PsA with axial involvement	TNFi preferred. When there is relevant skin involvement, IL-17 inhibitor may be preferred. IL-12/23i, Abatacept, apremilast, and tofacitinib not recommended.

Biologics include TNFi, IL-17i, IL-12/23i, abatacept. *PDE4i* Phosphodiesterase 4 inhibitors (apremilast), *JAKi* Janus kinase inhibitors (tofacitinib), *TNFi* TNF inhibitors, *IL-12/23i* IL-12/23 inhibitors, *IL-17 i* IL-17 inhibitors

Table 8.4 FDA-approved biologics for Pso and PsA

	FDA approved to treat psoriasis	FDA approved to treat psoriatic arthritis	Comments
Cimzia® (certolizumab pegol)	**X**	**X**	TNF inhibitor
Cosentyx® (secukinumab)	**X**	**X**	IL-17 inhibitor
Enbrel® (etanercept)	**X**	**X**	TNF inhibitor
Humira® (adalimumab)	**X**	**X**	TNF inhibitor
Ilumya™ (tildrakizumab)	**X**		IL-23 inhibitor
Remicade® (infliximab)	**X**	**X**	TNF inhibitor
Siliq[a]™ (brodalumab)	**X**		IL-17 inhibitor
Simponi® (golimumab)		**X**	TNF inhibitor
Skyrizi™ (risankizumab)	**X**		IL-23 inhibitor
Stelara® (ustekinumab)	**X**	**X**	IL-12/23 inhibitor
Taltz® (ixekizumab)	**X**	**X**	IL-17 inhibitor
Tremfya™ (guselkumab)	**X**		IL-23 inhibitor
Orencia™ (Abatacept)		**X**	T cell inhibitor Costimulation modulator

[a]Approved to treat adults when other psoriasis treatments fail to work or stop working. Skyrizi is approved in Japan for PsA

Table 8.5 Drugs effective in various domains of PsA

Disease domain	Drugs
Peripheral arthritis	MTX, SSZ, LEF, Tofa, Apremilast TNFi, IL-12/23i, IL-17i, Abatacept
Axial disease	TNFi, IL-17i
Dactylitis	MTX, SSZ, LEF, Tofa, Apremilast TNFi, IL-12/23i, IL-17i
Enthesitis	Tofa, Apremilast TNFi, IL-12/23i, IL-17i

MTX methotrexate, *SSZ* sulfasalazine, *LEF* Leflunomide, *Tofa* Tofactinib, *NSAIDs* nonsteroidal anti-inflammatory drugs, *TNFi* TNF inhibitors, *IL-12/23i* IL-12/23 inhibitors, *IL-17 i* IL-17 inhibitors

responding to NSAIDs. Dactylitis is first treated by csDMARDs. Refractory cases need biologics. Tofacitinib is indicated for patients with active PsA who have had a poor response or intolerance to methotrexate or other csDMARDs. Since monotherapy data in PsA is lacking, it is used in combination with methotrexate, sulfasalazine, or leflunomide. Tofacitinib should not be used in combination with biologic DMARDs. Tofacitinib has been shown to be effective in patients with inadequate response to TNFi. The usual dose is 5 mg twice daily or extended-release 11 mg once daily in combination with non-biologic DMARDs. Apremilast is used for PsA except for axial disease. The usual dose is 30 mg twice daily, built up slowly using the starter packs provided by the manufacturers. Despite a favorable safety profile, its efficacy is modest and considerably lower than biologics. It is not recommended for erosive disease because of a lack of data showing benefit in this patient population. Diarrhea, nausea/vomiting, loss of appetite, headache, or weight loss are common and may necessitate dose reduction/drug withdrawal.

8.4 Conclusions

PsA is a heterogeneous disease with multiple domains. The joint disease usually follows the skin disease. The clinical course of the two may be independent. The treatment has to be individualized according to the domain affected.

Suggested Reading

1. Coates LC, Kavanaugh A, Mease PJ, Soriano ER, Laura Acosta-Felquer M, Armstrong AW, et al. Group for Research and Assessment of Psoriasis and Psoriatic Arthritis 2015 treatment recommendations for psoriatic arthritis. Arthritis Rheumatol. 2016;68:1060–71.
2. Gossec L, Baraliakos X, Kerschbaumer A, de Wit M, McInnes I, Dougados M, et al. EULAR recommendations for the management of psoriatic arthritis with pharmacological therapies: 2019 update. Ann Rheum Dis. 2020;79:700–12.
3. Singh JA, Guyatt G, Ogdie A, Gladman DD, Deal C, Deodhar A, et al. Special Article: 2018 American College of Rheumatology/National Psoriasis Foundation Guideline for the treatment of psoriatic arthritis. Arthritis Rheumatol. 2019;71:5–32.
4. Ritchlin CT, Colbert RA, Gladman DD. Psoriatic arthritis. New Engl J Med. 2017;376:2095–6.

9 Reactive Arthritis

9.1 Introduction

Microbes and joints are interrelated in a variety of ways. From a teaching–learning perspective, infection-related arthritis can be divided into three broad groups:

(a) Septic or infectious arthritis (organism can often be cultured or isolated from the joint).
(b) Reactive arthritis (history of infection at a distant site in recent past, joint fluid is sterile).
(c) Para infectious arthritis (concurrent infection at another site triggering aseptic arthritis, e.g., Poncet's disease).

This chapter deals with Reactive arthritis (ReA), an acute aseptic nonsuppurative inflammatory arthritis that follows enteric or urogenital infections. The list of infections known to trigger ReA is relatively big. BCG instillation in the urinary bladder in bladder cancer can trigger ReA. BCG vaccination for the prevention of tuberculosis, however, has not been implicated. HIV infection is also associated with ReA. Rheumatic fever is also a type of reactive arthritis. However, traditionally most authorities prefer to use the term ReA for arthritis triggered by sexually acquired or enteric infections. ReA is included in the broad group of spondyloarthritides (SpA). Reactive arthritis was earlier referred to as *Reiter's disease* after Hans Reiter, who described arthritis, urethritis, and conjunctivitis in a German military officer after a bout of dysentery. *Reiter's disease or syndrome* may frequently occur in the absence of clinically apparent urethritis or conjunctivitis (incomplete Reiter's syndrome). As we move away from eponyms, the term "Reactive Arthritis" is now the preferred term.

9.2 Clinical Recognition and Investigations

ReA maybe post dysenteric or post venereal/sexually acquired. Intestinal infections are usually due to non-typhoidal Salmonella, Shigella, or Yersinia species. Sexually acquired ReA (SAReA) is caused by Chlamydia trachomatis and follows 1–4% of chlamydial urogenital infections. The onset is acute and begins 1–4 weeks after gastroenteritis or sexual exposure. The infection may be imperceptible. SAReA is more common in young men, while enteric infections affect both sexes equally. Nongonococcal urethritis is usually the first manifestation both in SAReA and post dysenteric ReA. Mild dysuria and penile discharge may go unnoticed by the patient. Women may have dysuria, vaginal discharge, and cervicitis/vaginitis. *Neisseria gonorrhoeae* may be found in the genital tract as it frequently coexists with chlamydia infection, but it does not cause reactive arthritis. Conjunctivitis may accompany or follow urethritis. Some patients develop acute anterior uveitis.

R. Handa, *Clinical Rheumatology*, https://doi.org/10.1007/978-981-33-4885-1_9

The joint manifestations are usually the last to appear after urethral and ocular inflammation has subsided. The arthritis is typically oligoarticular, asymmetric, and involves lower limb joints mainly. Sausage digits or dactylitis are typical of ReA (Fig. 9.1) and can easily be differentiated from fusiform swelling seen in RA. Heel pain and enthesopathy are characteristic. Low back pain may be present in some patients. Other extraarticular features include circinate balanitis (Fig. 9.2), keratoderma blennorrhagicum (Fig. 9.3), painless oral ulcers, and onycholysis. Nails do not show pitting, unlike psoriasis.

ReA is primarily a clinical diagnosis. "Incomplete forms" are observed more commonly than the classical triad. Many patients may have a clinically silent or asymptomatic triggering infection. ReA may be more severe and follow a protracted course in patients with symptomatic and bacterial culture positive triggering infections than those with asymptomatic triggering infection suggested only by serologic antibody testing. Arthritis usually lasts from 4 to 5 months in the majority of patients. Nearly 15–30% of the patients go on to have chronic, disabling arthritis. Recurrences are not uncommon. About 10% of patients develop spondylitis over 10–20 years.

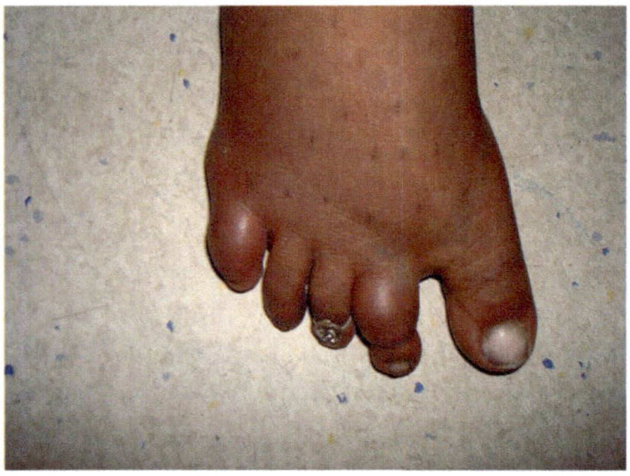

Fig. 9.1 Dactylitis in reactive arthritis

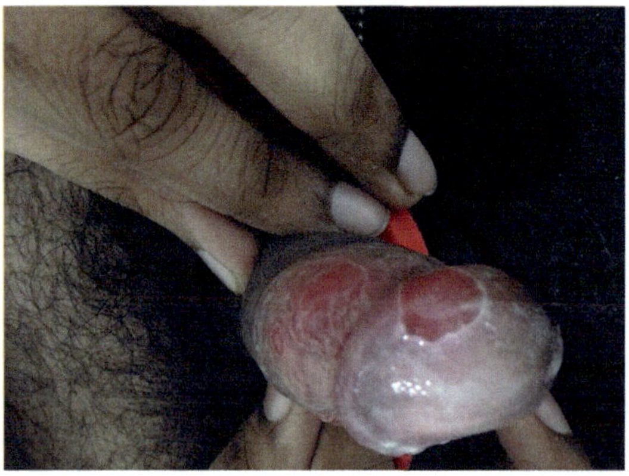

Fig. 9.2 Circinate balanitis in a young HLA B27 positive male with reactive arthritis

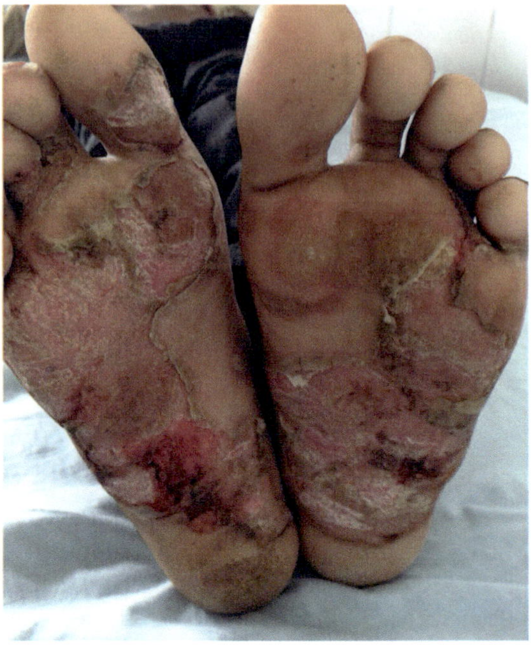

Fig. 9.3 Keratoderma blennorrhagicum

Investigations reveal a rise in acute phase reactants like ESR and CRP. The synovial fluid cell counts range from 5000/mm^3 to 50,000/mm^3. The dramatic onset of joint effusion with an angry-looking joint may raise suspicion of septic arthritis (pseudo-septic arthritis). However, synovial fluid cultures are sterile in contrast to septic arthritis. The synovial fluid sugar, in contrast to septic arthritis, is not significantly reduced. HLA B27 is positive in nearly 80% of Indian patients with ReA.

It is usually not possible to isolate the causative organism at the time ReA develops. The X-rays during the acute stage of ReA are usually normal except for soft tissue swelling. A fluffy periosteal reaction, if present, is characteristic. Bony erosions with joint space narrowing may be seen in chronic severe arthritis. Radiographic evidence of sacroiliitis is seen in 10% of patients during the acute stage and nearly 50% of chronic cases. The sacroiliitis is frequently unilateral. Syndesmophytes in ReA are asymmetric and nonmarginal in contrast to the marginal syndesmophytes seen in ankylosing spondylitis.

9.3 Management

NSAIDs form the cornerstone of therapy. In severe cases of acute ReA, when NSAIDs have been ineffective, a short course of steroids may be used. Prolonged oral corticosteroid therapy is not recommended. Intraarticular corticosteroids for the persistently active joint are helpful, provided septic arthritis has been ruled out. Painful enthesopathy or refractory plantar fasciitis may benefit from local corticosteroid injection. Sulfasalazine, methotrexate, or azathioprine have been tried in persistent arthritis. TNF inhibitor use is reserved for refractory cases.

Short-term antibiotic treatment does not influence the course of post-enteritic ReA. However, in cases of urogenital chlamydial infection in endemic areas, early treatment with antibiotics like lymecycline for several weeks leads to decreased subsequent development of ReA. Vigorous antibiotic treatment of chlamydia reinfections may reduce relapses of chlamydia induced ReA.

Skin lesions are treated with topical corticosteroids or keratinolytic agents like salicylic acid ointment. Retinoids/methotrexate are used for severe involvement. Acute anterior uveitis requires mydriatics and corticosteroids—local or systemic.

9.4 Conclusions

Reactive arthritis is a constituent of the spondyloarthritis group of diseases. Not all patients volunteer a history of preceding infection. In addition to arthritis, some patients may have dactylitis and prominent skin/eye manifestations. NSAIDs and DMARDs are used to treat this condition. Antibiotic treatment is of limited value.

Suggested Reading

1. Schmitt SK. Reactive arthritis. Infect Dis Clin North Am. 2017;31:265–77.
2. Castro Rocha FA, Duarte-Monteiro AM, Henrique da Mota LM, Matias Dinelly Pinto AC, Fonseca JE. Microbes, helminths, and rheumatic diseases. Best Pract Res Clin Rheumatol. 2020;34:101528

10 Seronegative Arthritis

10.1 Introduction

Seronegative arthritis is a challenging clinical problem that has long confronted rheumatologists. It is arthritis characterized by the absence of serologic markers (biomarkers/autoantibodies).

The definition is imprecise as the serologic workup in an individual can vary widely. This is akin to pyrexia or fever of unknown origin (PUO/FUO), which serves as the perfect analogy for seronegative arthritis. PUO is defined as a fever that remains undiagnosed within one week of hospital evaluation or three outpatient visits. The investigations are not explicitly spelled out and the investigative workup varies from center to center. Much in the same way, the definition of seronegative arthritis is influenced by and differs according to the investigations employed before declaring it seronegative.

The common biomarkers and the associated arthritides are listed in Fig. 10.1. For simplicity and unambiguity, it is preferable to define seronegative arthritis as a joint disease characterized by the absence of the classical autoantibody, namely the rheumatoid factor (RF). It is also important to reemphasize that not all patients with RF have rheumatoid arthritis (RA) since several conditions other than RA can be associated with a positive RF. With advances in the field of biomarkers and autoantibodies, it is likely that the universe of seronegative arthritis progressively shrinks. The entity of seronegative arthritis, as we know today, may cease to exist in times to come.

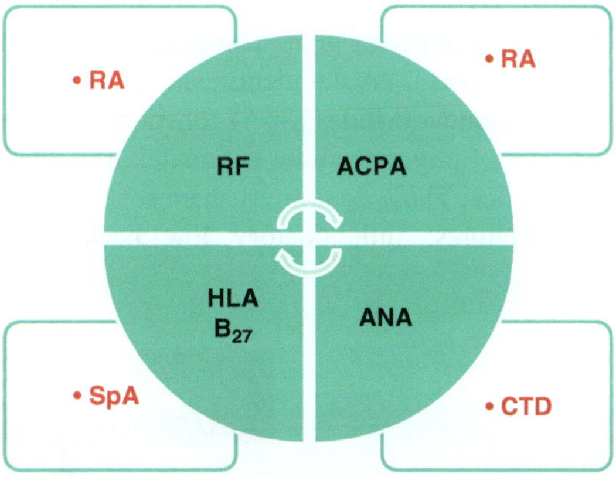

Fig. 10.1 Common biomarkers and associated arthritis. *RF* rheumatoid factor, *ACPA* anti citrullinated peptide antibody, *ANA* anti nuclear antibody, *RA* rheumatoid arthritis, *SpA* spondyloarthritis, *CTD* connective tissue disease

10.2 Approach to Seronegative Arthritis

Seronegative arthritis should be differentiated into inflammatory and noninflammatory. The important causes of noninflammatory seronegative arthritides are osteoarthritis and hypothyroidism. Inflammatory arthritides like RA are characterized by marked morning stiffness (>30 min), pain that improves on gently moving the joint, and elevated ESR/CRP. Noninflammatory arthritides are characterized by mild morning stiffness (<30 min), pain that worsens on joint movement, and normal acute phase response. Seronegative inflammatory arthritides can be divided into

R. Handa, *Clinical Rheumatology*, https://doi.org/10.1007/978-981-33-4885-1_10

monoarthritis (single joint involvement), oligoarthritis (2, 3, or 4 joints affected), and polyarthritis (≥ 5 joints). The important conditions in each category are listed in Fig. 10.2.

The involvement of a single joint should prompt the clinician to consider crystal arthropathy (like gout) or septic arthritis. *A good rule of the thumb is to consider every case of monoarthritis as* ***infection*** *of the joint unless proven otherwise* because untreated septic arthritis rapidly results in joint destruction. Serum urate is a useful and universally available biomarker for gout. It needs interpretation in light of the clinical context. Hyperuricemia alone is not sufficient to make a diagnosis of gout. The gold standard of gout diagnosis is crystal identification.

The spondarthritides (SpA) constitute the vast majority of oligoarthritides encountered in clinical practice. These conditions share several common features: inflammatory low back pain, asymmetrical, below the waist, large joint oligoarthritis, that is, asymmetric involvement of knees or ankles. HLA B27 positivity varies in the different entities, with patients of ankylosing spondylitis (radiographic axial SpA) showing HLA B27 in 90% of patients. However, it needs to be kept in mind that nearly 5–6% of the healthy north Indian population is HLA-B27 positive. Magnetic resonance imaging (MRI) is invaluable in clinching the diagnosis of non-radiographic SpA when HLA B27 is also negative.

Some conditions like gout can present as monoarthritis, oligoarthritis, or rarely even as polyarthritis. Similarly, juvenile idiopathic arthritis or psoriasis can have oligoarticular or polyarticular involvement.

The important seronegative inflammatory polyarthritides include seronegative RA, psoriasis, and the connective tissue diseases (CTDs). The absence of RF is seen in nearly 20% of

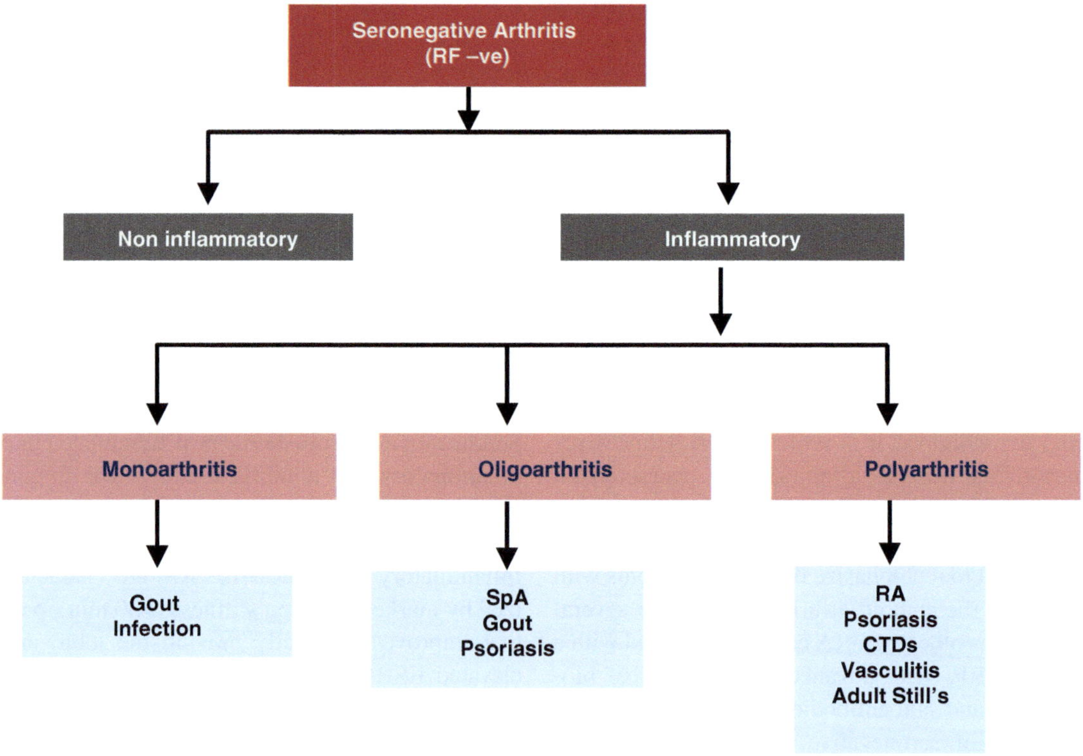

Fig. 10.2 Approach to seronegative arthritis. *RF* rheumatoid factor, *RA* rheumatoid arthritis, *SpA* spondyloarthritis, *CTD* connective tissue disease

patients with RA. The phenotype of seronegative RA is indistinguishable from seropositive RA. Psoriasis is an important cause of seronegative arthritis, especially that 15% of patients where arthritis precedes the skin lesions of psoriasis. Even with a background of skin psoriasis, patients may not volunteer a history of psoriasis because of the failure to link the skin with the joint condition. A search for psoriasis in hidden areas like around the umbilicus, natal cleft, etc. might point to a correct diagnosis. The CTDs demonstrate antinuclear antibodies (ANA) in the large majority of patients (Fig. 10.1). In addition to arthritis, fever, skin, and mucous membrane lesions, and multisystem involvement point toward the diagnosis. Patients with antineutrophil cytoplasmic antibody (ANCA) associated vasculitis occasionally have arthritis as a prominent and presenting symptom that gets labeled as seronegative arthritis. The evolution of clinical picture and ANCA, if present, point toward the correct diagnosis.

Conditions like adult Still's disease and classical polyarteritis nodosa are truly seronegative with no biomarkers save elevated acute phase reactants. Serum ferritin is used as a marker of inflammation in adult Still's disease. Cancer-associated arthralgias and arthritis also figure in the list of seronegative arthritides. Infective endocarditis is another mimic that can masquerade as seronegative arthritis.

The workup in seronegative arthritis is governed by the clinical presentation and physician judgment. Indiscriminate autoantibody panels are seldom useful. Imaging investigations complement blood investigations and need to be ordered selectively and rationally. Echocardiography and bone marrow examination may be needed in select cases.

10.3 Conclusions

Serologically bland arthritides without any autoantibodies or biomarkers are labeled as seronegative. There is no universally accepted definition. A thorough history and good physical examination enable the clinician to arrive at a working diagnosis in most instances. Investigations are meant to be *supplements to* and not *substitutes for* clinical judgment. The treatment should be supportive until the cause has been determined. Indiscriminate use of steroids is not recommended because they can mask symptoms and signs of the underlying disease process.

Suggested Reading

1. Handa R. Approach to seronegative arthritis. J Ind Acad Clin Med. 2003;4:190–2.

11 Adult Still's Disease

11.1 Introduction

Adult-onset Still's disease or simply put Adult Still's disease (ASD) is a rare, multisystem immuno-inflammatory disease characterized by daily (quotidian) high spiking fever, evanescent rash, and arthritis. The etiology is unknown. In the absence of a pathognomic test, the diagnosis requires careful exclusion of infections, malignancy, and other autoimmune rheumatic diseases. Treatment entails the use of nonsteroidal anti-inflammatory drugs (NSAIDs), corticosteroids, and other immunosuppressives/immunomodulators.

11.2 Clinical Features

The classical triad of ASD includes fever, arthritis, and rash. The fever generally exceeds 39 °C and exhibits a daily spike. Joint pains dominate the clinical picture and may take the form of arthralgia or arthritis. Both small and large joints can be affected in a symmetric, polyarticular fashion. Commonly involved joints include the knees, wrists, and ankles, although no joint is exempt. The joint pains may coincide with fever spikes. The rash may be quite elusive since the recognition of the textbook salmon-pink maculopapular rash is often tricky in dark-skinned individuals. This, coupled with its transient nature, makes skin rash the least appreciated feature in Indians. The rash is said to favor the trunk (Fig. 11.1). Face and distal extremities are rarely involved. In some patients, fever may be the only clinical symptom of ASD.

Other clinical features include myalgias, pharyngitis, hepatosplenomegaly, lymphadenopathy, and serositis. Renal and neurological complications have been described but are rare.

The clinical course may follow one of the three patterns: self-limited or monocyclic, intermittent or polycyclic, and chronic. Patients with monophasic or monocyclic ASD exhibit a disease course lasting weeks to months with a predominance of systemic features like fever along with rash, organomegaly, and serositis. There may be no recurrence after the disease has run its course in usually less than a year. Patients with polycyclic ASD continue to have multiple episodes of fever and/or arthritis of varying intervals. In between the episodes, the patient may appear normal with normal lab parameters. ASD patients with a chronic course behave more like chronic arthritis with a predominance of joint pains.

11.3 Classification Criteria

Given the lack of distinguishing features unique to this disease, several classification criteria have been proposed. Yamaguchi criteria proposed way back in 1992 are perhaps the best known (Table 11.1). These comprise four major and five minor criteria. Five or more criteria are required,

R. Handa, *Clinical Rheumatology*, https://doi.org/10.1007/978-981-33-4885-1_11

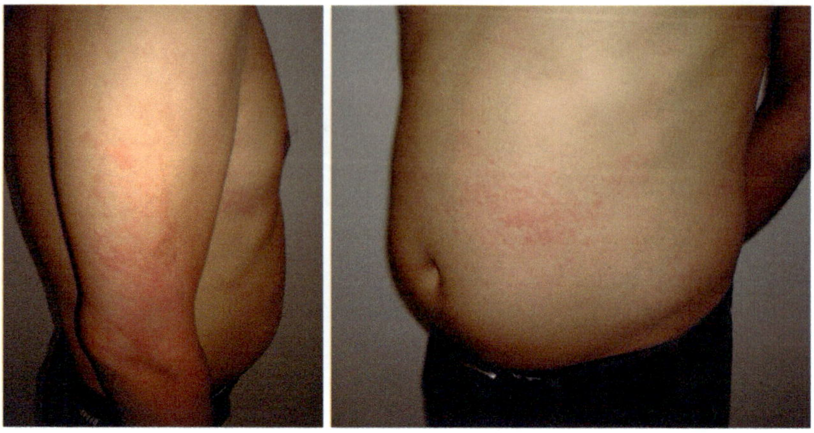

Fig. 11.1 Skin rash of Adult Still's Disease

Table 11.1 Yamaguchi criteria for Adult Still's Disease

Major criteria	
1.	Fever ≥ 39 °C (102.2 °F) lasting ≥1 week
2.	Arthralgias or arthritis lasting 2 weeks or longer
3.	Nonpruritic, evanescent, salmon-pink rash
4.	Leukocytosis (≥10,000 white cells per cubic millimeter) with granulocytosis (≥80%)
Minor criteria	
1.	Sore throat
2.	Lymphadenopathy
3.	Hepatomegaly or splenomegaly
4.	Abnormal liver function studies, particularly elevations in aspartate and alanine aminotransferase and lactate dehydrogenase
5.	Negative tests for antinuclear antibody and rheumatoid factor

of whom two or more must be major (sensitivity and specificity 90%). The Yamaguchi criteria are not valid in patients with cancer or infection.

11.4 Investigations

There are no pathognomonic laboratory abnormalities. The arthritis is seronegative, and autoantibodies like rheumatoid factor, antinuclear antibodies, etc. are typically absent. The blood picture reveals polymorphonuclear leukocytosis. Anemia of chronic disease is common. Other features of acute-phase response include high erythrocyte sedimentation rate (ESR), high C reactive protein (CRP), and thrombocytosis. A fall in ESR and the appearance of pancytopenia should arouse suspicion of macrophage activation syndrome, a known complication. Aminotransferase (AST and ALT) elevation is common. NSAID use may be a contributory factor in transaminitis.

Serum ferritin levels are grossly (usually more than fivefold) elevated. The levels parallel disease activity. The sensitivity of this laboratory marker is in excess of 80%. However, the specificity is <50% because very high ferritin levels are seen in other conditions like sepsis, leukemias, lymphomas, hemochromatosis, HIV, and macrophage activation syndrome. Glycosylated ferritin has been employed to increase specificity. Usually, 50–80% of ferritin is glycosylated. This fraction drops in inflammatory diseases. In ASD, glycosylated ferritin levels often fall below 20%. The glycosylated fraction is not useful in monitoring disease activity since levels remain low even after the control of disease activity.

Radiographs in early disease may be unremarkable. Patients with chronic arthritis may show erosive changes. Pericapitate ankylosis, if present, points toward ASD.

11.5 Diagnosis

The diagnosis of ASD is clinical and mandates careful ruling out of infectious, malignant, autoinflammatory, and autoimmune diseases. The disease may mimic rheumatoid arthritis (RA). However, carpal and pericapitate involvement are much more in ASD as compared to RA. Also, fever and leucocytosis are not a usual part of

RA. In the absence of any gold standard marker, there is no substitute for careful clinical judgment.

11.6 Treatment

No large trials exist. NSAIDs, especially naproxen, corticosteroids, and methotrexate, form the sheet anchor of treatment. Other agents that have been employed include leflunomide, cyclosporine, azathioprine, cyclophosphamide, sulfasalazine, intravenous immunoglobulins, etc. The treatment duration is prolonged, and the drugs are employed in doses similar to that for RA. IL-1 receptor antagonist (anakinra) is very useful in refractory ASD. Other biologics that have been tried include infliximab, etanercept, and tocilizumab. Emerging evidence dichotomizes ASD into two phenotypes: systemic and articular. The systemic form responds better to anakinra, while the phenotype dominated by arthritis may display a substantial response to tocilizumab. TNF inhibitors are thought to be less effective than tocilizumab.

11.7 Conclusions

Adult Still's disease is an inflammatory disease of unknown etiology. Systemic and articular symptoms dominate the clinical picture. Diagnosis entails the careful exclusion of malignant and infectious diseases. NSAIDs, disease-modifying drugs, and steroids are employed in the treatment with biologics reserved for refractory cases.

Suggested Reading

Efthimiou P, Paik PK, Bielory L. Diagnosis and management of adult onset Still's disease. Ann Rheum Dis. 2006;65:564–72.

Feist E, Mitrovic S, Fautrel B. Mechanisms, biomarkers and targets for adult-onset Still's disease. Nat Rev Rheumatol. 2018;14:603–18.

Yamaguchi M, Ohta A, Tsunematsu T, Kasukawa R, Mizushima Y, Kashiwagi H, et al. Preliminary criteria for classification of adult Still's disease. J Rheumatol. 1992;19:424–30.

12 Juvenile Idiopathic Arthritis

12.1 Introduction

Juvenile idiopathic arthritis (JIA) is the most common chronic rheumatic disease in children. It is an umbrella term embracing several entities with three cardinal features: disease onset before 16 years of age, arthritis persisting for 6 weeks or longer, and unknown etiology. Some of the earlier terms used include juvenile rheumatoid arthritis (JRA) and juvenile chronic arthritis (JCA). Currently, the preferred terminology is JIA.

The diagnosis of arthritis in children often gets delayed in developing countries because of the knee jerk tendency to label all joint pains in children as rheumatic fever. Physician ignorance and overreliance on antistreptolysin O (ASO) to the exclusion of clinical detail is responsible for this, at least in India. The differentiating points between rheumatic fever and JIA are tabulated in Table 12.1.

Table 12.1 Differentiating JIA (JRA) from rheumatic fever

	JIA (JRA)	Rheumatic fever
Pattern of arthritis	Additive, erosive	Migratory, non-erosive
Joints affected	Small + large	Large mainly
Extra-articular involvement	Uveitis	Carditis, chorea (in 75% cases)
Deformities	Common	Rare. If present, deformities are correctable-Jaccoud's arthropathy
Course	Slowly progressive	Self-limited (75% attacks subside in 6 weeks)
ESR	↑↑↑	↑
ECG	Normal	May be abnormal
Echocardiographic abnormalities	±	+++

12.2 Classification

The International League of Associations for Rheumatology (ILAR) has proposed classification criteria for JIA. The last revision in 2001 divides JIA into seven subtypes: systemic-onset JIA (sJIA), oligoarticular JIA, seropositive polyarticular JIA, seronegative polyarticular JIA, enthesitis-related arthritis (ERA), juvenile psoriatic arthritis (JPsA), and undifferentiated JIA. This classification aims to identify homogeneous, mutually exclusive disease subsets based on clinical and laboratory features seen in the first 6 months of illness. Oligoarthritis is the commonest JIA (50–80% cases) in Caucasian populations, while ERA is the commonest variety in India.

A move is underway to revise the ILAR classification. There was some confusion in the oligoarthritis category where these patients were also classified as RF-negative polyarthritis or as

R. Handa, *Clinical Rheumatology*, https://doi.org/10.1007/978-981-33-4885-1_12

psoriatic arthritis. It has therefore been proposed by the Pediatric Rheumatology International Trials Organization to group all these in a new category of early-onset, ANA-positive arthritis, independent of the number of joints involved or the presence of psoriasis. These preliminary criteria await formal validation.

12.2.1 Systemic Arthritis

This disease subtype affects both males and females with the same frequency and may occur at any time during childhood. The features include arthritis with, or preceded by, daily fever of at least 2 weeks' duration that is documented to be quotidian for at least 3 days, and accompanied by one or more of the following:

- Evanescent, nonfixed, erythematous rash
- Generalized lymph node enlargement
- Hepatomegaly and/or splenomegaly
- Serositis

The arthritis is usually symmetrical and polyarticular. It may come up much later in the disease course. Investigations reveal leukocytosis (with neutrophilia), thrombocytosis, increased erythrocyte sedimentation rate (ESR), and C reactive protein (CRP). Macrophage activation syndrome (MAS) is a well known, severe, life-threatening complication of this subtype. A change in the fever pattern from intermittent to continuous with fall in ESR, platelets, and fibrinogen, and an increase in ferritin, aminotransferases, and triglycerides may suggest MAS. Many children with MAS may have this complication at disease presentation and have no significant arthritis at this stage. This is an important consideration in the febrile cytopenic child, where elevated ferritin is an important clue to the underlying diagnosis.

12.2.2 Oligoarthritis

Oligoarthritis is the commonest subtype of JIA in Caucasians, usually seen in girls below 6 years. It is defined as arthritis that affects four or fewer joints during the first 6 months of disease. It predominantly involves the knees and ankles. Some patients present with knee monoarthritis. Two subcategories are recognized:

- Persistent oligoarthritis: Affects no more than four joints throughout the disease course
- Extended oligoarthritis: Affects a total of more than four joints after the first 6 months of disease

There is a high frequency of positive antinuclear antibody (ANA) and an increased risk of iridocyclitis. JIA-associated uveitis is typically silent and asymptomatic in contrast to the painful red eye in adults and children with HLA-B27 related acute anterior uveitis. The activity and severity of joint disease and uveitis may not parallel each other. Regular screening is mandatory. The risk stratification is related to ANA positivity and the age of onset of arthritis and is higher in children who have disease onset under 6 years of age.

12.2.3 Rheumatoid Factor-Positive Polyarthritis

Rheumatoid factor (RF)-positive polyarthritis is arthritis affecting five or more joints during the first 6 months of disease, in the presence of at least two positive tests for IgM RF performed at least 3 months apart. The clinical presentation is typically symmetric arthritis of the large and small joints of the upper and lower limbs. Rheumatoid nodules may be seen in nearly 30% of these children.

12.2.4 Rheumatoid Factor-Negative Polyarthritis

More common in girls, the arthritis in this subtype affects five or more joints. RF is negative. It is a heterogeneous category with three subgroups: The first resembles oligoarthritis JIA except for the number of joints involved. The arthritis is asymmetric, ANA is frequently positive, there is an increased risk of iridocyclitis, and association with HLA-DRB1*0801 is well known. Patients with the second subtype resemble adults with RF-negative RA. The arthritis is symmetric, involves large and small joints, and ANA is negative. The third subtype dubbed "dry synovitis" shows virtually no joint swelling but prominent stiffness, flexion contractures, and the worst prognosis. The last subcategory has been questioned and is likely to be a JIA mimic in patients with storage disorders, e.g., mucolipidoses where the child has joint contractures and not joint swellings that are seen in JIA.

12.2.5 Enthesitis-Related Arthritis

Enthesitis-related arthritis (ERA) afflicts boys older than 6 years and is characterized by HLA-B27, enthesitis, and arthritis. RF and ANA are absent. The arthritis is asymmetric, oligoarticular, and may involve the sacroiliac and spinal joints. A typical presentation is the child with a midfoot disease, a characteristic feature of this subcategory. Some children can present with an acute eye inflammation because of anterior uveitis. Fever is a feature reported in many children with ERA and has been seen in China and the Indian subcontinent.

12.2.6 Juvenile Psoriatic Arthritis

This subtype is defined by arthritis plus skin psoriasis. In the absence of psoriatic rash, two of the following are needed: dactylitis, nail pitting, onycholysis, or psoriasis in a first-degree relative.

12.2.7 Undifferentiated Arthritis

This subtype of JIA includes children who do not meet the criteria for any category or those who fit the criteria for more than one category.

12.3 Management

The management of JIA requires a multidisciplinary team and a holistic combination of pharmacologic interventions, physical and occupational therapy, and psychological support alongside patient education. Teacher sensitization is also important since children spend much of the time at school.

The treatment has to be individualized for each child and is guided by the following key points:

- The disease burden as assessed by the physician and parent.
- The prognostication feature of the joints involved, e.g., cervical spine, hip, and wrist disease indicate a poor outcome in the child with poly JIA.
- The presence of extra-articular problems in the child, e.g., severe uveitis and mild arthritis, would dictate the use of tumor necrosis factor inhibitors (TNFi) for the eyes.

Treatment modalities include nonsteroidal anti-inflammatory drugs (NSAIDs), intra-articular corticosteroid injections (IAS), systemic steroids, disease-modifying antirheumatic drugs (DMARDs), and biologics. IAS are employed primarily in children with oligoarthritis. Systemic steroids are used in systemic JIA (high fever unresponsive to NSAIDs, severe anemia, myocarditis or pericarditis, and MAS). Methotrexate (MTX) is the most widely used DMARD in JIA. Other drugs include leflunomide, sulfasalazine, and calcineurin inhibitors like cyclosporine.

Biologics used for systemic JIA include anakinra, canakinumab, rilonacept, and tocilizumab. TNFi and abatacept are recommended for systemic JIA patients with arthritis and without active systemic features. With arthritis in four joints or less, treatment comprises NSAIDs, IAS, methotrexate, and TNFi. Children with arthritis in five or more joints are managed like oligoarthritis with less emphasis on NSAIDs. Biologics in this group include TNFi, tocilizumab, abatacept, or rituximab, especially in RF-positive polyarticular JIA. TNFi is preferred in children with sacroiliitis.

The team should ideally involve a pediatric rheumatologist, physicians who are trained child specialists with specific training in rheumatic diseases that afflict the young. The aim of management of each child with JIA is to treat the child early, within 12 weeks of disease onset, objectively assess the child at each visit with the aim of attaining remission without long-term steroids, which are very detrimental for the growing skeleton.

12.4 Conclusions

Children are not miniature versions of adults. Pediatric rheumatic diseases are distinctly different from their adult counterparts. They have a distinct phenotype, many a time a different genotype and treatment considerations may vary from adults. JIA is no exception to this rule. It embraces all forms of arthritis that begin before the age of 16 years, persists for more than 6 weeks, and where the etiology is of unknown cause. The treatment paradigm includes NSAIDs, steroids, DMARDs, and biologics and has to be individualized.

Acknowledgment The author would like to thank Dr. Sujata Sawhney for her inputs and critical review of this manuscript.

Suggested Reading

Beukelman T, Patkar NM, Saag KG, Tolleson-Rinehart S, Cron RQ, DeWitt EM, et al. American College of Rheumatology recommendations for the treatment of juvenile idiopathic arthritis: initiation and safety monitoring of therapeutic agents for the treatment of arthritis and systemic features. Arthritis Care Res (Hoboken). 2011;63:465–82.

Cimaz R, Marino A, Martini A. How I treat juvenile idiopathic arthritis: a state of the art review. Autoimmun Rev. 2017;16:1008–15.

Ferrara G, Mastrangelo G, Barone P, La Torre F, Martino S, Pappagallo G, et al. Methotrexate in juvenile idiopathic arthritis: advice and recommendations from the MARAJIA expert consensus meeting. Pediatr Rheumatol Online J. 2018;16(1):46.

Martini A, Ravelli A, Avcin T, Beresford MW, Burgos-Vargas R, Cuttica R, et al. Toward new classification criteria for juvenile idiopathic arthritis: first steps, Pediatric Rheumatology International Trials Organization International Consensus. J Rheumatol. 2019;46:190–7.

Ravelli A, Consolaro A, Horneff G, Laxer RM, Lovell DJ, Wulffraat NM, et al. Treating juvenile idiopathic arthritis to target: recommendations of an international task force. Ann Rheum Dis. 2018;77:819–28.

13 Connective Tissue Diseases: The Concept and Approach

13.1 Introduction

The term connective tissue disease (CTD) refers to a group of similar yet different autoimmune multisystem rheumatic diseases common in women and characterized by the presence of antinuclear antibodies (ANA). While different authors use this term differently, with some including rheumatoid arthritis, myositis, and vasculitides under this umbrella term, most experts list four diseases under this category (Fig. 13.1). This is indeed the concept that is used in this book. Systemic lupus erythematosus (SLE) is the flagship CTD and perhaps the most well studied. However, in terms of commonality, Sjogren's syndrome is perhaps far more common than lupus but goes under-recognized.

The concept of CTD owes much to the pioneering work of Paul Klemperer, a pathologist working at the Mount Sinai school of Medicine in New York. He and his colleagues first proposed the concept of "collagen vascular diseases" in 1941 to explain the involvement of diverse and distant organ involvement in lupus, years before the discovery of the LE cell. As it became apparent that collagen is but one component of the connective tissue, the term CTD gained widespread acceptance and persists to this day. The description of the LE cell in 1948 by Malcolm Hargraves in the bone marrow of a patient with lupus led to subsequent use of this test as a marker for SLE. The LE phenomenon referred to a neutrophil that phagocytoses the liberated nuclear

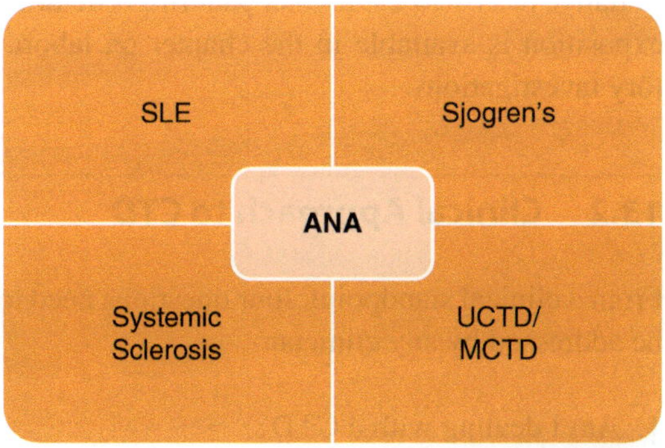

Fig. 13.1 Spectrum of connective tissue diseases. *ANA* anti nuclear antibody, *SLE* systemic lupus erythematosus, *UCTD/MCTD* undifferentiated/mixed connective tissue disease

material of another leukocyte. This was the forerunner of the ANA test. The LE cell test is now obsolete. The ANA test, which owes a lot to the seminal work by Eng Tan and Henry Kunkel, has undergone refinements.

Currently, the HEp2 substrate derived from Human epithelial type 2 (HEp-2) cells, originating from a human laryngeal carcinoma, is used. Slide-based ANA testing earlier used rodent tissue (stomach, liver, and/or kidney) as the substrate. Drawbacks of rodent substrate were small cell size, a lack of dividing cells (mitotic), and low antigen expression that made interpretation of patterns difficult. The advantages of HEp2 include a large nucleus, better antigen expression, and abundant mitotic cells facilitating pat-

R. Handa, *Clinical Rheumatology*, https://doi.org/10.1007/978-981-33-4885-1_13

tern recognition. More recently, HEp-2000®, a cell line transfected with the cDNA for overexpression of the SSA/Ro antigen, is used. Automated systems for image acquisition and interpretation of indirect immunofluorescence patterns are increasingly being employed.

ANA is actually a test that detects autoantibodies to all cellular antigens and not the nucleus alone. Thus, there is a concerted move to use the all-encompassing term of anti-cellular (AC) antibodies. The breathtaking advancement in this field is baffling for many clinicians. The International Consensus on ANA Patterns (ICAP) initiative has listed 29 distinct patterns. A detailed exposition is available in the chapter on laboratory investigations.

13.2 Clinical Approach to CTD

From a clinical standpoint, four questions need to be addressed by any clinician:

1. Am I dealing with a CTD?
2. What is the type of CTD?
3. How should I investigate the patient?
4. How should I treat this patient?

13.3 How to Recognize CTD?

Clinical recognition of CTD requires a high index of suspicion because of heterogeneity of presentation and multiplicity of organs involved like the skin, mucous membranes, joints, lungs, kidneys, central and/or peripheral nervous system, heart, gastrointestinal tract, etc. To make matters complex, the organ involvement may be in isolation or combination and may be sequential or simultaneous. Constitutional features of fever, fatigue, anorexia, and weight loss are common. A clinician should suspect CTD in the following situations:

- Multisystem involvement especially in young women
- Inflammatory polyarthritis with additional features like fever, prominent mucocutaneous involvement, active urine sediment, cytopenias, and neuropsychiatric features (the presence of these features make RA less likely)
- FUO (Fever of unknown origin)
- Unexplained renal failure/nephrotic syndrome
- Polyserositis
- Mononeuritis multiplex
- Psychosis in a young female
- Picture of ITP (idiopathic thrombocytopenic purpura) with splenomegaly.
- Raynaud's phenomenon
- Palpable purpura
- Parotid enlargement
- Generalized lymphadenopathy
- Sicca symptoms
- Photosensitive rash
- Pulmonary renal syndrome
- Dry cough and breathlessness suggestive of interstitial lung disease

This is not meant to be a comprehensive listing but rather an attempt to list some of the common modes of presentation. Despite the myriads of presentations, patterns are often recognizable that permit bedside diagnosis. Paul Klemperer, with remarkable prescience, had said that the term is liable to misuse as a wastepaper basket term for "*maladies with puzzling clinical and anatomic features*," precisely what we should take care to avoid. CTDs are not meant to be diagnoses of exclusion (per exclusionem) but diagnoses of inclusion instead, prospectively entertained and systematically confirmed.

13.4 Type of CTD

The phenotype of lupus or Sjogren's or SSc may be apparent from the very beginning, or symptoms may gradually accumulate over some time. A young woman with alopecia, photosensitive malar rash, inflammatory polyarthritis, and positive ANA can be diagnosed as SLE at the bedside. In the same context, Raynaud's, skin thickening, and positive ANA point toward systemic sclerosis (SSc) while sicca features with a positive ANA point toward Sjogren's syndrome. However, in real life, a textbook description of the disease may either not be present initially or may never develop. A picture which is highly suggestive of CTD but does not allow precise categorization into a definite phenotype is labeled as undifferentiated (UCTD). Overlap of different CTDs may exist. Mixed connective tissue disease (MCTD) is a variety of this overlap syndrome.

13.5 Criteria and Classification of CTDs

The clinical spectrum of multisystem CTDs can be very variegated and pleomorphic. Even within a system, the presentation can be variable, e.g., neuropsychiatric lupus. The clinical heterogeneity is mirrored by serologic heterogeneity. This spawns the need for criteria that have evolved in response to the fact that most systemic rheumatic diseases lack a single pathognomonic or distinguishing feature. Features like arthritis, morning stiffness, fever, Raynaud's phenomenon, skin rash are common to several diseases. Raynaud's phenomenon (Table 13.1) is a common cause of referral to a rheumatologist. Also, many of the features do not occur concurrently but sequentially. When present in a particular combination and specific laboratory investigations, these clinical features help identify a specific disease and are termed "criteria."

Criteria are of several different types: classification criteria, prognostic criteria, response criteria, diagnostic criteria, etc. Classification criteria help differentiate patients with a particular disease from patients with a potentially confusing condition and the normal population (case definition). For example, criteria for SLE would help differentiate lupus from another inflammatory polyarthritis like RA. Classification criteria do not address the issue of whether the patient has a disease but instead try to address the issue of what disease the patient has. "Classification" criteria apply to groups and are more specific than "diagnostic" criteria, which are applied to individuals and are more sensitive. Classification criteria serve several useful purposes:

- Provide uniformity for patients being included in epidemiological studies and trials
- Facilitate comparison between different centers
- Provide a lingua franca for scientific communication

To add to the complexity, criteria do constantly evolve as knowledge advances. For example, SLE criteria were first proposed in 1971, revised in 1982, and further revised in 1997. These were followed by the Systemic Lupus International Collaborating Clinics classification criteria (SLICC) criteria in 2012. The newest is the European League Against Rheumatism/ American College of Rheumatology classification criteria for systemic lupus erythematosus published in 2019.

However, at the bedside, the role of classification criteria is somewhat limited. For example, a patient with a malar rash and strongly positive ANA would be diagnosed as lupus on the bedside while such a patient would not be classified as SLE on account of failure to fulfill the requisite number of criteria. Criteria accrual takes time. In general, diagnostic criteria for CTDs do not exist because there is no gold standard for making a diagnosis. Making a diagnosis is a complex process that integrates history, physical examination, and laboratory investigations into evidence-based clinical decision-making. Diagnosis making cannot be constrained by a lack of classification criteria, especially since several individuals with a CTD may not initially or ever meet the classification criteria. The fact that an individual does not meet the classification criteria for a particular CTD does not exclude that diagnosis at the bedside.

Table 13.1 Causes of Raynaud's phenomenon

• Raynaud's disease
• Connective Tissue Diseases: SSc, MCTD, UCTD, SLE, RA
• Drugs: amphetamines, clonidine, ergot, bleomycin
• Structural: athero-emboli, thoracic outlet, Buerger's
• Occupational
• Hematologic: cryoglobulins, paraproteins, cold agglutinin
• Misc: Hypothroidism, CRPS, paraneoplastic

SSc systemic sclerosis, *SLE* systemic lupus erythematosus, *UCTD/MCTD* undifferentiated/mixed connective tissue disease, *RA* rheumatoid arthritis, *CRPS* complex regional pain syndrome

Similarly, therapeutic decisions in an individual patient should not be governed or fettered solely by fulfillment or lack of fulfillment of criteria.

13.6 Implications for a Clinician

From the foregoing discussion, it is clear that classification criteria serve a relatively limited role in clinical decision-making and diagnosis at the bedside. The clinician should aim to delineate the organ involvement in every patient with CTD by a thorough physical examination and judicious use of investigations. Therapy is directed according to organ involvement. For example, the arthritis of CTD, whether SLE or SSc, would be treated similarly with hydroxychloroquine, methotrexate, or sulfasalazine in addition to NSAIDs. Similarly, the nephritis of lupus or vasculitis would warrant corticosteroids and additional immunosuppressives in a broadly similar, if not identical, fashion. Treatment decisions should never be postponed or delayed pending classification.

13.7 Investigations in a Patient Suspected of Having CTD

These may be divided into three categories:

1. ANA which serves as serologic evidence of a CTD
2. ANA subsets
3. Other investigations to assess organ involvement like complete blood counts, urinalysis, imaging, echocardiography, kidney biopsy, nail fold capillaroscopy (NFC), minor salivary gland biopsy, etc.

CTDs are characterized by the presence of ANA (Table 13.2). Indirect immunofluorescence (IIF) continues to be the gold standard for the detection of ANA. ELISA is less sensitive for the detection of ANA but lends itself to automation and greater throughput for the laboratory. IIF is operator dependent and requires skilled laboratory personnel. ANA reporting should ideally mention the titer, pattern, and intensity of fluorescence. Since low titer ANA is seen in nearly 5% of healthy young women, interpretation of autoantibody results should always be in the context of the clinical picture. A positive ANA does not mean CTD and a negative ANA does not exclude CTD. High titers are less likely to be false-positive. The patterns reflect the target antigens and possible disease associations. Repeat testing of ANA in a CTD patient who has tested positive once is not recommended.

Table 13.2 ANA positivity in different connective tissue diseases

Connective Tissue Disease (CTD)	ANA positivity
SLE	>99%
Sjogren's	90%
Systemic sclerosis	95%
Mixed CTD	100%
Undifferentiated CTD	100%

ANA subsets should be ordered only in patients who test positive for screening ANA. Ideally, all positive fluorescent ANAs should be followed by antigen-specific immunoassays. Line immunoblot tests have become widely available for the semiquantitative determination of IgG antibodies against various nuclear antigens like nRNP/Sm, Sm, SS-A, Ro-52, SS-B, Scl-70, PM-Scl, Jo-1, centromere protein B, PCNA, dsDNA, nucleosomes, histones, ribosomal P-proteins, AMA M2, etc. The purified antigens are deposited as bands onto nitrocellulose strips, and the bound antibodies are detected after staining by an enzyme-catalyzed substrate reaction. This test is also referred to as an extractable nuclear antigen (ENA) panel.

Some ANA subsets like dsDNA (sensitivity 50–60%) and Sm (sensitivity 30%) are highly specific for SLE and should not be used as a screening test. The primary utility is in confirmation of the diagnosis of lupus in ANA positive individuals. Also, dsDNA levels generally correlate with disease activity, especially in lupus nephritis. In an occasional patient, the dsDNA levels may not parallel disease activity, the so-called clinico-serologic discordance. In such cases, the dictum is to treat the patient and not chase the dsDNA levels.

Other investigations like complete blood counts, kidney and liver function tests, and urine examination are carried out in all patients. Urine examination is mandatory in all patients with CTD at every hospital visit to detect kidney involvement, which is mostly asymptomatic. Despite being paucisymptomatic, kidney involvement is the primary determinant of outcome and should be diligently sought in every patient. Tests like NFC, kidney biopsy, nerve conduction studies, etc. are ordered either to determine the CTD phenotype or disease extent.

13.8 Treatment Considerations in CTD

Since CTDs are multisystem diseases with remitting and relapsing course, the treatment has to be individualized for every patient. Since young women are the primary patient population, reproductive issues assume importance. The following factors are considered (Fig. 13.2):

(a) Organs involved
(b) The extent of organ involvement
(c) Disease activity
(d) Disease damage
(e) Reproductive issues
(f) Patient preference
(g) Long-term safety of treatments
(h) Cost

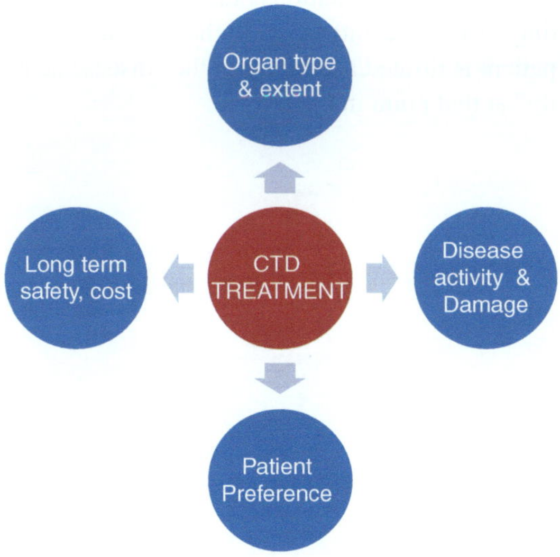

Fig. 13.2 Key treatment considerations

Organ involvement and the extent of involvement play an important role in deciding treatment. For example, pleuritis in lupus is treated very differently from active neuropsychiatric lupus. Similarly, photoprotection and hydroxychloroquine (HCQ) may suffice for mild malar rash in lupus, while an extensive rash may need additional agents like corticosteroids or mycophenolate mofetil (MMF). In the same context, Class II lupus nephritis and Class III nephritis are treated in a very different fashion. Since CTDs affect women, contraception choices and drug selection have to factor in several vital aspects. To illustrate this further, oral pills are best avoided in antiphospholipid syndrome. HCQ, low dose steroids, azathioprine, and calcineurin inhibitors (CNIs) can be used during pregnancy and lactation, although some experts advise caution while the infant is breastfed while on CNIs. Methotrexate, cyclophosphamide, MMF, and rituximab are contraindicated during pregnancy and lactation. Safety concerns have led to a curtailment in the use of cyclophosphamide, while cost precludes the widespread use of rituximab in many resource-limited settings. Patient education, as in other chronic illnesses, is crucial in CTDs. Associated problems like blood pressure, lipids, electrolytes, seizures, anemia, osteoporosis, etc. need as much attention as the primary disease. Tight blood pressure control, aggressive correction of dyslipidemia, and bone protection with appropriate agents, if needed, are important. The concept of disease activity and disease damage in CTD is discussed in greater detail below.

13.9 Assessing Disease Activity in CTD

The aggressiveness of therapy in any CTD should match the disease activity. Assessment of disease activity refers to the determination of the extent to which the immuno-inflammation of CTD is contributing to the clinical setting at a particular point in time and the likelihood that it will produce diseases-related morbidity or mortality. It is analogous to the concept of "tumor burden" in oncologic disease. The change in CTD activity helps a clinician to decide whether the CTD is improving or worsening. Disease activity is assessed by a thorough clinical examination and by using laboratory parameters. The single most important laboratory investigation is urinalysis for proteins and sediment (casts and cells). Proteinuria can be easily quantified and tracked. The urine sediment is also inexpensive and universally available. Other laboratory variables used include C3/C4 levels, dsDNA levels, platelet counts, and total white cell count (TLC). ESR and CRP, being nonspecific, are not very helpful. Repeated ANA testing has no clinical utility as the titers of ANA do not correlate with disease activity. A number of standardized scoring systems have been developed to provide a more reproducible and quantitative assessment of disease activity.

13.10 Differentiating Disease Activity from Disease Damage

Crucial to CTD management is the concept of differentiating 'activity' from 'damage'. 'Disease activity' refers to ***reversible*** manifestations while 'damage' refers to ***nonreversible*** charges present for at least 6 months, which are not related to active inflammation. Disease severity is an amalgam of both activity and severity (Fig. 13.3). The following examples will help to clarify this further. A patient of SSc with active interstitial lung disease (alveolitis on HRCT) would benefit from steroids and MMF/cyclophosphamide. On the other hand, in advanced interstitial fibrosis, these therapies would be counterproductive. It would be best to consider supportive treatment or lung transplantation, if warranted. Similarly, myocarditis in SLE would require aggressive immunosuppression, while cardiomyopathy, once it has developed, would be best treated with diuretics and vasodilators rather than immunosuppressives. In the same context, lupus nephritis Class III and IV warrant aggressive immunosuppression, which is contraindicated in class VI (glomerulosclerosis). Patients in Class VI are best treated with renal replacement therapy (dialysis/transplantation) rather than aggressive immunosuppression. Validated damaged indices are available.

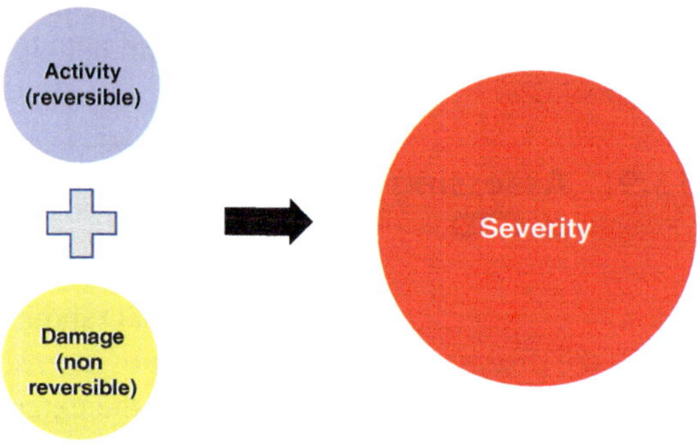

Fig. 13.3 Cardinal concepts in CTD

13.11 Conclusions

Physician awareness holds the key to early diagnosis in CTDs. Investigations are employed to confirm the diagnosis and assess organ involvement. The disease course is punctuated by remissions and relapses. The management of a CTD has to be ***individualized*** for every patient. The drug treatment is determined mainly by individual disease manifestations rather than the primary diagnosis. The intensity of therapy in a given patient is titrated according to the "disease activity" at that point in time.

14 Systemic Lupus Erythematosus

14.1 Introduction

Systemic Lupus Erythematosus (SLE) is the prototypic connective tissue disease encountered in clinical practice. It is a multisystem disorder that can involve any organ. Therefore, patients present to a variety of specialties like dermatology, internal medicine, hematology, nephrology, neurology, or pulmonology apart from rheumatology. Remissions and relapses punctuate the disease course. The management of SLE needs to be individualized for every patient. The drug treatment is determined mostly by specific organ involvement rather than the primary diagnosis. Antimalarials, nonsteroidal anti-inflammatory drugs (NSAIDs), and corticosteroids form the sheet anchor of treatment. Azathioprine, mycophenolate mofetil, tacrolimus, and cyclophosphamide are employed to treat major organ involvement like nephritis. Biologic therapies used for treatment include rituximab and belimumab. Comorbidities like hypertension, dyslipidemia, atherosclerosis, and osteoporosis need to be sought and adequately treated. Satisfactory disease control and reasonable quality of life are possible in the majority of patients.

14.2 Clinical Recognition

Constitutional features like fever, fatigue, anorexia, and weight loss are common in SLE. Arthritis and arthralgias are seen in an overwhelming proportion of patients (>90%). Indeed, inflammatory arthritis that resembles rheumatoid arthritis with the additional features of fever, oral ulcers, Raynaud's, photosensitive rash, or active urine sediment should alert the clinician to the possibility of SLE (Figs. 14.1 and 14.2). The skin involvement in SLE can assume three forms: acute cutaneous lupus erythematosus (ACLE), subacute cutaneous lupus erythematosus (SCLE), and chronic cutaneous lupus erythematosus (CCLE). The classic malar rash sparing the nasolabial folds represents ACLE (Fig. 14.3). SCLE typically presents as psoriasiform or annular erythematous plaques on the neck, upper trunk, shoulders, or forearms. The discoid lupus erythematosus (DLE) is the most common form of CCLE, accounting for more than three-fourths of the cases. About 20–25% of patients with SLE can develop DLE lesions. Over time 5–10% of patients with DLE may develop clinical features of SLE. Other forms of CCLE include lupus erythematosus tumidus, lupus panniculitis or profundus, chilblain lupus, etc. Nonspecific skin lesions like vasculitis may occur in SLE (Fig. 14.4).

Serosal involvement can take the form of pleural or pericardial effusion. Ascites is much less common. Some patients may present with lymphadenopathy, interstitial lung disease, pulmonary hypertension, or alveolar hemorrhage. Cytopenias are common. Renal involvement, most often asymptomatic, can occur in nearly 60% of patients. Neuropsychiatric involvement

R. Handa, *Clinical Rheumatology*, https://doi.org/10.1007/978-981-33-4885-1_14

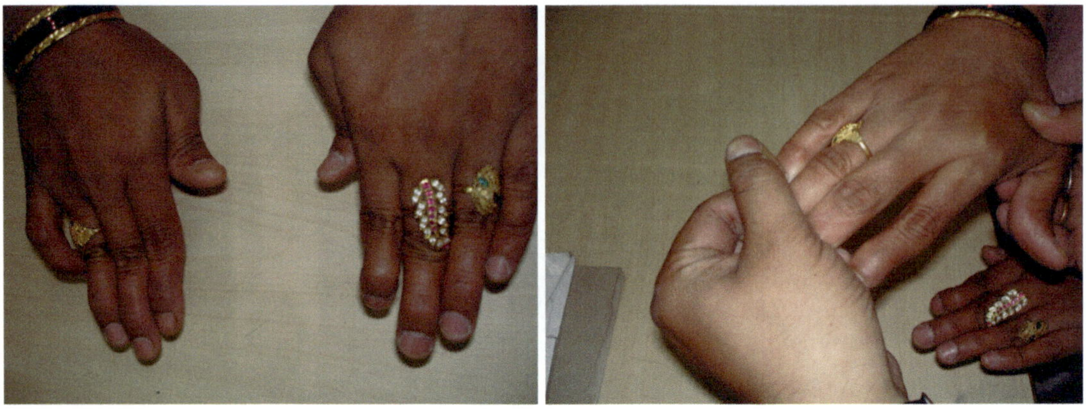

Fig. 14.1 Jaccoud's arthritis in SLE (correctable deformity)

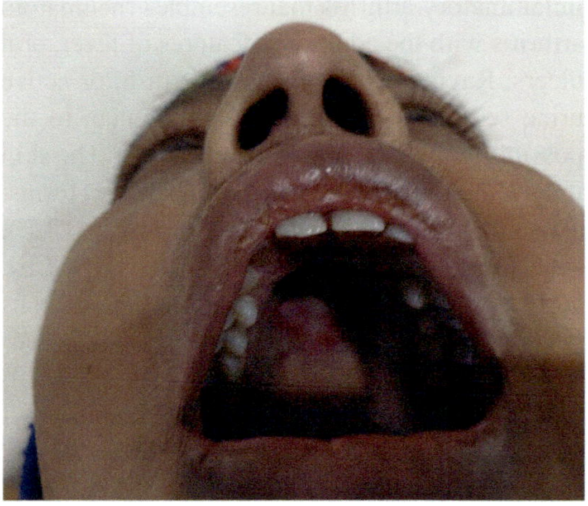

Fig. 14.2 Oral ulcers in SLE

of SLE can be quite diverse and lead to neurologic and psychiatric manifestations like cognitive dysfunction, stroke, delirium, psychosis, seizures, or peripheral neuropathy. SLE women with antiphospholipid syndrome may present to the obstetrician with recurrent pregnancy loss.

The diagnosis is clinico-serologic, that is, pattern recognition of characteristic constellations of symptoms and signs supported by serology.

14.3 Investigations

Antinuclear antibodies are used as the first serologic investigation in a patient with suspected lupus. The method of choice is indirect immunofluorescence (IIF). A positive test may or may not confirm SLE and needs clinical correlation. A negative ANA virtually rules out SLE because ANA-negative SLE is very rare in clinical practice (<5% of patients). With the use of HEp-2000® cells transfected to hyper express the 60kD SS-A/Ro antigen, the frequency of ANA-negative SLE is even lower. Once positive, there is no need to repeat ANA. Rarely, SLE patients after years of treatment may become seronegative.

ANA is a generic term for antibodies that target a variety of nuclear (cellular) antigens. ANA-positive individuals may need confirmation of the antigen type by determining antibodies to ENA-"extractable nuclear antigen." The important ones include Ro, La, Sm, RNP, Scl-70, and Jo1. Anti-ENA should be ordered only in ANA-positive individuals. Other investigations include C3 and C4, antiphospholipid antibodies, lupus anticoagulant, dsDNA levels, Coombs test, etc.

CBC, ESR, CRP, urine routine, liver, and kidney function tests are done at the initial presentation and then periodically. Urine examination is the single most crucial test to pick up kidney disease. The presence of proteinuria and/or active urine sediment should alert the clinician to the possibility of lupus nephritis (LN). Active urinary sediment is defined as >5 RBCs per high-power field (HPF) and/or cellular casts where none previously existed. Proteinuria should be quantified by spot urine protein creatinine ratio and 24-h urine protein estimation. There is a good correlation between 24-h proteinuria and random protein creatinine ratio

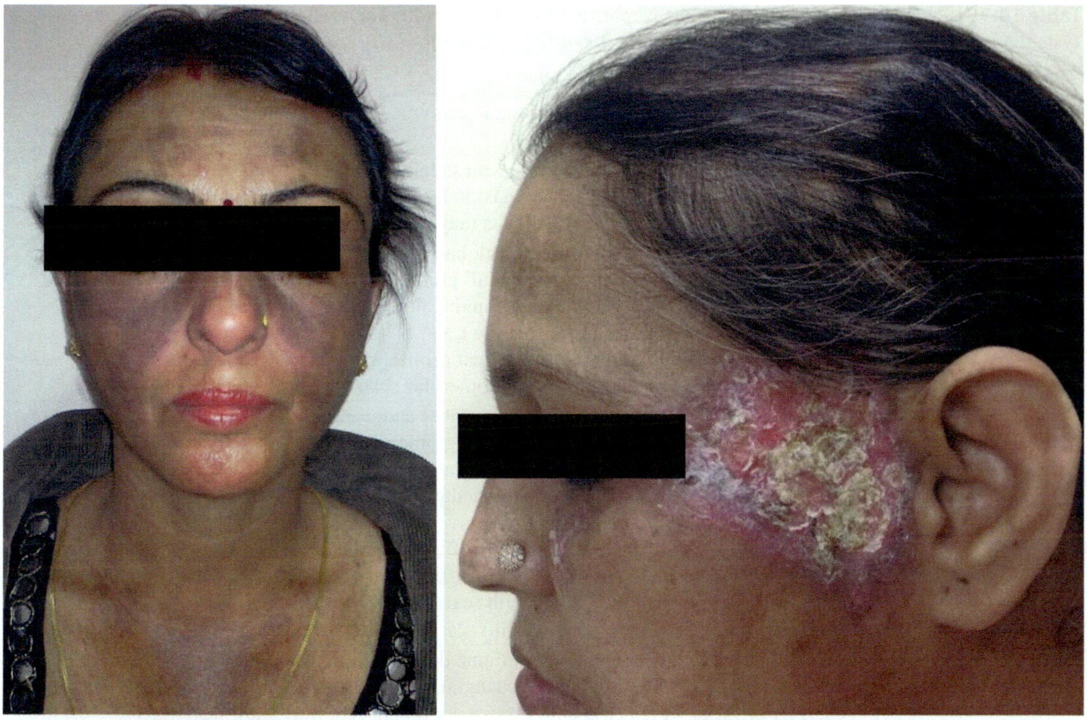

Typical rash sparing nasolabial folds

Discoid lupus

Fig. 14.3 Cutaneous manifestations of SLE

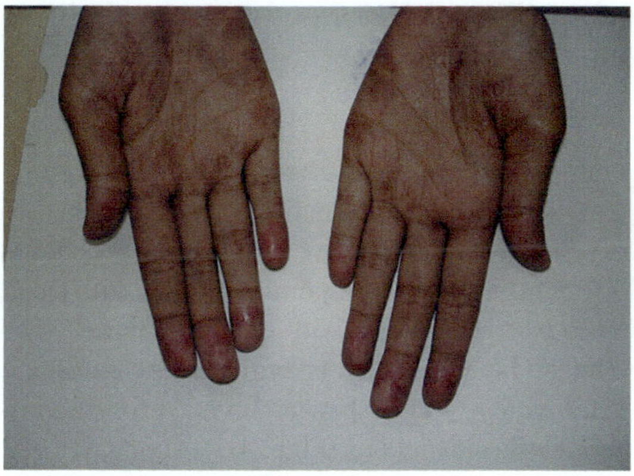

Fig. 14.4 Lupus non-specific skin disease

Box 14.1 Indications of Kidney Biopsy in SLE

- Urinary protein excretion greater than 500 mg daily
- Active urinary sediment (five or more red blood cells per high-power field and/or cellular casts)
- Serum creatinine level greater than 1.3 mg/dl unexplained by another mechanism
- Suspected class transformation may need re-biopsy

among patients with LN. However, this correlation may be poor when proteinuria is less than 500 mg/day.

A kidney biopsy is recommended in all patients with SLE who develop renal involvement (urinary protein excretion greater than 500 mg/day, active urinary sediment $\geq$5 red blood cells per high-power field and/or cellular casts, or rising serum creatinine that cannot be explained by another mechanism) (Box 14.1). It should be subjected to immunofluorescence and electron microscopy in addition to light microscopy. The International Society of Nephrology (ISN)/Renal Pathology Society (RPS) classify the glomerular pathology of lupus into six different classes with subcategorizations based upon activity and chro-

Table 14.1 ISN/RPS classification of Lupus Nephritis (Weening JJ, et al. The classification of glomerulonephritis in systemic lupus erythematosus revisited. Kidney Int 2004; 65: 521–530)

Class	Definition
Class I Minimal mesangial LN	Normal glomeruli by LM, but mesangial immune deposits by IF.
Class II Mesangial proliferative LN	Purely mesangial hypercellularity (≥3 mesangial cells per mesangial region in 3 μ thick section) of any degree or matrix expansion by LM, along with mesangial deposits. Few subepithelial or subendothelial deposits may be visible by IF or EM, but not by LM.
Class III Focal LN	Active or inactive focal, segmental or global endocapillary or extracapillary glomerulonephritis involving <50% of all glomeruli, typically with focal subendothelial immune deposits, with or without mesangial alterations. III (A): active lesions; focal proliferative LN III (A/C): active and chronic lesions; focal proliferative and sclerosing LN III (C): chronic inactive lesions with glomerular scars; focal sclerosing LN
Class IV Diffuse LN	Active or inactive diffuse, segmental or global endocapillary or extracapillary glomerulonephritis involving ≥50% of all glomeruli, typically with diffuse subendothelial immune deposits, with or without mesangial alterations. IV-S[a] (A): active lesions; diffuse segmental proliferative LN IV-G[b] (A): active lesions; diffuse global proliferative LN IV-S[a] (A/C): active and chronic lesions; diffuse segmental proliferative and sclerosing LN IV-G[b] (A/C): active and chronic lesions; diffuse global proliferative and sclerosing LN IV-S[a] (C): chronic inactive lesions with scars; diffuse segmental sclerosing LN IV-G[b] (C): chronic inactive lesions with scars; diffuse global sclerosing LN
Class V Membranous LN	Global or segmental subepithelial immune deposits or their morphological sequelae by LM and by IF or EM, with or without mesangial alterations. May occur in combination with class III or IV, in which case both classes are diagnosed. May show advanced sclerosis
Class VI Advanced Sclerotic LN	≥90% of glomeruli globally sclerosed without residual activity

EM electron microscopy, *IF* immunofluorescence, *LM* light microscopy, *LN* lupus nephritis

[a]Diffuse segmental LN indicates that 50% or more of the involved glomeruli have segmental lesions (that is, glomerular lesions involving less than 50% of the glomerular tuft)

[b]Diffuse global LN indicates that 50% or more of the involved glomeruli have global lesions (that is, glomerular lesions involving 50% or more of the glomerular tuft)

nicity of the lesions by light microscopy (Table 14.1). Overlaps and class transformation are well known.

NB: In patients with an elevated serum creatinine level but no proteinuria or haematuria, causes of acute kidney injury like NSAIDs, CNIs, RAAS blockers, dehydration should be ruled out.

NSAIDs= Nonsteroidal anti-inflammatory drugs, CNI=calneurin inhibitor, RAAS= Renin–angiotensin–aldosterone system

14.4 Classification Criteria for SLE

The variegated and pleomorphic clinical spectrum of SLE can make diagnosis challenging in some patients. There is no single pathognomonic or distinguishing clinical feature. Apart from multiple system involvement, even within a system, the presentation can be variable, e.g., neuropsychiatric lupus. Also, the disease behaves differently at different points in time, with quiet periods interspersed with periodic flares. The clinical heterogeneity is mirrored by serologic heterogeneity. This spawns the need for classification criteria in lupus (Fig. 14.5). The ACR 1982 criteria, revised in 1997, required 4 out of 11 criteria. The latest in the classification criteria are the 2019 European League Against Rheumatism/ American College of Rheumatology (EULAR/ ACR) Classification Criteria for Systemic Lupus Erythematosus. The obligatory entry criterion is a positive ANA at a titer of ≥1:80 on HEp-2 cells or an equivalent positive test at least once. There is a point system that gives varying weight to each of the 22 criteria clustered into seven clinical and three immunologic domains (Fig. 14.6).

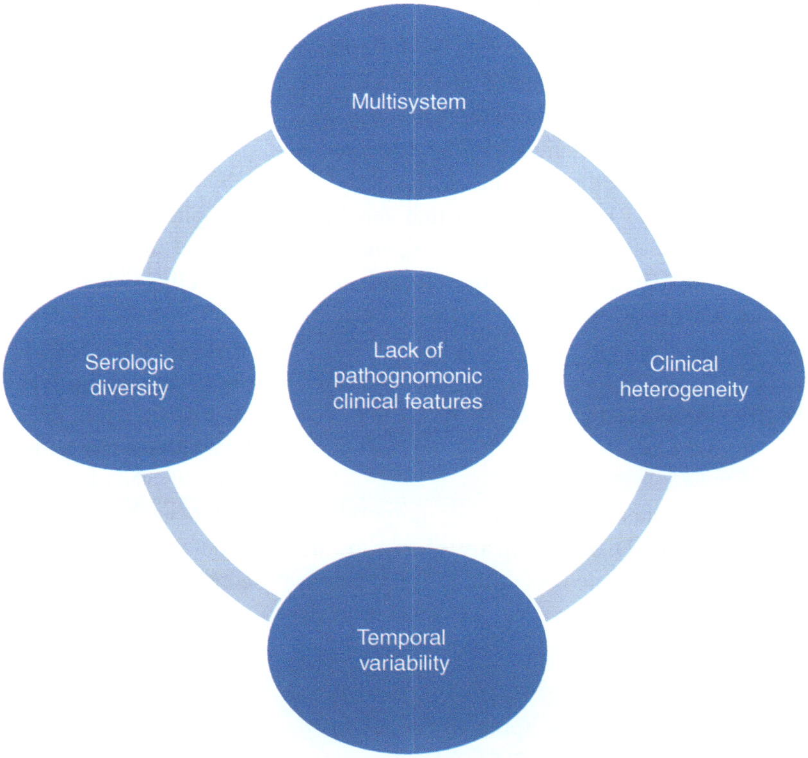
Multisystem
Serologic diversity
Lack of pathognomonic clinical features
Clinical heterogeneity
Temporal variability

Fig. 14.5 Need for classification criteria in SLE

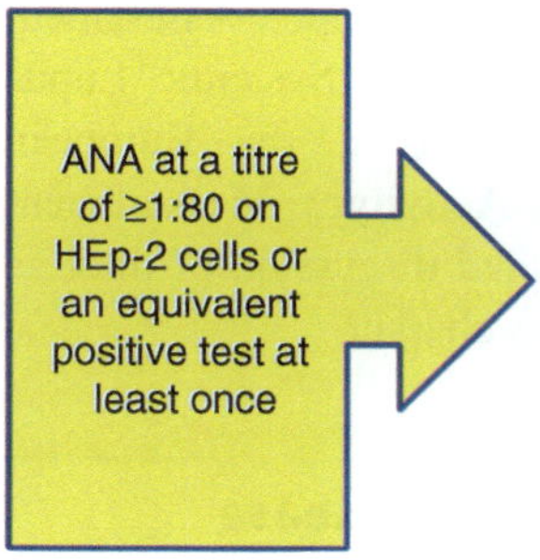

Clinical domains	Points
Constitutional domain	
Fever	2
Cutaneous domain	
Nonscarring alopecia	2
Oral ulcers	2
Subacute cutaneous or discoid lupus	4
Acute cutaneous lupus	6
Arthritis domain	
Synovitis in at least two joints or tenderness in at least two joints, and at least 30 min of morning stiffness	6
Neurologic domain	
Delirium	2
Psychosis	3
Seizure	5
Serositis domain	
Pleural or pericardial effusion	5
Acute pericarditis	6
Hematologic domain	
Leukopenia	3
Thrombocytopenia	4
Autoimmune hemolysis	4
Renal domain	
Proteinuria >0.5g/ 24 hr	4
Class II or V lupus nephritis	8
Class III or IV lupus nephritis	10

Immunologic domains	Points
Antiphospholipid antibody domain	
Anticardiolipi IgG >40 GPL or anti-β2GP1 IgG >40 units or lupus anticoagulant	2
Complement protenis domain	
Low C3 or low C4	3
Low C3 and low C4	4
Highly specific antibodied domain	
Anti-dsDNA antibody	6
Anti-Smith antibody	6

10

Martin Aringer et al. Ann Rheum Dis 2019;78:1151-1159

Fig. 14.6 SLE classification criteria 2019

A patient needs to score at least 10 points to be classified as SLE. Some caveats in the application of these criteria are listed in Box 14.2. The new criteria have a sensitivity of 96.1% and specificity of 93.4%, compared with 82.8% sensitivity and 93.4% specificity of the ACR 1982/1997 criteria. It has to be pointed out that sensitivity and specificity are reciprocally related, and specificity can be increased only at the expense of sensitivity, a trade-off that has to be finely balanced.

14.5 Assessing Disease Activity in SLE

The clinical course of SLE exhibits temporal variability (Fig. 14.7). The intensity of therapy in a given patient is titrated according to the "disease activity" at that point in time. Assessment of disease activity refers to the ascertainment of inflammation in a particular organ at that point in time. It helps the clinician to track whether SLE is improving or worsening. Disease activity is assessed by a physical examination and by using laboratory parameters like ESR, CRP, hemoglobin, platelet counts, total white cell count (TLC), amount of proteinuria, and urine sediment (casts and cells). Other laboratory variables used include C3/C4 levels, dsDNA levels, and antinucleosome antibodies. ESR and CRP, being nonspecific, may not be very helpful. Repeated ANA testing has no clinical utility as the titers of ANA do not correlate with disease activity. Falling complement and rising dsDNA levels suggest active disease, especially nephritis (Fig. 14.8). In an occasional patient, the dsDNA levels may not parallel disease activity, the so-called clinico-serologic discordance. Treatment should not be escalated in serologically active but clinically quiescent patients. In such cases, the dictum is to treat the patient and not chase the dsDNA levels. A number of standardized scoring systems have been developed to provide a more reproducible and quantitative assessment of lupus activity. Herein each clinical/laboratory variable, e.g., arthritis, alopecia, psychosis, proteinuria, is given a weighted score. Examples of scoring systems include the Systemic Lupus Erythematosus Disease Activity Index-2K (SLEDAI-2K), British Isles Lupus Assessment Group (BILAG), the Revised Systemic Lupus Activity Measure (SLAM-R), the European Consensus Lupus Activity Measurement (ECLAM), etc. A detailed discussion of these is beyond the scope of this chapter.

Box 14.2 Caveats while applying the 2019 classification criteria for SLE

- At least one clinical criterion is required.
- Criterion is not counted if an explanation other than SLE is more likely.
- Occurrence of a criterion on at least one occasion is sufficient.
- Criteria need not occur simultaneously.
- Within each domain, only the highest weighted criterion is counted toward the total score.

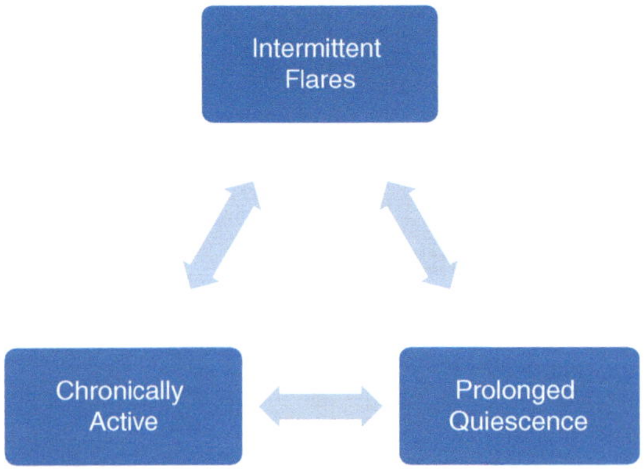

Fig. 14.7 Clinical course of SLE

14.6 Differentiating Disease Activity from Disease Damage

Crucial to the management of SLE is the concept of differentiating "lupus activity" from "damage" due to SLE. "Disease activity" refers to *reversible* manifestations while "damage" refers to *nonreversible* charges present for at least 6 months, which are not related to active inflammation. The following examples will help to clarify this fur-

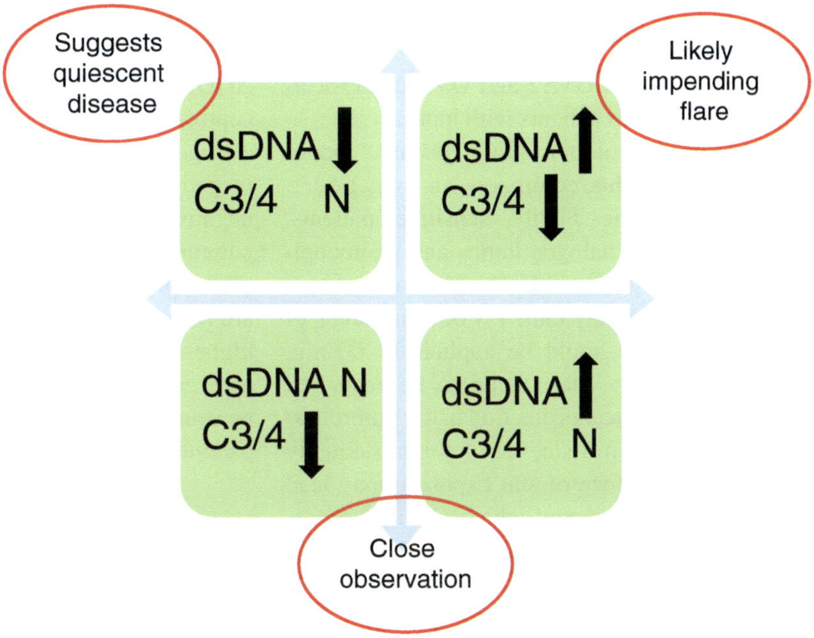

Fig. 14.8 Serologic variability in SLE

ther. Active lupus nephritis Class III and IV warrant aggressive immunosuppression, which is contraindicated in class VI (glomerulosclerosis). Patients in Class VI are best treated with renal replacement therapy (dialysis/transplantation) rather than aggressive immunosuppression. In the same context, myocarditis in SLE merits aggressive immunosuppression while cardiomyopathy, once developed, would be best treated with diuretics and other decongestive measures rather than high doses of immunosuppressives. Disease activity and damage may coexist in the same patient making treatment decisions difficult. The renal activity and chronicity can be assessed on a kidney biopsy and scores assigned (activity index 0–24 and chronicity index 0–12). Validated damage indices are available. The Systemic Lupus International Collaborating Clinics American College of Rheumatology damage index (SLICC/ACR-DI) is widely used.

14.7 Treat to Target in SLE

Treat to Target is a principle that is firmly entrenched in the management of several diseases like diabetes and hypertension. Rheumatologists have enthusiastically embraced it as we move from subjective impressions to objective disease assessments. Low disease activity and goal-driven treatment are the buzz words in the lexicon of the present-day rheumatologist. Starting with rheumatoid arthritis, the concept of treat to target has recently been extended to SLE. The target is remission or low disease activity.

14.8 General Measures

Patient education, as in other chronic illnesses, is essential in SLE. Smokers should be counseled to quit smoking. There are no specific dietary dos and don'ts. Regular exercise is vital as a part of general fitness.

Photoprotection is an integral part of treatment. Sunlight is known to induce or exacerbate cutaneous and systemic lupus erythematosus. Ultraviolet light is categorized into three major groups according to wavelength: UVA (320–400 nm), UVB (290–320 nm), and UVC (200–290). Initially, only UVB was thought to be a concern for lupus patients. It is now believed that UVA can also trigger photosensitivity. This has practical implications because ordinary glass and many sunscreens do not protect against UVA irradiation. Of UVA components, UVA1 does not influence photosensitivity. It is UVA2, which is photobiologically important for lupus patients. Thus, the current evidence suggests that UVA2 and UVB can exacerbate skin disease in patients with lupus.

Apart from outdoor sun exposure, indoor exposure from lights, computers, etc. may be detrimental in some highly sensitive patients. Incandescent and halogen lamps and photocopiers may emit significant UVA, while unshielded fluorescent bulbs may emit UVB. Sunscreens of SPF 30 or more should be applied 30–60 min before going out. These need to be reapplied every 4–6 h. Physical protection using umbrellas/caps, shades, and full-sleeved clothing is equally important. Avoidance of sun exposure may lead to vitamin D deficiency, which should be corrected if present.

14.9 Infections and Immunization in SLE

Infectious diseases continue to be a major contributor to mortality in patients with rheumatic disorders such as SLE. These need early and aggressive treatment. There is no evidence to support routine antibiotic prophylaxis before invasive procedures like dental work, genitourinary instrumentation, etc. in patients with lupus. Immunizations with influenza and pneumococcal vaccine are recommended. The details are available in the chapter on immunization. Glucocorticoids or other immunosuppressive agents may blunt the antibody response in lupus. Live vaccines (e.g., measles, mumps, rubella, polio, varicella, etc.) are not recommended in patients on immunosuppressives, including high-dose glucocorticoids. Country-specific guidelines, if available, should be followed.

14.10 Pregnancy and Contraception

Given the fact that lupus affects young women, these issues assume great importance. Pregnancy is best avoided during active disease, and women with SLE should be counseled to consider pregnancy only after the disease has been quiescent for at least 6 months. An intrauterine device (IUD) is considered a safe and effective contraceptive option for most patients with SLE. The estrogen–progestin contraceptives may be used in patients with stable low disease activity and negative antiphospholipid antibodies (aPLs). In patients with high disease activity and/or positive aPLs, progestin-only contraceptives and IUDs are recommended. Progestin-only pills may have higher rates of discontinuation due to unscheduled erratic bleeding. Gynecologist advice may be sought to individualize treatment according to patient preference.

14.11 Major and Minor Organ Involvement in SLE

Since SLE can affect any organ, it is clinically useful to categorize patients into those with ***major organ*** involvement and those with ***minor organ*** involvement. Therapy is directed accordingly. Minor involvement includes serositis, mucocutaneous, musculoskeletal, or constitutional symptoms. The major manifestations include lupus nephritis neuropsychiatric SLE, significant cytopenias, and interstitial lung disease. The concept is not meant to undermine the importance of organs like the skin, which may have a major impact on the patient's life. Instead, it is used to help the clinician determine the appropriate steroid dose in a given patient. In general, patients with minor organ involvement of lupus can be treated with NSAIDs and hydroxychloroquine. If needed, corticosteroids are given in relatively small doses (prednisolone 0.25–0.5 mg/kg/day). On the other hand, major organ involvement necessitates the use of high-dose corticosteroids (prednisolone 1 mg/kg/day) initially often with immunosuppressives (Fig. 14.9). Patients with minor organ involvement may also need high-dose corticosteroids during disease flare. In the same vein, once patients with major organ involvement go into quiescence, the corticosteroids should be tapered to a maintenance dose. Contrary to popular perception, corticosteroids can indeed be stopped in many patients with lupus.

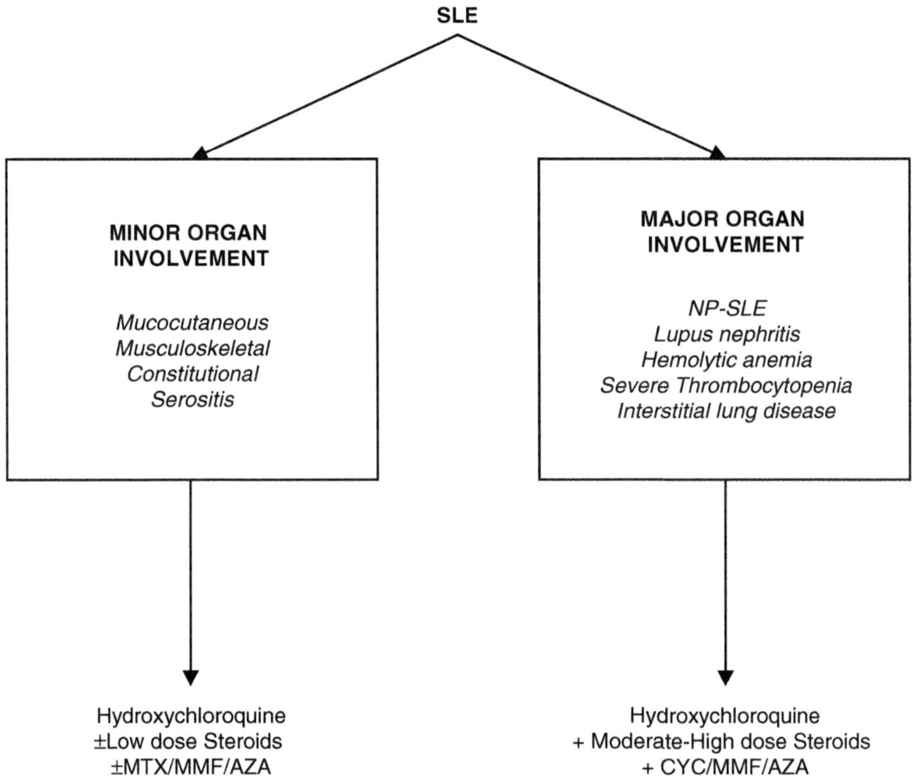

NP-SLE = Neuropsychiatic SLE;MMF = Mycophenolate mofetil; Steroids = Prednisolone; CYC= Cyclophosphamide; MTX= Methotrexate, AZA= Azathioprine

After initial disease control, the dose/duration of corticosteroid therapy has to be individualised. Not all minor organ involvement requires steroids. Conversely major organ involvement after induction can be managed with lower doses.Major flares in minor organs may need MTX/MMF/AZA

Fig. 14.9 Approach to management of SLE

14.12 Drugs Used to Treat SLE

The various drugs used to treat SLE include NSAIDs, antimalarials, corticosteroids, and immunosuppressives (Table 14.2). The type and severity of clinical features guide treatment (Fig. 14.9). A brief outline of the various drugs used is given below:

14.12.1 NSAIDs

Nonsteroidal anti-inflammatory drugs are used to combat musculoskeletal symptoms, fever, fatigue, and mild serositis. In equipotent doses, all NSAIDs are similar in efficacy, although side effects differ. Also, in a given patient, the response to an individual NSAID may vary markedly.

Table 14.2 Drugs used in the treatment of SLE

Drug	Used for	Side effects	Remarks
NSAIDs	Musculoskeletal, serositis, constitutional	Renal, gastrointestinal, blood dyscrasias, neuropsychiatric	Selected patients require gastric protection with proton pump inhibitors
Hydroxychloroquine	Mucocutaneous, musculoskeletal, serositis, constitutional, plasma glucose, and cholesterol decreased, aPL decreased	Mainly ocular toxicity. Can cause skin rash, myopathy, psychosis	Safe in pregnancy. Regular ocular screening (see text)
Corticosteroids	Benefit almost all manifestations of SLE	Weight gain, hirsutism, Cushingoid habitus, cataract, hypertension, diabetes, osteonecrosis, osteoporosis, infections.	Use the minimum possible dose for the shortest time possible. Taper slowly.
Methotrexate	Arthritis, serositis, skin rash, fever	Hepatic toxicity, cytopenias, hair loss, mucositis	Monitor LFT. May also be used as a steroid-sparing agent. Use concomitant folic acid.
Cyclophosphamide	Lupus nephritis, CNS lupus, refractory thrombocytopenia, ILD	Nausea, vomiting, bone marrow suppression, bladder toxicity, gonadal failure, malignancy	Use reserved for major organ involvement. Intermittent pulses are preferable to daily oral.
Azathioprine	Major organ involvement	Bone marrow suppression, transaminitis, malignancy	May be used for its steroid-sparing effect. Safe in pregnancy
Mycophenolate mofetil	Major organ involvement	Gastrointestinal toxicity, bone marrow suppression	An important alternative to cyclophosphamide in severe lupus nephritis
CNI (calcineurin inhibitors)	Major organ involvement	Hirsutism, hypercholesterolemia, gingival hyperplasia, nephrotoxicity, HT, glucose intolerance, hyperkalemia	Used as part of multi-target therapy (steroids+MMF+CNI)

What works for one patient may not work for the other patient. Therefore, NSAID selection is based on patient preference, dosing frequency, and side-effect profile. NSAIDs may cause acute interstitial nephritis, acute tubular necrosis, or membranous nephropathy. NSAID-induced renal injury in SLE needs to be differentiated from lupus nephritis. Similarly, NSAIDs may be responsible for neuropsychiatric features like headache, dizziness, aseptic meningitis, etc. which need differentiation from neuropsychiatric involvement in SLE.

14.12.2 Antimalarials—The Anchor Drugs for Lupus

Hydroxychloroquine (HCQ) has virtually replaced chloroquine in the treatment of lupus. The therapeutic efficacy of both agents is similar, but HCQ is preferred because of greater ocular safety. Antimalarials benefit serositis, cutaneous, musculoskeletal, and constitutional symptoms of SLE. Data from non-randomized studies have suggested favorable effects of antimalarials on various other SLE outcomes, such as a reduction of flares, prevention of damage accrual, and a possible reduction in mortality risk. In addition, HCQ has been shown to favorably alter risk factors for atherosclerotic disease by reducing cholesterol and glucose levels. Titers of antiphospholipid antibodies decline with HCQ treatment. In pregnant women, HCQ decreases lupus activity without harming the baby. Despite being economical and effective, antimalarials are underutilized in the treatment of SLE. All patients with lupus should receive HCQ unless there are specific contraindications.

The usual daily dose of HCQ is 5 mg/kg of real body weight. Hydroxychloroquine is a well-tolerated drug. Some patients may experience nausea and skin hyperpigmentation. Ocular toxicity, while being the most serious adverse effect, is uncommon. It may take the form of keratopathy, ciliary body involvement, lens opacities, and retinopathy. Deposits of the antimalarial drugs on the cornea are related to high daily doses. This effect is more common with chloroquine as compared to HCQ. The corneal deposits do not affect vision but may cause transient halos or heightened light sensitivity. These reverse on drug discontinuation. Rarely, antimalarials may lead to accommodation problems or cataracts. The ocular toxicity of concern is retinopathy, seen more with chloroquine than HCQ. While no completely safe dosage is identified, daily HCQ consumption of 5.0 mg/kg of real body weight or less is associated with a low risk for up to 10 years—the prevalence of retinal toxicity remains less than 2% within the first 10 years of use but rises to almost 20% after 20 years of use. Commonly accepted risk factors include dose >5 mg/kg/day real body weight, cumulative dose of >1000 g of HCQ, duration of treatment >5 years, renal or liver dysfunction, preexisting retinopathy, elderly individuals, concomitant tamoxifen use, and the presence of macular disease.

All patients on HCQ need ophthalmic examination. Amsler's grid is considered obsolete and fundus examination is deemed insensitive. The main aim of doing a baseline fundus is to rule out preexisting maculopathy. By the time fundus changes become apparent, it may be too late to do anything. The ethos is for modern screening to discern retinopathy before it is visible in the fundus. The primary screening tests employed currently are automated visual fields and spectral-domain optical coherence tomography (SD-OCT). Early OCT changes are often asymptomatic and may not progress if HCQ is discontinued. Traditionally HCQ retinal toxicity has been recognized as manifesting in the parafoveal retina, and hence 10-2 automated visual field is recommended as it tests the visual field on 10° to either side of the fovea. It has been pointed out that in the Asian population, retinopathy manifests in the perifoveal region (>7° from the fovea), and therefore one might need wide-angle screening using 24-2 or 30-2 visual fields to examine beyond the central macula. Our own studies have shown a parafoveal and a mixed pattern (para and perifoveal pattern) in Indian patients. Therefore, we recommend wide-angle visual fields so as not to miss peripheral, extra macular (perifoveal) lesions.

Spectral-domain optical coherence tomography (SD-OCT) is slowly becoming widely available. It reveals disruption, or complete loss, of the outer nuclear layer, external limiting membrane, inner/outer segment junction, and retinal pigment epithelium (RPE) in the parafoveal region. Bilateral parafoveal outer retinal and RPE atrophy with central sparing has been termed the "flying saucer sign." Other modalities include fundus autofluorescence (FAF) and multifocal electroretinogram (mfERG).

The screening frequency during the first 5 years of treatment should be individualized based upon the assessment of risk. Annual screening is recommended after 5 years for patients on acceptable doses and without major risk factors.

14.12.3 Corticosteroids

Corticosteroids are beneficial in most of the lupus manifestations. Prednisolone is preferred over long-acting steroids such as betamethasone/dexamethasone except in pregnancy with fetal complete heart block where the latter are used since prednisolone does not cross the placental barrier. In emergent and life-threatening situations, methylprednisolone pulses may be used (1 g intravenous infusion daily for 3–5 days). In most patients, steroids can be tapered and even discontinued once the disease is quiescent for a prolonged period. However, some patients of SLE have a *minimum corticosteroid threshold*—a reduction of steroid dose below this threshold leads to a lupus flare. Such patients may need life-long corticosteroids. In general, SLE maintenance treatment should aim for the lowest glucocorticoid dosage needed to control disease, and if possible, glucocorticoids should be withdrawn altogether (Box 14.3). There is no convincing data to show the greater benefit or safety of methylprednisolone or deflazacort.

Box 14.3 Corticosteroids in SLE

- Steroid exposure (dose and duration) should be kept to a minimum.
- Not all patients of SLE need steroids.
- Steroid requirement may go up or down. Disease in remission may not need steroids. Flares may require institution or escalation of steroids.
- "Minor organ" lupus may require low steroid doses (prednisolone 0.25 mg/KBW/day or less) while "major organ" involvement may need moderate to high doses (prednisolone 0.5–1 mg/KBW/day), when active.
- Many patients with minor organ lupus may not need corticosteroids.
- Major organ involvement, when quiescent, can well be managed by low dose steroids or no steroids.
- The induction dose of 1 mg/KBW per day of prednisolone is not sacrosanct. Modest doses of 30–60 mg/day may suffice even in patients weighing more than 60 kg.

14.12.4 Immunosuppressives in SLE

In general, these agents are indicated in patients with major organ SLE. Patients with severe organ or life-threatening manifestations like renal and central nervous system are treated with an initial period of intensive immunosuppressive therapy (induction therapy). Intermittent monthly boluses of intravenous cyclophosphamide (CYC) have been the standard treatment. However, side effects, including gonadal failure, infection, and secondary malignant disease, have led to alternative regimens/agents. The Eurolupus regimen (six pulses of 500 mg cyclophosphamide intravenously every 2 weeks) provides the opportunity to treat patients with lupus nephritis effectively with lower doses of cyclophosphamide and reduced infection risk (Fig. 14.10). Most centers now use it in preference to the older regimen recommended by the US National Institutes of Health (monthly intravenous cyclophosphamide 750 mg/m^2 body surface area for 6 months, followed by intravenous cyclophosphamide every 3 months for 2 years).

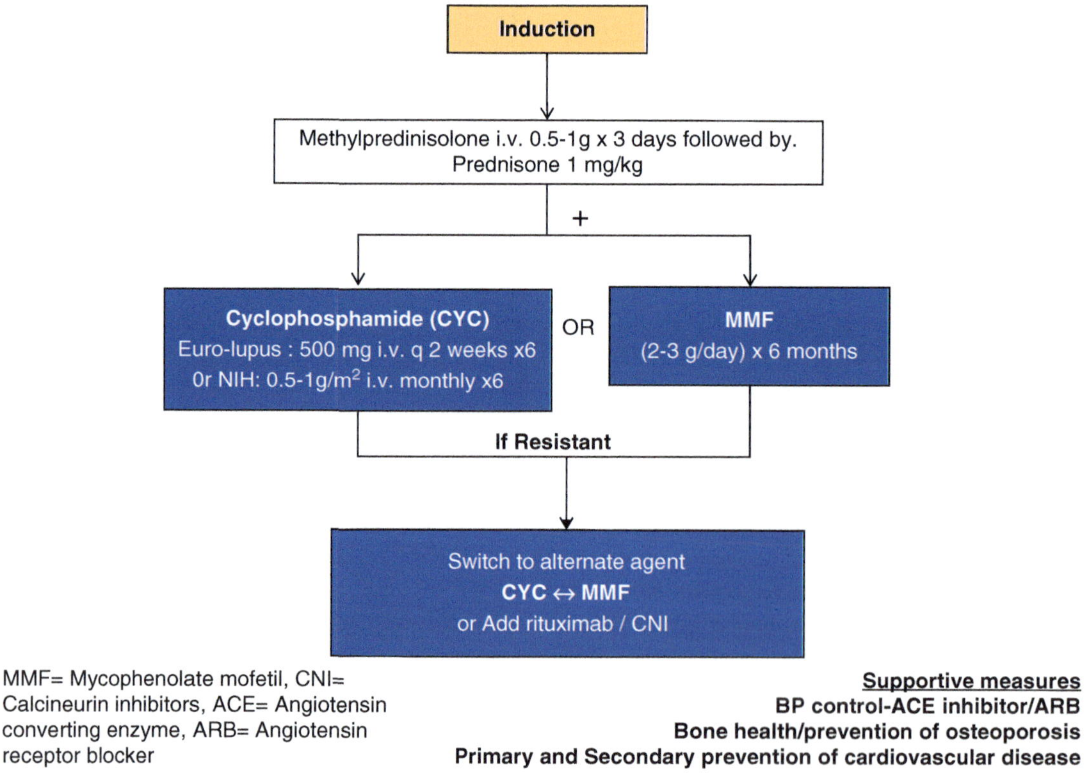

Fig. 14.10 Treatment of proliferative lupus nephritis

The growing disenchantment with cyclophosphamide is because of fear of gonadal toxicity, bone marrow suppression, and increased cancer (bladder cancer, acute myeloid leukemia, nonmelanoma skin cancer) in patients, especially with cumulative doses >36 g. A daily dose of 100 mg for 1 year translates into a dose of 36 g/year. Daily oral CYC is seldom, if ever, used in Rheumatology practice these days because daily oral CYC is associated with an increased risk of both hemorrhagic cystitis and bladder cancer, in a dose- and/or duration-dependent fashion. The hemorrhagic cystitis with cyclophosphamide treatment is associated with an increased risk of bladder cancer. The intravenous pulse administration delivers a lesser dose, carries a low risk of cystitis, and probably also of bladder cancer. Some centers use oral or intravenous 2-mercaptoethanesulfonate sodium (MESNA) in patients receiving oral or pulse intravenous CYC. MESNA binds to acrolein, a toxic metabolite of CYC rendering it nontoxic. The evidence for use of MESNA in preventing cystitis is derived largely from its use with ifosfamide in patients with cancer and may not be applicable to rheumatic diseases. There is no definite evidence that it prevents bladder cancer in humans. Adequate hydration to ensure good diuresis is recommended in all patients receiving pulse CYC. Antiemetic therapy is routinely administered with intravenous cyclophosphamide.

Mycophenolate in doses of 2–3 g/day has emerged as an important alternative to CYC. Rituximab is another agent employed for induction. For lupus nephritis, following induction therapy, at least 3 years of immunosuppressive maintenance treatment is recommended to optimize outcomes. The treatment of lupus nephritis is outlined in Table 14.3 and Fig. 14.10.

Apart from cyclophosphamide and mycophenolate, methotrexate, azathioprine have been used in clinical settings where lupus activity fails to respond completely to steroids or for their steroid-sparing effect. Methotrexate given weekly (oral dose ranging from 7.5 to 25 mg) is used to treat the arthritis of SLE and as a steroid-sparing agent in patients requiring large doses. Azathioprine, given orally in doses of 2–3 mg/KBW, is used to treat major organ lupus, especially in young women where gonadal toxicity is a major concern while using cyclophosphamide. In an effort to reduce drug toxicity, azathioprine has also been used as a maintenance agent after induction of remission with cyclophosphamide. Azathioprine can be used during pregnancy and lactation. Intravenous immunoglobulin (IVIG) is occasionally used to control acute bleeding associated with lupus thrombocytopenia or rapidly increase the platelet count to allow for splenectomy or emergency surgery. Belimumab is used in patients with active musculoskeletal or cutaneous SLE that is unresponsive to standard treatment with glucocorticoids or other immunosuppressive agents. It is presently not recommended for use in severe active lupus nephritis or severe active CNS disease. Calcineurin inhibitors like cyclosporine or tacrolimus are used as part of multi-target therapy.

Table 14.3 Management of lupus nephritis (classes according to the International Society of Nephrology/Renal Pathology Society Classification)

Class I	RAAS blockade
Class II	RAAS blockade CNI or steroids in patients with podocytopathy and urinary protein excretion ≥3 g daily
Class III	See Fig. 14.9
Class IV	
Class V	RAAS blockade Nephrotic range proteinuria: steroids and CNI or MMF or CYC or AZA
Class VI	CKD management Avoid high-dose corticosteroids/immunosuppressives

Renin–angiotensin–aldosterone system (RAAS) blocking agents

CYC cyclophosphamide, *MMF* mycophenolate mofetil, *CNI* calneurin inhibitor (cyclosporine or tacrolimus), *AZA* azathioprine

14.13 Comorbidities

Associated problems like hypertension, hyperlipidemia, anemia, osteoporosis, antiphospholipid syndrome, pulmonary hypertension, etc. need as much attention as the primary disease. Atherosclerosis has emerged as a major challenge in SLE. According to the current paradigm, inflammation plays a major role in atherosclerosis. Lupus being a prototype systemic inflammatory disease is associated with accelerated atherosclerosis, and our data, utilizing carotid intimo-medial thickness as a surrogate marker for atherosclerosis, reveals that this problem is widespread in Asian Indian patients with SLE. Tight blood pressure control, use of ACE inhibitors and/or angiotensin receptor blockers, aggressive correction of dyslipidemia, and bone protection with calcium, vitamin D, and bisphosphonates if needed is important. Fever in SLE mandates a diligent search and treatment for an infection.

14.14 Conclusions

SLE is a challenging disorder because of its clinical diversity, serologic complexity, multiple comorbidities, and variable natural history. Advances in understanding the pathobiology of lupus have changed the therapeutic landscape of this disease. Several drugs are available, and many more are in the pipeline. The need of the hour is to strike a balance between efficacy, patient preference, and safety.

Suggested Reading

Dadhaniya NV, Sood I, Patil A, Mallaiah U, Upadhyaya S, Handa R, et al. Screening for hydroxychloroquine retinal toxicity in Indian patients. In: J Clin Rheum.; 2020.

Fanouriakis A, Kostopoulou M, Alunno A, Aringer M, Bajema I, Boletis JN, et al. 2019 update of the EULAR recommendations for the management of systemic lupus erythematosus. Ann Rheum Dis. 2019;78:736–45.

Fanouriakis A, Kostopoulou M, Cheema K, Anders HJ, Aringer M, Bajema I, et al. 2019 Update of the Joint European League Against Rheumatism and European Renal Association-European Dialysis and Transplant Association (EULAR/ERA-EDTA) recommendations for the management of lupus nephritis. Ann Rheum Dis. 2020;79:713–23.

Gordon C, Amissah-Arthur MB, Gayed M, Brown S, Bruce IN, D'Cruz D, et al. British Society for Rheumatology Standards, Audit and Guidelines Working Group. The British Society for Rheumatology guideline for the management of systemic lupus erythematosus in adults. Rheumatology (Oxford). 2018;57(1):e1–e45.

Muangchan C, van Vollenhoven RF, Bernatsky SR, Smith CD, Hudson M, Inanç M, et al. Treatment algorithms in systemic lupus erythematosus. Arthritis Care Res (Hoboken). 2015;67:1237–45.

van Vollenhoven RF, Mosca M, Bertsias G, et al. Treat-to-target in systemic lupus erythematosus: recommendations from an international task force. Ann Rheum Dis. 2014;73:958–67.

15 Sjogren's Syndrome

15.1 Introduction

Connective tissue diseases (CTDs) are characterized by remarkably diverse clinical features bound by the common thread of autoantibodies, notably the antinuclear antibody (ANA). While lupus is the flagship CTD, others are no less important but often go unrecognized. Sjogren's syndrome (SS) is the commonest CTD in clinical practice, far more common than lupus. In fact, the frequency may approximate or even exceed that of rheumatoid arthritis. Earlier reports of its rarity in India have not been borne out by subsequent clinical experience. Despite being common, Sjogren's syndrome is uncommonly diagnosed. Patients with SS frequently present to the ophthalmologist with dry eyes. Others present to the dentist with accelerated dental decay or to the dermatologist with purpura. Most are never investigated further and receive only symptomatic treatment without a diagnosis of SS. Patients with arthralgias and low-level rheumatoid factor positivity are erroneously labeled as rheumatoid arthritis (RA). The unfounded assumption that SS is rare and physician unfamiliarity are the major contributors to this inability to connect dots and delay in diagnosis. Cross-disciplinary consultation with ophthalmologists, dentists, pulmonologists, etc. is invaluable in improving the quality of care in what can be a frustrating condition for the patient.

SS may occur in isolation (primary Sjogren's syndrome) or in association with other autoimmune diseases such as RA, systemic lupus erythematosus, scleroderma, or dermatomyositis (secondary Sjogren's syndrome).

15.2 Clinical Recognition

The classical clinical triad of SS comprises dryness of the mouth and eyes, fatigue, and pain. Dry eyes and dry mouth are ubiquitous in clinical practice and may remain unnoticed by the patient or be attributed to contact lenses, dry/dusty environment, poor dental hygiene, etc. The first caregiver is usually a non-rheumatologist like the ophthalmologist or dentist who may overlook the possibility of systemic disease. Many patients do not volunteer a history of dry mouth. A direct question like "do you have dryness in the mouth?" may evoke a negative reply. However, they may readily give a history of difficulty in swallowing dry food and the inability to eat food without water or liquids. It is rewarding to ask a history of accelerated dental decay, which may need capping/tooth replacement at a young age. Extensive caries, or caries at atypical sites, or reduced saliva pool should arouse suspicion of SS (Figs. 15.1 and 15.2). This is often a surrogate for salivary hypofunction. Hyperlobulation and fissuring of the tongue are characteristic changes associated with salivary hypofunction in patients with SS.

A dry mouth is not necessarily a painful mouth. Pain should prompt a search for candida. Oral candidiasis is frequent and may manifest as

R. Handa, *Clinical Rheumatology*, https://doi.org/10.1007/978-981-33-4885-1_15

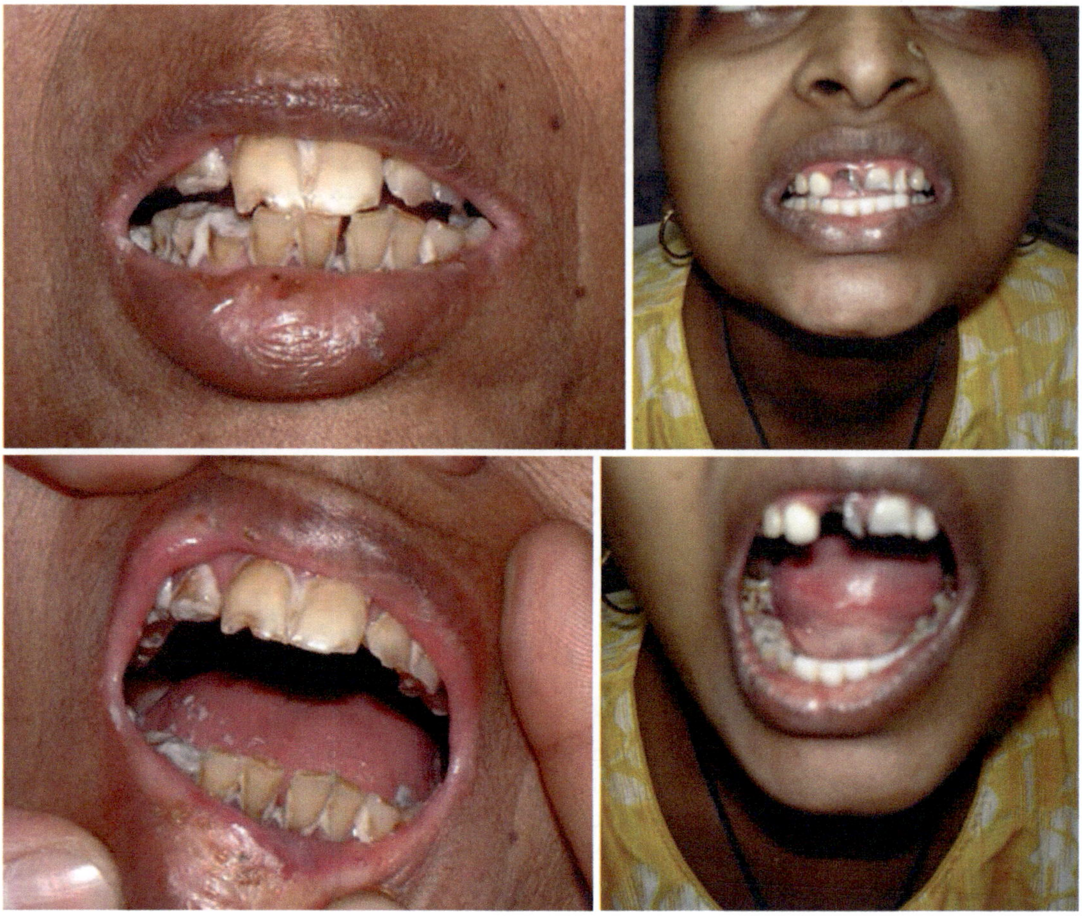

Fig. 15.1 Teeth in Sjogren's syndrome

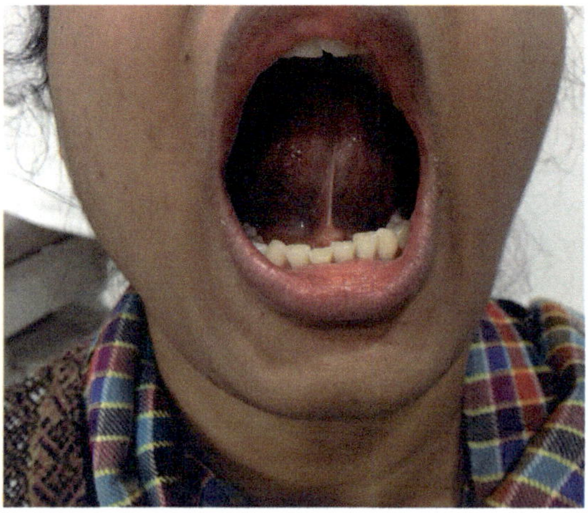

Fig. 15.2 Reduced salivary pool in Sjogren's syndrome

papillary atrophy, angular cheilitis, or erythematous changes of the hard palate or lichen planus like changes in buccal recess. Treatment with antifungals can be very gratifying.

Table 15.1 Differential diagnosis of dry mouth

• Sjögren's syndrome
• Drugs (anticholinergics, diuretics, anxiolytics, antihypertensives, or antihistamines)
• Diabetes mellitus
• Mouth breathing, nasal obstruction
• Head and neck irradiation
• Dehydration/summers
• Psychological factors

Dry mouth has several causes apart from Sjogren's syndrome (Table 15.1). A given patient may have more than one cause that should be sought and addressed.

Dry eye may go unnoticed by the patient. Patients describe eye symptoms in a variety of ways: dryness, grittiness, scratchiness, irritation,

Table 15.2 Dry eye—causes

Environmental causes
• Dry, dusty environment
• Low ambient humidity
Evaporative dry eye
• Contact lens use
• Disorders of lid aperture
• Drugs (e.g., isotretinoin)
• Vitamin A deficiency
• Allergic conditions
Aqueous deficient dry eye
• Sjogren's syndrome
• Aging
• Lacrimal gland obstruction
• Graft versus host disease
• Radiation therapy
Other causes
• LASIK and refractive surgery

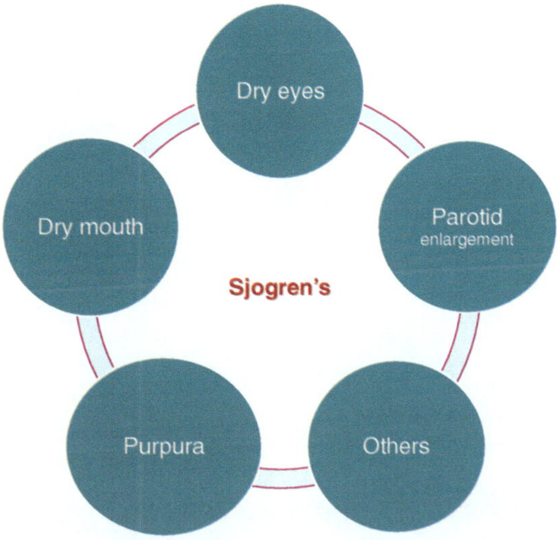

Fig. 15.3 Clinical spectrum of Sjogren's syndrome

burning, watering, soreness, desire to rub eyes, and eye fatigue. Patients may report pain evoked by exposure to wind, light, and temperature extremes. Some routinely use lubricant drops and often fail to mention this to the doctor while describing their rheumatic complaints. Sjogren's syndrome is not the only cause of dry eyes.

Dry eye is a common disorder with multiple causes listed in Table 15.2. A patient with SS may have other interrelated, overlapping causes, which too should be tackled. There is a poor correlation between objectively measured signs and patient-reported symptoms of dryness. Schirmer's test and salivary flow rates often do not parallel patient symptoms.

There is more to Sjogren's syndrome than sicca symptoms (Fig. 15.3). It is a systemic disease. Sjogren's may be associated with parotid, lacrimal, or submandibular gland swelling (Fig. 15.4). Table 15.3 lists the differential diagnosis of enlarged parotids. Palpable purpura may be the presenting feature in some patients (Fig. 15.5). In the setting of palpable purpura, hypergammaglobulinemia should alert a clinician to the possibility of SS. Hypergammaglobulinemia is found in 20–40% of patients. Cryoglobulinemia occurs in 10–15% of patients with SS and may be associated with leukocytoclastic vasculitis and hypocomplementemia. Systemic involvement may include interstitial lung disease (commonest type is nonspecific interstitial pneumonitis), kidney involvement (tubulointerstitial nephritis, renal distal tubular acidosis (Fig. 15.6), membranoproliferative glomerulonephritis secondary to cryoglobulinemia, etc.), or peripheral neuropathy. The neurologic disease may take the form of pure sensory neuropathy or mononeuritis multiplex. Hypokalemic paralysis may be the first manifestation. Patients with SS are at an increased risk for non-Hodgkin B cell lymphoma. In some patients, sicca features or rheumatic manifestations are rather minimal. The extra-rheumatic complaints may dominate the clinical picture, e.g., interstitial lung disease. Such patients are labeled as lung dominant CTD or interstitial pneumonia with autoimmune features (IPAF).

The incidental discovery of heart block in the fetus during pregnancy may draw attention to the presence of ant-Ro (SSA) and anti-La (SSB) antibodies in the mother who may be totally asymptomatic. Some women are found to have serology suggestive of SS after they deliver babies with congenital heart block. Such women may never evolve into SS or develop symptoms after years to decades. The risk of congenital heart block in Ro-positive mothers is only 1–3%. With one child having heart block, the risk in subsequent pregnancies approximates 15%.

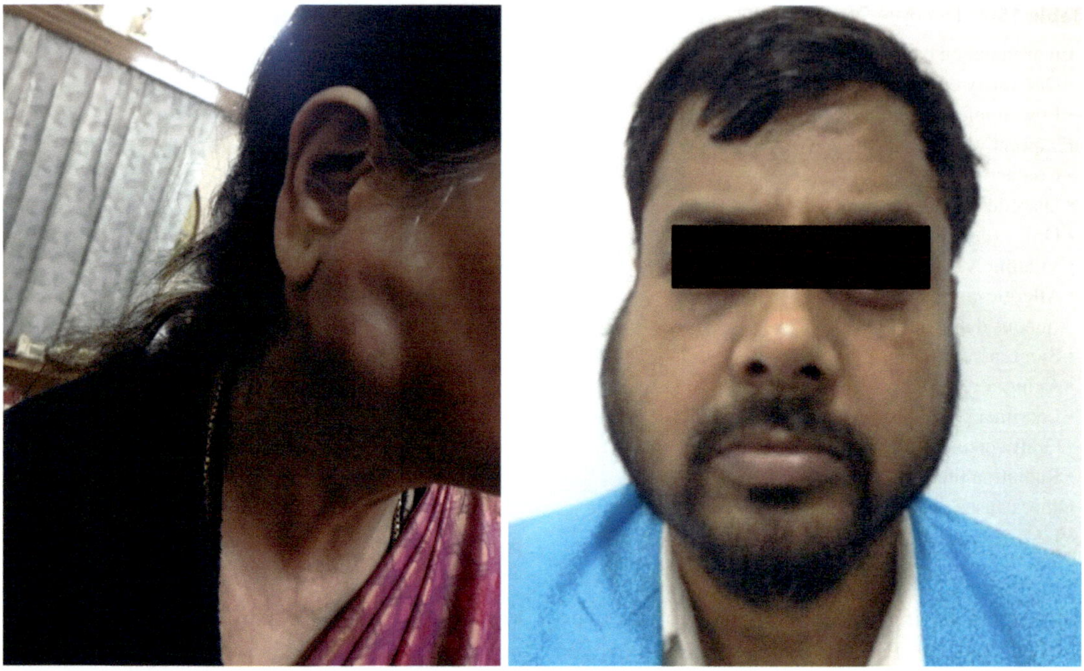

Fig. 15.4 Parotid enlargement in Sjogren's syndrome

Table 15.3 Differential diagnosis of parotid swelling

• Infections: Mumps, HIV, EBV
• Metabolic: Diabetes, Cushing's syndrome, hypothyroidism, hypertriglyceridemia
• Alcohol
• Tumors
• Sialolithiasis, ductal stenosis
• Sjogren's syndrome, systemic lupus erythematosus, sarcoidosis
• IgG4-related disease

HIV human immunodeficiency virus, *EBV* Epstein virus disease

15.3 Investigations

Routine investigations may reveal elevated ESR and CRP, anemia of chronic inflammation, and elevated globulins with reversal of the albumin globulin ratio. Urinalysis may show mild proteinuria and white cell casts.

Schirmer's test is used for the assessment of dry eye. It measures the 5-min wetting of a standardized strip of filter paper placed in the lower lateral fornix of the eyelid. Schirmer test is sup-

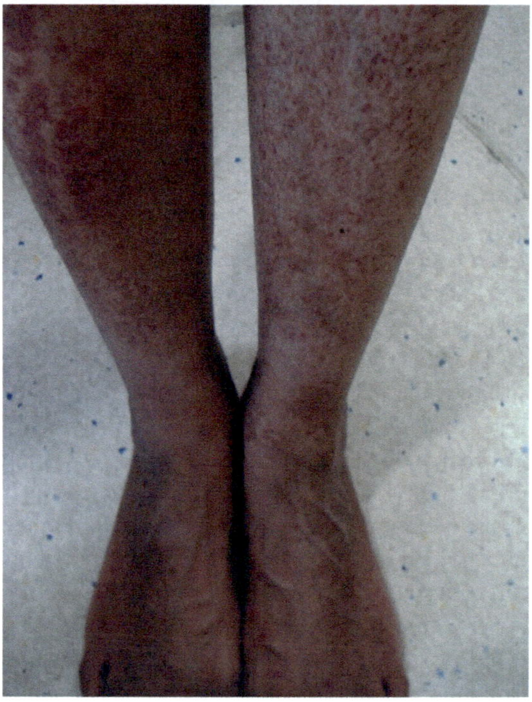

Fig. 15.5 Hypergammaglobulinemic purpura in Sjogren's syndrome

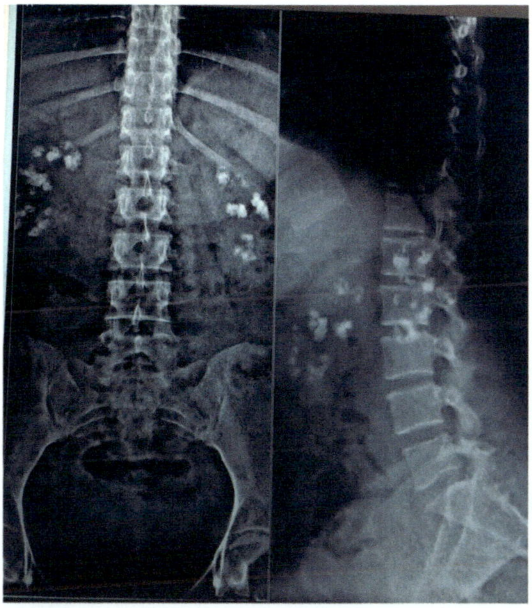

Fig. 15.6 Nephrocalcinosis in a patient with Sjogren's syndrome and distal renal tubular acidosis

portive of SS when wetting measures 5 mm or less in either eye. However, this stringent cutoff value decreases the sensitivity of the test in patients with mild SS. Also, test results decline with age, and therefore, the test may not be appropriate for older individuals. A normal Schirmer's test does not rule out SS.

Ocular staining is done using fluorescein and lissamine green. Fluorescein stains corneal epithelium and is used to detect defects in the corneal epithelium, while lissamine green stains devitalized conjunctival cells. Rose Bengal stains conjunctiva but is less used because it is more irritating. Tear break up time is a test done for an evaporative dry eye, and a value <10 s is considered abnormal.

The serology in Sjogren's syndrome can be quite variable (Table 15.4). Autoantibodies in SS include ANA (~90% patients), anti-Ro [SSA] (70–80%) and anti-La [SSB] (30–40%) antibodies. Rheumatoid factor is seen in 40–60% of patients. Antibodies to dsDNA are absent unless there is an overlap with lupus.

Table 15.4 Autoantibodies in Sjogren's syndrome

Autoantibody	Frequency
Antinuclear antibody	~90%
Rheumatoid factor	40–60%
Ro (SSA)	70–80%
La (SSB)	30–40%

In Sjogren's syndrome, both anti-Ro 52 and 60 are seen in nearly the same frequency. Isolated anti-Ro 52 is more common in inflammatory myositis

Labial (Minor Salivary Gland) Biopsy is an easy, rewarding, and yet underutilized procedure in SS. Minor salivary gland biopsy is required for definitive evaluation of patients with suspected SS who lack both anti-Ro/SSA and anti-La/SSB antibodies or have equivocal serologic test results. An adequate biopsy should contain at least 6–7 minor salivary glands. SS is pathologically characterized by focal lymphocytic sialadenitis (tightly aggregated clusters or foci of lymphocytes containing 50 or more cells) surrounding a duct in a 4 mm^2 area of gland tissue. The approximate density of the lymphocytic foci in the tissue is called a "focus score." One important caveat is that lymphocytic foci should be considered a feature of SS-related focal lymphocytic sialadenitis only if they are adjacent to normal-appearing mucous acini. This is because lymphocytic foci are also seen in glands damaged due to ductal obstruction. Serologically negative patients should not be labeled as SS based on loosely worded pathology reports like "consistent with Sjogren's syndrome." Minor salivary gland biopsy has 38–82% sensitivity and approximately 85–94% specificity for Sjögren syndrome. Although very safe, a biopsy may cause persistent lip numbness in up to 2% of patients.

Other investigations include a kidney biopsy or a skin biopsy. Small fiber neuropathy may require a skin biopsy.

Referral to a rheumatologist may be necessary to confirm the diagnosis in patients with suggestive clinical features but equivocal or negative serologies, refractory disease, patients with systemic involvement, or when biologics are contemplated.

15.4 Treatment

A multidisciplinary approach is needed. Treatment of SS entails the use of muscarinic agonists (pilocarpine hydrochloride and cevimeline hydrochloride) for the treatment of oral and ocular dryness. Pilocarpine is available as a 5-mg tablet, and the dose is gradually escalated to thrice or four times daily as tolerated. The maximum daily dose is 30 mg. The main adverse effect is sweating, which can be minimized by a gradual escalation of the dose. Cevimeline (dose 30 mg thrice daily p.o.) is not available in India. These agents help oral symptoms more than the eye. Meticulous dental hygiene, brushing after every major meal, physical stimuli for salivation like sugar-free chewing gum, and oral sprays help in oral symptom relief. Eye dryness needs lubricating drops, cyclosporine eye drops, or punctal occlusion. Moisturizers are used for skin dryness. Women may need lubricants for vaginal dryness.

Hydroxychloroquine is often used for arthralgias, arthritis, and purpura. Severe organ manifestations are treated with corticosteroids and immunosuppressive agents like methotrexate, mycophenolate mofetil, azathioprine, cyclophosphamide, or rituximab.

15.5 Conclusions

Sjogren's syndrome is neither exotic nor esoteric. It is common but challenging because of its clinical heterogeneity and the need for dialog between various subspecialties. Rheumatologists, given their familiarity with and expertise in tackling multisystem disorders, are uniquely placed to handle this disease.

Suggested Reading

Clayton JA. Dry eye. N Engl J Med. 2018;378:2212–23.

Fischer A, Antoniou KM, Brown KK, Cadranel J, Corte TJ, du Bois RM, et al. "ERS/ATS Task Force on Undifferentiated Forms of CTD-ILD". An official European Respiratory Society/American Thoracic Society research statement: interstitial pneumonia with autoimmune features. Eur Respir J. 2015;46:976–87.

16 Systemic Sclerosis

16.1 Introduction

Systemic sclerosis (SSc) or scleroderma is an uncommon connective tissue disease characterized by fibrosis, vasculopathy, and immunologic abnormalities (Fig. 16.1). The word "scleroderma" reflects the predominant involvement of the skin (Greek *skleros*—hard, *derma*—skin). The preferred nomenclature is "systemic sclerosis" because it highlights the disease's multisystem nature that often extends beyond the skin. Even though the term "scleroderma" should be restricted to cases where the disease is confined to the skin, it continues to enjoy widespread usage, and many a time is used interchangeably with SSc. The terminology of PSS or "progressive systemic sclerosis" has been abandoned because not all cases are progressive. Sir William Osler's description of generalized SSc cannot be bettered "one of the most terrible of all human ills…to wither slowly… and be 'beaten down and marred and wasted' until one is literally a mummy, encased in an ever-shrinking, slowly contracting skin of steel, is a fate not pictured in any tragedy, ancient or modern."

16.2 Classification

The disease can be classified into localized and generalized varieties depending on whether it is confined to the skin and subcutaneous structures or is multisystem (Fig. 16.2). Localized disease is commoner in children and can be categorized into morphea (disease confined to the skin) and linear scleroderma (where subcutaneous structures are also affected). Morphea may be further subdivided into localized or generalized depending on whether the plaques of skin induration are few or widespread. Linear scleroderma may occur on the limbs. A variant affecting the face and scalp (midline or parasagittal) is termed "en coup de sabre" in an apparent reference to a sword's stroke.

Generalized SSc may be limited cutaneous (lcSSc) or diffuse cutaneous (dcSSc), as depicted in Table 16.1). In the former, skin involvement is confined to the face and distal to elbows/knees. In contrast, skin involvement proximal to elbows/knees and truncal involvement is seen in diffuse cutaneous SSc. CREST syndrome is a variant of limited cutaneous SSc with Calcinosis, Raynaud's phenomenon, Esophageal dysmotility, Sclerodactyly, and Telangiectasias. This term is rarely used these days because of its inability to describe the disease burden in this group of patients fully. Some patients do not show skin thickening but have typical autoantibodies and internal organ involvement (sine scleroderma). Systemic sclerosis may exist along with other rheumatic diseases like rheumatoid arthritis, myositis, and SLE (overlap syndrome).

R. Handa, *Clinical Rheumatology*, https://doi.org/10.1007/978-981-33-4885-1_16

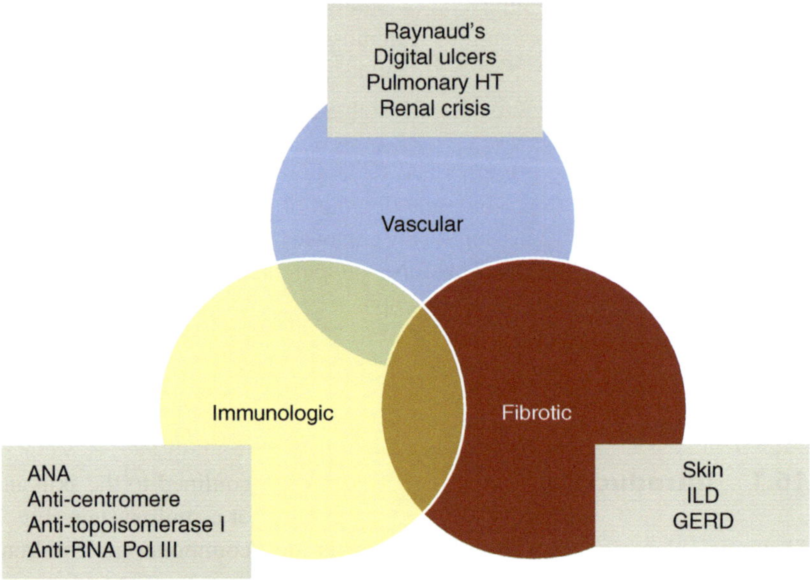

Fig. 16.1 Pathomechanistic Troika of SSc and organs affected. *ILD* interstitial lung disease, *GERD* gastroesophageal reflux disease, *HT* hypertension

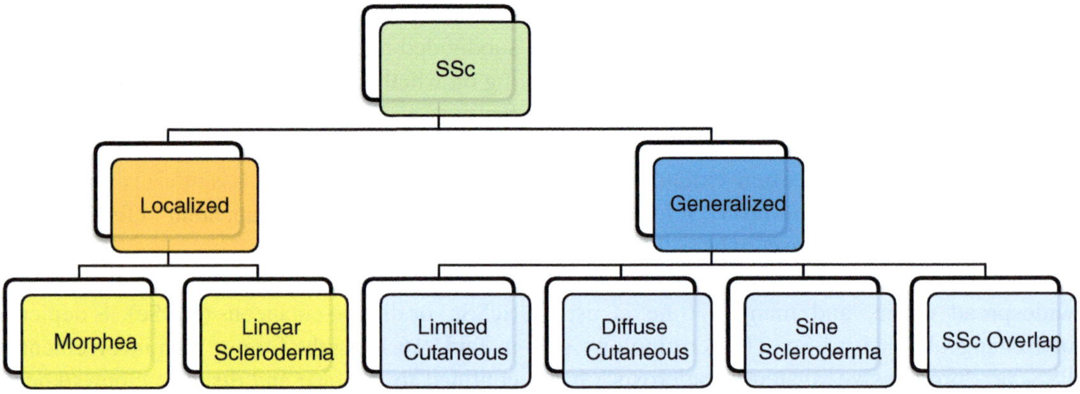

Fig. 16.2 Spectrum of systemic sclerosis

16.3 Clinical Features and Investigations

Localized scleroderma may take the form of morphea or linear scleroderma (Figs. 16.3 and 16.4). In contradistinction to generalized SSc, Raynaud's phenomenon and internal organ involvement are not encountered. However, the rate of progression and extent of damage is variable in different patients, and some overlap may exist between localized scleroderma and generalized SSc. The skin lesions in morphea are more common on the trunk and legs as compared to acral parts. The lesions of linear scleroderma are dermatomal in distribution, can cross joint lines, and may result in disfiguring growth defects.

Most patients with generalized SSc present with Raynaud's phenomenon. Raynaud's phenomenon (RP) is an episodic digital ischemia provoked by exposure to cold. This history may not be forthcoming in patients residing in parts of the country where the climate is tropical and warm throughout the year. RP can be precipitated by asking the patient to immerse hands in a bowl

Table 16.1 Classification of systemic sclerosis

Type	Phenotype	Autoantibodies
Limited cutaneous	Skin thickening distal to elbows and knees. May involve face and neck. Trunk spared. Calcinosis and telangiectasia commoner than diffuse cutaneous. Raynaud's phenomenon predates skin involvement by several years. Renal involvement, pulmonary fibrosis rare. Isolated pulmonary arterial hypertension may occur after several years of disease onset.	Anticentromere antibodies in 60–80% of patients
Diffuse cutaneous	Skin thickening extends proximally to elbows and knees. Truncal involvement present. Raynaud's phenomenon accompanies or comes up within a year of onset of skin changes. Pulmonary, renal, gastrointestinal involvement common.	Antitopoisomerase antibodies (Scl-70) in 40–45% patients Anti-RNA polymerase III in 4–25% of patients
Systemic sclerosis sine scleroderma	No skin thickening but typical visceral organ involvement. Serologic abnormalities, even in the absence of skin involvement.	ANA, antitopoisomerase antibodies (Scl-70) or anticentromere antibodies[a]
Systemic sclerosis Overlap	Skin thickening and other systemic sclerosis features combined with another autoimmune rheumatic disease like lupus, rheumatoid, or myositis	Antibodies to u1RNP and PM-Scl (variable frequency)

[a]All these patients exhibit scleroderma-related antibodies in varying combinations. The diagnosis cannot be entertained in absence of serologic evidence of SSc

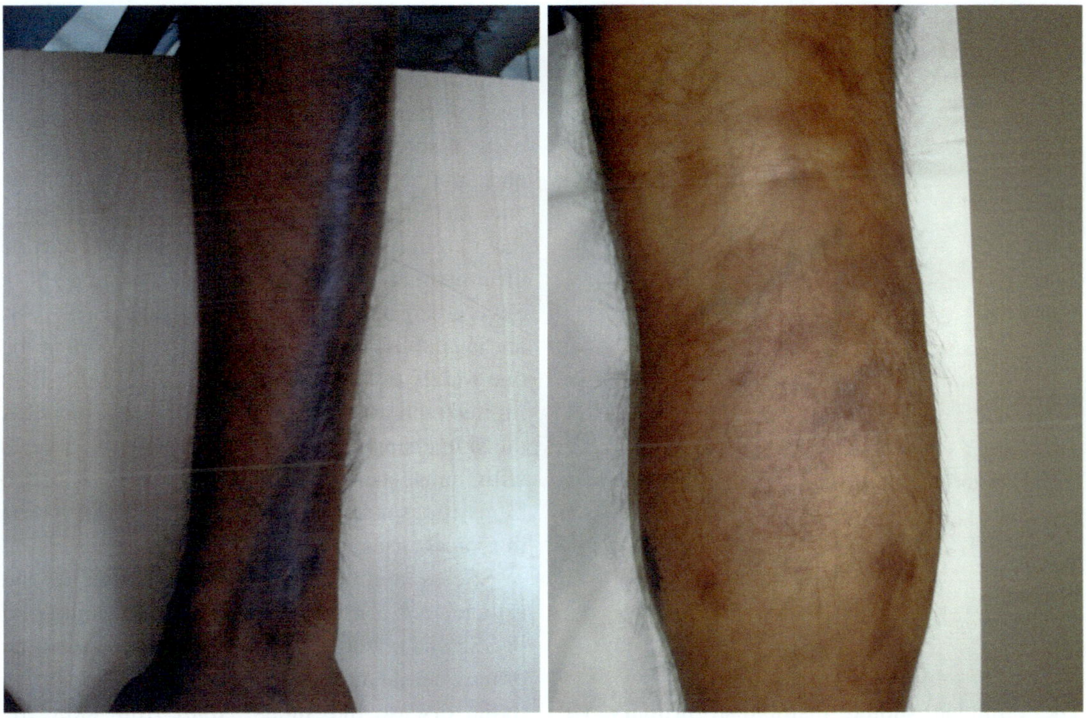

Fig. 16.3 Morphea

of cold water. There are three classical stages of RP: pallor, cyanosis, and suffusion. The pallor results from arterial vasospasm, the cyanosis is due to deoxygenation of static venous blood, and the redness is because of reactive hyperemia on the return of blood flow. Some patients have associated pain or tingling. Not all three phases may be apparent, and not all digits may be affected.

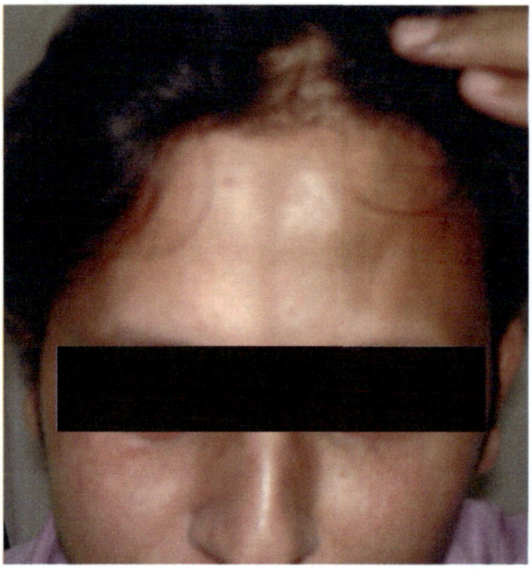

Fig. 16.4 Linear scleroderma

Table 16.2 Differentiating primary Raynaud's phenomenon from secondary Raynaud's

	Primary Raynaud's (Raynaud's disease)	Secondary Raynaud's
Age at onset	Younger age	Older age (exception juvenile systemic sclerosis)
Symmetry	Symmetric	Maybe asymmetric
Severity	Mild	May be severe
Tissue loss	Nil	Finger pits, pulp loss, digital ulcers, gangrene
Family history	Usually positive	Usually negative
Antinuclear antibody	Absent	Present
Nail fold capillaroscopy	Normal	Abnormal

The clinician should distinguish primary RP (Raynaud's disease) from RP secondary to SSc. Factors in favor of secondary Raynaud's are the onset of RP in young children or after the age of 45 years, particularly intense attacks, digital ulceration, and asymmetric involvement of digits (Table 16.2). Investigations helpful in this differentiation include antinuclear antibodies (ANA) and nail fold capillaroscopy. The latter may show capillary proliferation, drop out, or hemorrhages (Fig. 16.5). The presence of ANA and nail fold capillary abnormalities suggests secondary RP. Raynaud's may go unnoticed or unreported by the patient for years.

Skin changes commonly bring the patient to medical attention in SSc. These include skin tightening, change in color of skin (hyperpigmentation or depigmentation), or difficulty in mouth opening. In the early stage, the patients may complain of puffiness of the hands and feet. This edematous phase lasts a few weeks or months. Later, the skin slowly becomes thickened and tethered to underlying structures. In fingers, this is termed sclerodactyly. The skin changes in SSc extend proximal to the metacarpophalangeal joints. In advanced disease, the taut hidebound skin makes diagnosis easy. Other dermatologic features include ulcers over bony prominences, extrusion of calcium from ulcers, flexion contractures, stretched, shiny skin with loss of creases, pitting scars and loss of volar pads, resorption of digits, puckering of mouth, and "nutmeg" or "salt and pepper" like appearance due to depigmentation and sparing of pigment around hair follicles. Telangiectasia may be prominent in some patients (Figs. 16.6 and 16.7). Several scoring systems to quantify skin sclerosis are available. Modified Rodnan skin score is the one widely used. Skin changes progress slowly in limited cutaneous SSc. In diffuse cutaneous SSc, the skin changes progress rapidly over 3–5 years with subsequent softening and atrophy. Skin biopsy does not add much diagnostic information in typical cases.

SSc is a multisystem disease. Fatigue and asthenia are common. However, fever is unusual in SSc and should prompt a search for infection, or may herald an overlap with another connective tissue disease like lupus. Apart from skin, the brunt is borne by the gastrointestinal tract, kidneys, lungs, and heart. Gastrointestinal tract involvement is common and manifests as difficulty in swallowing solids due to esophageal dysmotility and gastroesophageal reflux disease (GERD). The latter may present with a cough. Small bowel disease hypomotility can lead to

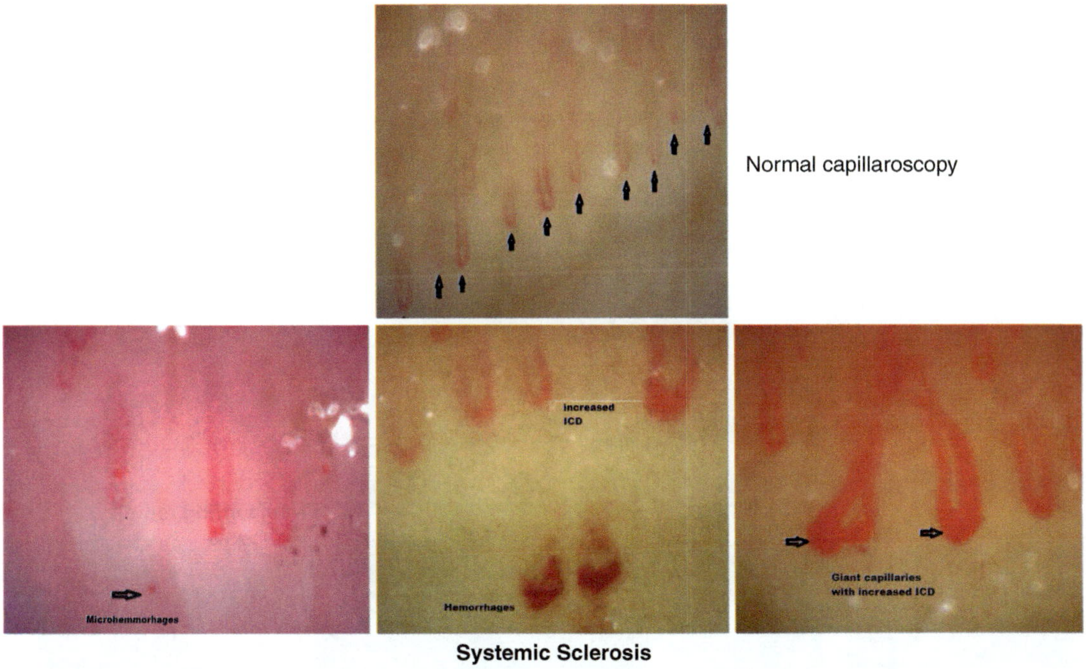

Fig. 16.5 Nailfold capillaroscopy in SSc

malabsorption, small intestinal bacterial overgrowth (SIBO), and pseudo-obstruction. Constipation often results from recto-sigmoid hypomotility.

Pulmonary disease is a significant contributor to mortality (Fig. 16.8). The common presenting symptoms are breathlessness, especially on exertion and dry cough. Cough, a common problem in SSc, can be due to multiple factors like GERD, interstitial lung disease (ILD), pulmonary hypertension, or angiotensin-converting enzyme (ACE inhibitors). Aspiration pneumonitis can contribute to pulmonary symptoms. Hemoptysis is rare in SSc unless there is a superadded infection. Chest auscultation may be unremarkable or show features of ILD by way of bilateral basal velcro crepitations. Radiographs in the early stage may be normal and are an insensitive method of detecting early lung disease. Later, these reveal reticulonodular shadowing more pronounced at the lung bases (Fig. 16.9). High-resolution computerized tomography (HRCT) of the chest is the investigative modality of choice to detect early ILD. As many as 50% of patients with dcSSc and 25% of patients with lcSSc develop ILD. The presence of antitopoisomerase antibodies (Scl-70) is strongly associated with the development of ILD. The HRCT chest shows different patterns which often give a clue to the histologic type. Nonspecific interstitial pneumonitis (NSIP) pattern is the commonest followed by usual interstitial pneumonitis (UIP). The NSIP pattern has a more favorable outcome compared with the UIP pattern. HRCT findings of NSIP include ground-glass opacities in a peripheral distribution and traction bronchiectasis. The involvement tends to be subpleural and symmetrical with an apico-basal gradient. Predominant or exclusive upper lobe involvement or purely unilateral disease makes the diagnosis of NSIP less likely. Honeycombing is rare with NSIP. UIP shows bibasilar reticular opacities associated with traction bronchiectasis and the development of honeycombing. Volume loss is seen in advanced disease. The extent of fibrosis on HRCT is used to stage SSc-ILD (limited disease is <20% while extensive disease is >20%).

Pulmonary function test (PFT) abnormalities show a restrictive pattern and may precede radiographic changes. The key points are tabu-

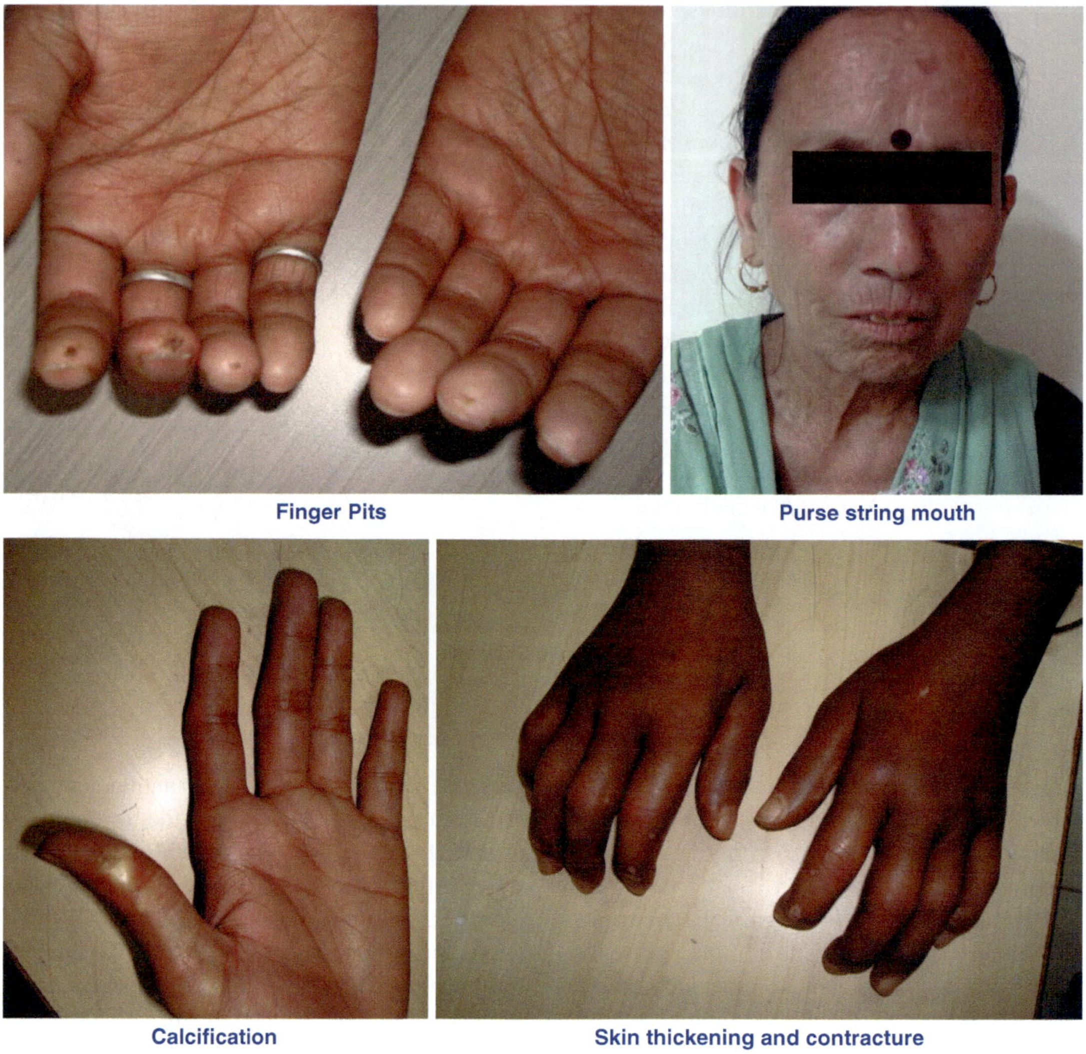

Fig. 16.6 Skin manifestations of SSc

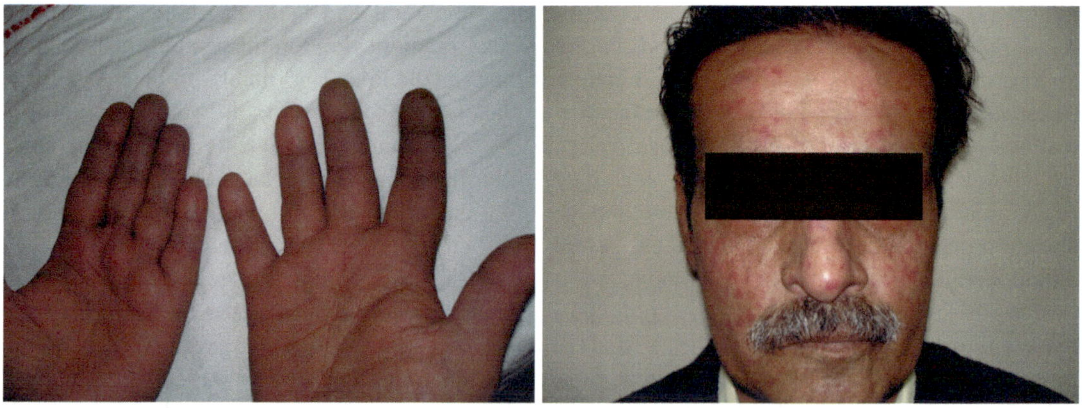

Fig. 16.7 Telangiectasia in SSc

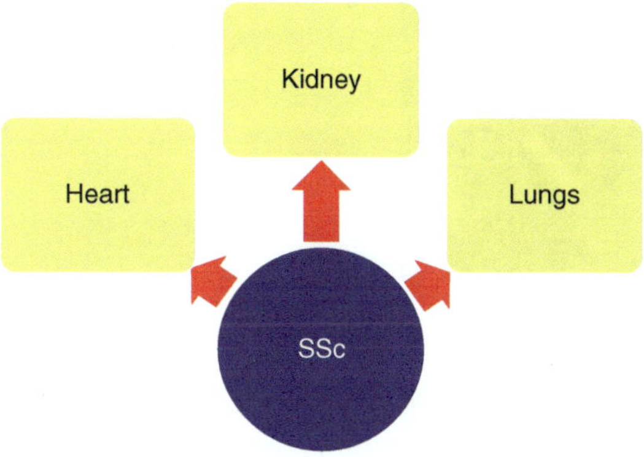

Fig. 16.8 Organs influencing prognosis and outcome in SSc

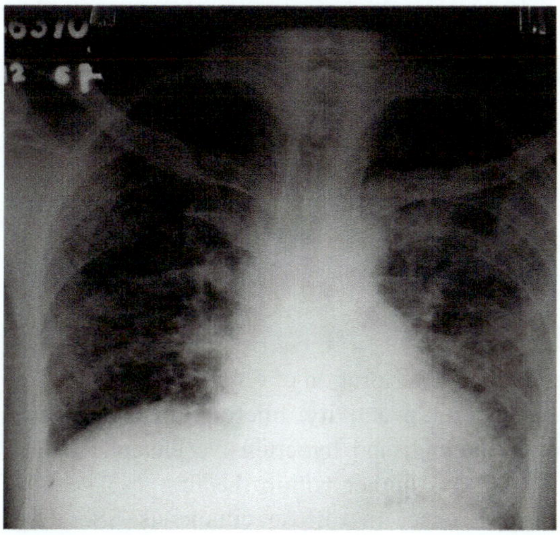

Fig. 16.9 Interstitial lung disease in SSc

> **Box 16.1 Pulmonary Function Testing (PFT) in SSc**
>
> - Patient cooperation is essential in the proper performance of PFT.
> - Spirometry alone is insufficient in the workup of patients with ILD. A full PFT study comprising spirometry, lung volumes, and diffusion capacity is required.
> - Spirometry reveals a reduction of the forced expiratory volume in one second (FEV_1) and forced vital capacity (FVC). The FEV_1/FVC ratio is normal suggesting a restrictive defect.
> - Lung volumes reveal a reduction in total lung capacity (TLC), functional residual capacity (FRC), and residual volume (RV).
> - Diffusion capacity—The single-breath diffusion capacity for carbon monoxide (DLCO) is a sensitive screening test for ILD. Reduction in DLCO is the earliest abnormality in patients with SSc. Apart from ILD, reduced DLCO may be seen in pulmonary hypertension, smokers, thromboembolic disease.
> - Minor alterations in PFT are not uncommon. In significant disease, the values are usually <70% of predicted.
> - FVC and DLCO go hand in hand in pulmonary fibrosis. In pulmonary hypertension, there is a disproportionately greater or isolated decline in DLCO. The ratio of FVC%/DLCO% is useful in the differential diagnosis.
> - PFT should be obtained every 6 months in diffuse SSc for 3 years and thereafter every year. Sicker patients may need more frequent monitoring.

lated in Box 16.1. The 6-min walk test (6MWT) is widely used as a measure of exercise performance to determine the distance walked (meters) and the degree of oxygen desaturation. Despite widespread usage, the utility in SSc is limited as the distance covered does not discriminate well between patients with and without lung involvement due to musculoskeletal and peripheral vascular problems common in SSc.

Some patients may have minimal or no skin involvement and present with ILD as the predominant or only manifestation. Investigations may throw up the characteristic antibodies and/or capillaroscopic features of SSc. Such a phenotype is variously labeled as SSc sine scleroderma, Lung dominant Connective Tissue Disease, or Interstitial Pneumonia with Autoimmune Features (IPAF).

Pulmonary arterial hypertension (PAH), another important contributor to mortality, often

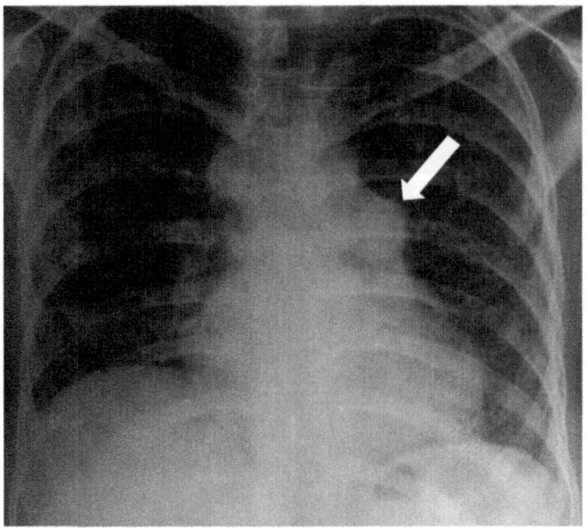

Fig. 16.10 Pulmonary hypertension and interstitial lung disease in long standing SSc

goes unrecognized and undertreated. It is seen in 10–15% of patients, especially those with long-standing lcSSc. It can also occur in dcSSc. Symptoms include dyspnea, tiredness, palpitations, chest pain, syncope, and cough. There may be no warning symptoms. PAH may be isolated or occur in conjunction with ILD (Fig. 16.10). The outcome in SSc-associated PAH is said to be worse than isolated idiopathic PAH. All patients should be routinely screened for PAH by Doppler echocardiography yearly. Doppler echo provides pulmonary artery systolic pressure (PASP) or the tricuspid regurgitant jet velocity (TRV), where PASP = 4 $(TRV)^2$. However, tricuspid regurgitation is absent in about 15–20% of patients, and PAH may be missed in up to 30% of cases. Right heart catheterization is the gold standard for evaluating PAH. N-terminal pro Brain Natriuretic Peptide (NT-proBNP) levels are also employed as a biomarker for PAH in SSc. It is to be noted that myocardial dysfunction in SSc may also contribute to the elevation of BNP. Factors suggesting PAH include RV systolic pressure >40 mm Hg (RVSP is the same as PA systolic pressure in the absence of PA obstruction); Mean PA pressure >25 mm Hg at rest or >30 mm Hg with exercise; DLCO <60% predicted; FVC/DLCO ratio >1.4; BNP >140 pg/ml; TRV >2.9 m/s (Table 16.3).

Renal disease is currently not a significant cause of mortality due to the use of ACE inhibitors. Features of renal crisis include abrupt onset of hypertension, hypertensive retinopathy >grade III, rapid deterioration of renal function, elevated plasma renin activity, microangiopathic hemolytic anemia, and hypertensive encephalopathy. The risk is higher within the first 2–3 years of disease onset in diffuse cutaneous SSc. High doses of prednisolone can precipitate a renal crisis. Nearly 10% of patients have a normotensive renal crisis. Scleroderma renal crisis is rarely encountered even in major centers in India. Whether this reflects an ethnic difference is not known? Proliferative glomerulonephritis and interstitial nephritis are uncommon in SSc.

Table 16.3 PFT abnormalities in pulmonary hypertension and pulmonary fibrosis

	Pulmonary hypertension	Pulmonary fibrosis	Mixed picture
DLCO	Reduced	Reduced	Reduced
FVC	Normal	Reduced	Reduced
FVC/DLCO ratio	>1.4	<1.4	1.4–1.8

Other clinical features of SSc include arthritis, which may be similar to rheumatoid arthritis. Distal interphalangeal joints can be affected. Acro-osteolysis may be apparent on radiographs in longstanding disease (Fig. 16.11). Tendon friction rubs may be palpable in some patients with diffuse cutaneous SSc.

Immunologic abnormalities in SSc include the presence of autoantibodies. ANA is detected in >95% of patients with SSc (Table 16.4). Specific antinuclear antibodies in SSc are antitopoisomerase 1 (earlier called anti-Scl 70) antibodies, anticentromere antibodies, and anti-RNA polymerase III antibodies. These antibodies have very high specificity but modest sensitivity. Also, these autoantibodies are nearly always mutually exclusive. It is extremely rare to find them together in the same patient. Antibodies to RNA polymerase III connote rapidly progressive skin involvement as well as increased risk for renal crisis. Nearly one-fourth of the patients exhibit rheumatoid factor. Overlap patients may show anti-PM-Scl and anti-u1RNP.

The differential diagnosis of SSc includes toxic oil syndrome, bleomycin-induced fibrosis, scleromyxedema, scleredema adultorum of Buschke, Type 1 diabetes mellitus, and amyloidosis. The hand and feet are usually spared in scleredema. Careful attention to clinical detail, including history and relevant investigations, facilitates differential diagnosis in most instances.

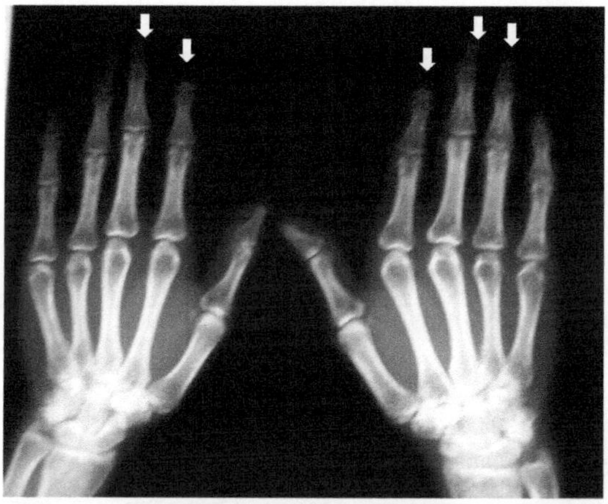

Fig. 16.11 Acro-osteolysis

16.4 Treatment

Despite major advances in the treatment of renal crisis, PAH, GERD, etc., SSc can be a difficult disease to treat because of the nonavailability of real disease-modifying drugs. Physical measures like protection against cold and the use of gloves/socks etc. may be sufficient to treat Raynaud's in limited cutaneous SSc. Drugs that potentiate or cause vasoconstriction like clonidine, beta-blockers, ergot derivatives, etc. should be avoided. Smokers should be encouraged to give up tobacco. Topical nitroglycerin may help. The mainstay of drug treatment for Raynaud's phenomenon is calcium channel blockers like nifedipine and amlodipine. Nifedipine dose may range from 30 to 90 mg/day according to tolerance, while amlodipine doses range from 5 to 20 mg/day. Low doses are employed, to begin with, and then up titrated according to response and blood pressure. Practical problems encountered include worsening of GERD, fall in blood pressure, headache, or pedal edema. Alternative agents include the phosphodiesterase type 5 (PDE) inhibitors like sildenafil, tadalafil, or vardenafil. Other agents that help include alpha-adrenergic blockers like prazosin, ACE inhibitors like captopril, enalapril, etc., angiotensin receptor blockers like losartan and endothelin receptor antagonists like bosentan. Fluoxetine, a selective

Table 16.4 Autoantibodies in systemic sclerosis

Antibody	ANA pattern on immunoflorescence	Frequency
ANA	Depends on the specific ANA present	>95%
Anticentromere	Centromere	60–80% of patients with limited cutaneous SSc and in <4–5% of patients with diffuse cutaneous SSc
Antitopoisomerase I (Scl 70)	Speckled	40–45% of patients with diffuse cutaneous SSc and in <10% of patients with limited cutaneous SSc
Anti-RNA Pol III	Fine speckled nucleolar	4–20% of patients with diffuse cutaneous SSc
Anti-u1RNP	Speckled	5–10% of patients with limited cutaneous SSc. Also present in SSc overlap
Anti-PM-Scl	Nucleolar	Frequency variable. Present in SSc overlap

ANA antinuclear antibody

serotonin reuptake inhibitor, and pentoxifylline have also been tried.

Digital ulcers are treated with vasodilators, dressings, topical or oral antibiotics if an infection is present, and analgesics in case of pain. Pentoxifylline and cilostazol are often tried with disappointing results. Severe acute digital ischemia or impending gangrene are medical emergencies requiring hospitalization and prostaglandin infusion through an infusion pump. Iloprost (a prostacyclin analog) is used in doses ranging from 0.5 to 2.0 ng/kg/min over 6 h for 3–7 days. The ampoule contains 50 μg in 0.5 ml and is not easily available in India. Alprostadil injection (500 μg in 1 ml) is available in India. The dose varies from 6 to 10 ng/kg/min and has to be individualized and carefully monitored. Sympathectomy is reserved for severe, refractory cases. There is no strong evidence to support low-dose aspirin or long-term anticoagulation in patients with digital ischemia. Digital ulcers can prove quite difficult to treat.

Morphea lesions are managed with topical medications (steroids or tacrolimus) or phototherapy. Systemic treatment with methotrexate and steroids is used for generalized progressive morphea. Systemic treatment is best withheld in limited, nonprogressive disease. Skin manifestations in lcSSc may be managed by topical emollients like vaseline for symptomatic relief. In dcSSc, low-dose corticosteroids (10 mg prednisolone daily or less) are prescribed for the early edematous phase of skin disease. In general, since progression is rapid in early disease, treatment requirements may be more in the initial 3–4 years. The treatment of skin disease also takes into account other organ involvement (Fig. 16.12). Methotrexate (15–25 mg/week) and mycophenolate mofetil (MMF) (2–3 g/day) are employed. For patients with significant arthritis or myositis, methotrexate is preferred. With ILD accompanying skin involvement, MMF is preferred. Cyclophosphamide is reserved for progressive skin disease refractory to MTX or MMF, or very severe rapidly progressive distressing skin thickening. IVIG and rituximab are used as salvage regimens. Results with antifibrotic agents like D-penicillamine, colchicine, tocopherol, human relaxin have been disappointing. Pruritus requires antihistamines. The treatment of calcinosis is frustrating. Drugs and procedures like

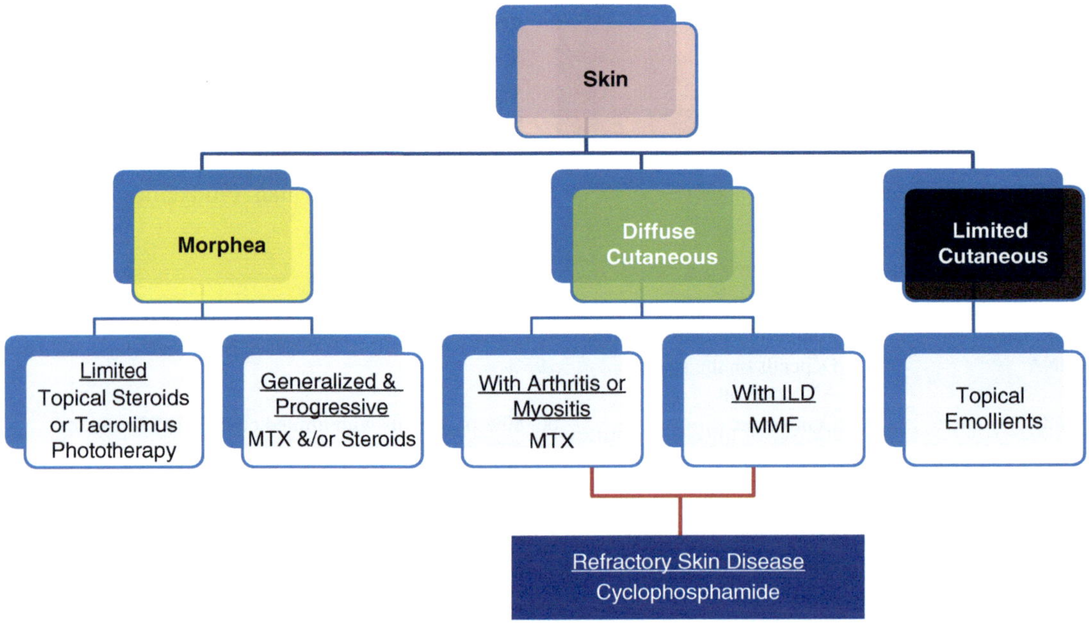

Fig. 16.12 Treatment of skin disease in SSc

warfarin, colchicine, probenecid, bisphosphonates, diltiazem, minocycline, aluminum hydroxide, surgical extirpation, and carbon dioxide lasers have been used for calcinosis with little success.

Proton pump inhibitors (PPI) like omeprazole, pantoprazole are employed to treat GERD. Difficult disease may require twice-daily PPI therapy or an H2 receptor antagonist. Prokinetics like domperidone, mosapride, itopride are used to treat esophageal dysmotility. Refractory disease is better treated by short-acting formulation before each meal rather than extended-release preparations used once a day. The mainstay of treatment of SIBO is antibiotic therapy.

Many patients with SSc-ILD have minimal symptoms with stable or slowly progressive disease. The decision to institute treatment has to balance treatment efficacy, which at best is modest, and treatment side effects, which at worst can be considerable. Table 16.5 gives a general idea of who should be treated. This is an indicative listing and by no means meant to be a substitute for physician judgment. Asymptomatic patients with long disease duration and only PFT abnormalities that remain stable may need observation without intervention. Most guidelines recommend mycophenolate mofetil (MMF) as the first choice (Fig. 16.13). The target dose of MMF is between 2 and 3 g/day in two divided doses. PPIs interfere with MMF absorption and should be spaced at least 2 h from MMF. Many experts prefer MMF over cyclophosphamide (CYC) because of the concern of side effects. CYC can be given as daily oral (2 mg/kg/day) dose or monthly intravenous pulses (15 mg/kg/month or 0.6 g/m^2/month). Intravenous pulses (15 mg/kg) once a month for 6 months are used more often

Table 16.5 Identifying patients who need treatment for SSc-ILD

Recent disease	Symptomatic patients with limited or diffuse SSc within 4–6 years of disease onset
Progressive disease	Progressive decline in FVC or DLCO by ≥10% in the preceding 6–12 months
Significant disease	FVC% predicted ≤70% at the time of presentation
Extensive disease	HRCT showing fibrosis >20% of the lung
Clinical decision	Patients who are symptomatic and who in physician judgment have progressive disease

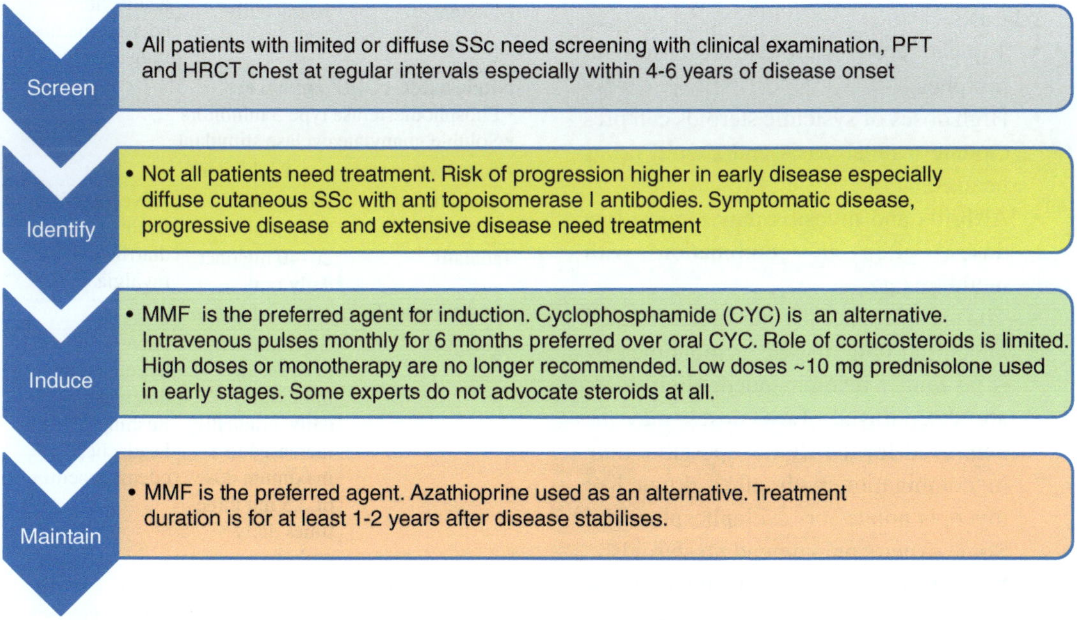

Fig. 16.13 Approach to SSc-ILD

than oral cyclophosphamide, again to minimize side effects with oral cyclophosphamide. Azathioprine is an alternative immunosuppressive agent in patients who do not tolerate MMF or cyclophosphamide. Methotrexate is usually not used to treat SSc-ILD. Pirfenidone is thought not to be of major use. There is a growing tendency to use minimal steroids (<10 mg prednisolone daily) or no steroids. High-dose steroids are actively discouraged. Steroid monotherapy is also discouraged (Box 16.2). Nintedanib is added to the treatment in those patients where ILD is progressing despite MMF or CYC. Occasionally it is used as monotherapy in patients intolerant to MMF and CYC. The usual dose of nintedanib is 150 mg twice daily. Diarrhea is the commonest adverse effect. There is no benefit to skin thickening. Rituximab is also used as a second-line agent to treat SSc-ILD. The optimal duration of treatment of SSc-ILD is unknown but extends to at least 1–2 years after attaining stability. The prognosis in SSc-associated ILD is better than idiopathic interstitial fibrosis. Lung transplantation can be considered in refractory disease.

Box 16.2 Corticosteroids in Systemic sclerosis

- Topical corticosteroids are used in morphea.
- High doses of systemic steroids can precipitate a renal crisis and should never be used.
- Arthritis and myositis may require low doses, often in combination with methotrexate.
- The use of corticosteroids in SSc-related interstitial lung disease as monotherapy is no longer recommended. High doses are discouraged. Low doses may be employed for the shortest possible time in combination with other drugs like mycophenolate or cyclophosphamide. Some experts recommend no steroids.
- Steroids have no role in the treatment of SSc related pulmonary hypertension.

PAH is another critical determinant of outcome in SSc. The severity of PAH does not parallel the severity of skin disease or activity of SSc. Corticosteroids, immunosuppressives, and anticoagulants have virtually no role in the treatment of SSc PAH. This is different from SLE, where experts recommend a trial of steroids and immunosuppressives for pulmonary hypertension. PAH treatments target three signaling pathways: the prostacyclin pathway, the nitric oxide pathway, and the endothelin pathway (Table 16.6). The treatment takes into account the WHO class, as outlined in Table 16.7. Patients in WHO functional class I do not require pharmacologic intervention but surveillance. In class II and III, the current consensus is to start treatment with a combination of drugs from two different classes, typically an oral endothelin receptor antagonist and a phosphodiesterase inhibitor like ambrisentan and tadalafil. Patients with WHO functional class IV are given a parenteral prostanoid with an

Table 16.6 Drugs to treat PAH in SSc

Endothelin receptor antagonists		
Bosentan	62.5–125 mg twice daily oral	Adverse effects: dizziness, flushing, upset stomach, headache, edema, anemia, transaminitis
Ambrisentan	5–10 mg daily oral	
Macitentan	10 mg daily oral	
Nitric oxide-cGMP enhancers • Phosphodiesterase type 5 inhibitors • Soluble guanylate cyclase stimulant		
Phosphodiesterase type 5 inhibitors		
Sildenafil	20 mg thrice daily oral	Adverse effects: flushing, diarrhea, myalgia
Tadalafil	20–40 mg once daily oral	
Soluble guanylate cyclase stimulant		
Riociguat	An initial dose of 0.5–1 mg three times daily, gradually increased to a maximum dose of 2.5 mg three times daily oral.	Adverse effects: hypotension, dizziness, flushing, headache, edema, anemia
Others: Prostacyclin pathway agonists like epoprostenol, iloprost, treprostinil, selexipag, etc.		

cGMP cyclic guanosine monophosphate

Table 16.7 World Health Organization (WHO) functional classification for pulmonary hypertension

Class	WHO functional classification
I	Patients with pulmonary hypertension but no limitation of physical activity. Ordinary physical activity does not cause undue fatigue, dyspnea, chest pain, or heart syncope.
II	Patients with pulmonary hypertension resulting in slight limitation of physical activity. Patients are comfortable at rest. Ordinary physical activity results in undue fatigue, dyspnea, chest pain, or heart syncope.
III	Patients with pulmonary hypertension resulting in marked limitation of physical activity. They are comfortable at rest. Less than ordinary physical activity causes undue fatigue, dyspnea, chest pain, or heart syncope.
IV	Patients with pulmonary hypertension resulting in an inability to carry on any physical activity without symptoms. Dyspnea and/or fatigue present even at rest. Symptoms worsen on physical activity.

oral drug. Agents from the same class are usually not combined, e.g., riociguat and PDE5 inhibitors are usually not combined because of fear of hypotension. Lung transplantation is reserved for refractory SSc-PAH.

Scleroderma renal crisis is an emergency. ACE inhibitors like captopril, enalapril are drugs of choice. While controlling blood pressure, care must be taken to prevent hypovolemia due to sudden, marked vasodilatation of the constricted vascular bed, which can compromise renal perfusion. The goal is to bring blood pressure under control within 72 h. Intravenous nitroprusside is used in patients with central nervous system involvement. Dialytic support may be needed. Recovery in renal function can be slow, and improvement has been reported even after 2–3 years. This should be factored in before deciding regarding renal transplantation. Life long ACE therapy is recommended in these patients.

Autologous stem cell transplantation is reserved for selected patients with early, severe, progressive dcSSc who have moderate (but not end-stage) internal organ involvement refractory to standard treatment.

16.5 Course and Prognosis

The course is unpredictable. The prognosis in limited SSc is relatively better than diffuse SSc. The 5- and 10-year survival rates in limited SSc are 90% and 75%, while for diffuse SSc, these are 70% and 55% approximately. Major causes of death include pulmonary fibrosis and pulmonary hypertension.

16.6 Conclusions

Systemic sclerosis is a challenging disorder because of multiple organ involvement in a multitude of ways. Treatment is based on organ involvement and disease activity. PAH and lung fibrosis are the major determinants of outcome.

Suggested Reading

Denton CP, Hughes M, Gak N, Vila J, Buch MH, Chakravarty K, et al. BSR and BHPR guideline for the treatment of systemic sclerosis. Rheumatology (Oxford). 2016;55:1906–10.

Galie N, Humbert M, Vachiery JL, Gibbs S, Lang I, Torbicki A, et al. 2015 ESC/ERS Guidelines for the diagnosis and treatment of pulmonary hypertension: the Joint Task Force for the Diagnosis and Treatment of Pulmonary Hypertension of the European Society of Cardiology (ESC) and the European Respiratory Society (ERS): endorsed by Association for European Paediatric and Congenital Cardiology (AEPC), International Society for Heart and Lung Transplantation (ISHLT). Eur Heart J. 2016;37:67–119.

Hoffmann-Vold AM, Maher TM, George PM, Philpot EE, Ashrafzadeh A, Barake R, et al. The identification and management of interstitial lung disease in systemic sclerosis: evidence-based European consensus statements. Lancet Rheumatol. 2020;2:e71–83.

Kowal-Bielecka O, Fransen J, Avouac J, Becker M, Kulak A, Allanore Y, et al. Update of EULAR recommendations for the treatment of systemic sclerosis. Ann Rheum Dis. 2017;76:1327–39.

Lynch BM, Stern EP, Ong V, Harber M, Burns A, Denton CP. UK Scleroderma Study Group (UKSSG) guidelines on the diagnosis and management of scleroderma renal crisis. Clin Exp Rheumatol. 2016;34(Suppl 100):106–9.

17 Undifferentiated Connective Tissue Disease, Mixed Connective Tissue Disease, and the Overlap Syndromes

17.1 Introduction

Connective tissue diseases (CTDs) are characterized by multisystem involvement, persistent inflammation, and autoantibodies. The clinical features are diverse and, yet, there is unity among diversity, signifying that the concept of CTD remains valid more than 70 years after it was initially mooted. Clinical features common to these immunoinflammatory conditions include arthritis, rash, Raynaud's phenomenon, serositis, nephritis, myocarditis, etc. The ethos behind this term was to highlight the overlapping clinical features of these diverse illnesses and not evoke a single nosological entity with several different manifestations, e.g., lupus, scleroderma, etc. Unfortunately, many clinicians find the nosologic conundrum baffling and, unable to appreciate the subtle nuances, use the term undifferentiated CTD or mixed CTD loosely, vaguely, or even interchangeably. This chapter briefly explains the concept of undifferentiated CTD (UCTD), mixed CTD (MCTD), and the overlap syndromes.

17.2 Nomenclature (UCTD or MCTD or Overlap Syndrome)

The CTDs may present with signs and symptoms that allow categorization into a defined disease entity like systemic lupus erythematosus (SLE) or systemic sclerosis (SSc) or Sjogren's syndrome from the word go. However, on several occasions, the clinical features may suggest a CTD but defy categorization into any defined entity. The term undifferentiated connective tissue disease (UCTD) is used in such a situation. The term *forme fruste* (French, "crude, or unfinished, form") is applied to an atypical or attenuated manifestation of a disease or syndrome, with the implications of incompleteness, partial presence, or aborted state. The concept of UCTD is something similar. The literature is also replete with a plethora of terms: lupus-like, lupus variant, borderline SLE, latent, incipient, incomplete, or possible lupus. The UCTDs, over a period of time, may evolve into a defined syndrome or stay undifferentiated or disappear (Fig. 17.1). This usually happens in the first few years of disease onset.

UCTD is a label that can be applied only after exercising due diligence. Antinuclear antibody (ANA) is a very sensitive test and should be ordered only if the pre-test probability of CTD is high. Indiscriminate ANA testing in every patient with vague rheumatic complaints is likely to lead to the erroneous label of UCTD (false-positive UCTDs). To obviate this problem, criteria have been proposed for UCTD:

1. Signs and symptoms suggestive of a CTD, but not fulfilling criteria for a defined CTD
2. Positive ANA on two separate measurements
3. Disease duration of at least 3 years

R. Handa, *Clinical Rheumatology*, https://doi.org/10.1007/978-981-33-4885-1_17

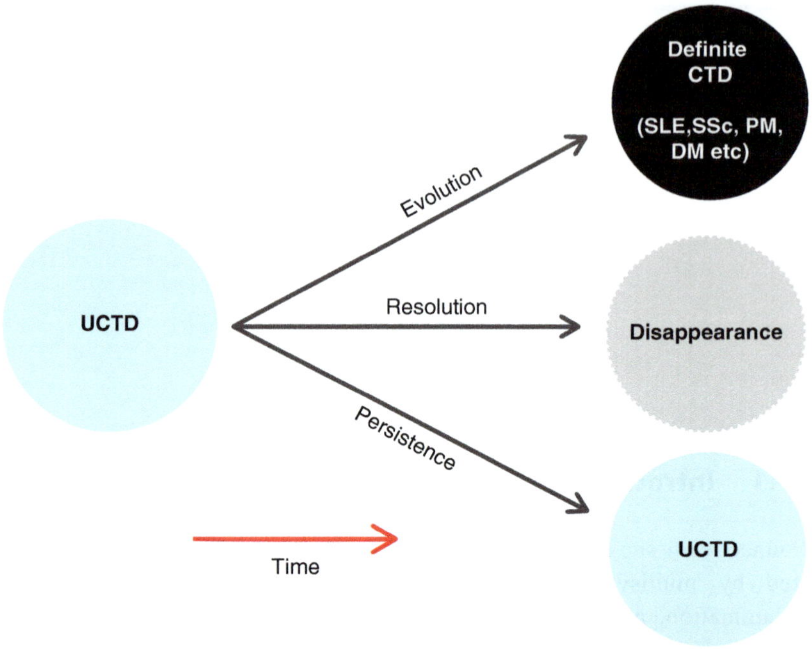

Fig. 17.1 Outcome of undifferentiated connective tissue diseases (UCTD). *CTD* connective tissue disease, *SLE* systemic lupus erythematosus, *SSc* systemic sclerosis, *PM* polymyositis, *DM* dermatomyositis

Nearly 25% of patients with systemic rheumatic diseases exhibit features of two or more diseases when the term overlap syndrome is used. RA and SLE overlap is not uncommon and is termed "rhupus." The term "sclerodermatomyositis" is used to designate the hybrid of systemic sclerosis and dermatomyositis. The clinical features may develop simultaneously or sequentially. The most well defined of these overlap syndromes is MCTD first enunciated in 1972. MCTD has features of SLE, scleroderma, and polymyositis. The concept of MCTD has evoked much debate, with some authorities questioning the existence of MCTD as a separate disease entity.

MCTD is a term employed for a subset of overlap syndrome characterized by antibodies against ribonucleoproteins (anti-U1snRNP). The defining feature of MCTD is these antibodies, and it needs to be emphasized that MCTD is a label given only when serology demonstrates high titer antibodies against U1snRNP. MCTD is a disease that can be suspected clinically but has to be confirmed serologically. It stands to reason that all patients with MCTD can be included under the broad label of overlap syndrome, but not all patients with overlap syndrome have MCTD (Fig. 17.2). Also, anti U1snRNP are not restricted to MCTD. Patients with SLE, SSc, and myositis may exhibit these antibodies in varying percentages. Several criteria sets have been proposed for MCTD, which only serve to highlight the confusion amongst experts (Tables 17.1 and 17.2).

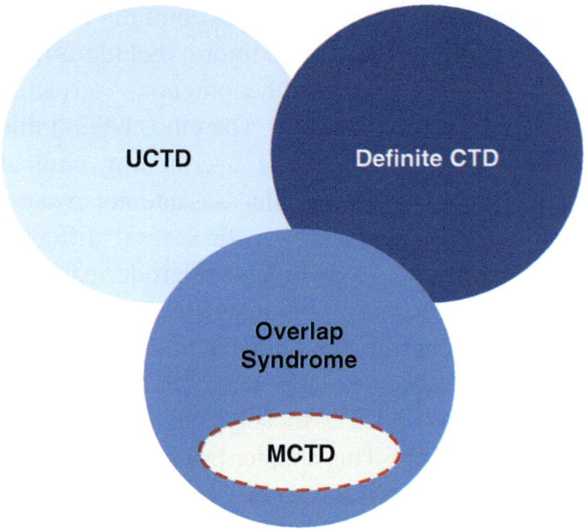

Fig. 17.2 Spectrum of connective tissue diseases

Table 17.1 Alarcon Segovia's criteria for MCTD

(A) Serological criteria
Anti-RNP antibodies with a hemagglutination titer of ≥1:1600
(B) Clinical criteria
1. Swollen hands
2. Synovitis
3. Myositis
4. Raynaud's phenomenon
5. Acrosclerosis

MCTD is present if criterion A is accompanied by three or more clinical criteria—one of which must include synovitis or myositis

Reference: Alarcón-Segovia D, Villarreal M. Classification and diagnostic criteria for mixed connective tissue disease. In: Kasukawa R, Sharp GC, editors. Mixed connective tissue disease and anti-nuclear antibodies. Amsterdam: Elsevier Science Publishers B.V. (Biomedical Division); 1987. pp. 33–40

Table 17.2 Kahn's criteria for MCTD

(A) Serological criteria
High titer anti-RNP corresponding to a speckled ANA of ≥1:1200 titer
(B) Clinical criteria
1. Swollen fingers
2. Synovitis
3. Myositis
4. Raynaud phenomenon

MCTD is present if criterion A is accompanied by the Raynaud's phenomenon and two or more of the three remaining clinical criteria

Reference: Kahn MF, Appelboom T. Syndrome de Sharp. In: Kahn MF, Peltier AP, Mayer O, Piette JC, editors. Les maladies systémiques. 3rd. Paris: Flammarion; 1991. pp. 545–56

MCTD patients start with constitutional features like fatigue, myalgias, arthralgias, and fever. Over a period of time, the typical phenotype with Raynaud phenomenon, hand edema, puffy fingers, and/or prominent synovitis becomes apparent. The initial suggestion was that MCTD follows a benign course. However, this notion was dispelled by subsequent studies, which revealed that only a third of the patients with MCTD had a benign course. One-third of the patients pursued an aggressive course while one-third improved with immunosuppressive therapy that was needed long term.

17.3 Treatment

Hydroxychloroquine, steroids, and methotrexate are employed akin to their usage in RA or SLE. No large trials are available. The treatment has to factor in the individual organ affected in a given patient. Hydroxychloroquine is offered to all patients. Methotrexate is added for arthritis. Corticosteroids help almost all manifestations but should be used sparingly. Nephritis, pulmonary hypertension, etc. if present are treated like in SLE.

17.4 Conclusions

UCTD is a disease entity with clinico-serologic features of an autoimmune rheumatic disease that cannot meet the criteria of a defined CTD. Overlap syndromes are a hybrid of two or more rheumatic diseases. MCTD is a variety of overlap syndrome defined by anti-U1snRNP. Classification criteria are available for MCTD. The delineation of organ involvement in these CTDs is far more important than labels. Clinicians should refrain from floundering in semantic depths or nosologic debates. The focus ought to be on the patient rather than descriptive labels! The dictum in clinical rheumatology is "treat the patient and not to chase the classification criteria."

Suggested Reading

John KJ, Sadiq M, George T, Gunasekaran K, Francis N, Rajadurai E, et al. Clinical and immunological profile of mixed connective tissue disease and a comparison of four diagnostic criteria. Int J Rheumatol. 2020:9692030. https://doi.org/10.1155/2020/9692030.

LeRoy EC, Maricq HR, Kahaleh MB, Bashar Kahaleh M. Undifferentiated connective tissue syndromes. Arthritis Rheum. 1980;23:341–3.

Mosca M, Neri R, Bombardieri S. Undifferentiated connective tissue diseases (UCTD): a review of the literature and a proposal for preliminary classification criteria. Clin Exp Rheumatol. 1999;17:615–20.

18 Antiphospholipid Syndrome

18.1 Introduction

Antiphospholipid syndrome (APS) is a systemic autoimmune disease characterized serologically by antiphospholipid antibodies (aPL) and clinically by recurrent venous or arterial thrombosis and/or late pregnancy loss (Fig. 18.1). APS has emerged as an important hypercoagulable state. The word itself is a misnomer because the antibodies are not against the phospholipids but instead target the plasma proteins which bind to anionic phospholipids. Lupus anticoagulant, a cardinal laboratory feature of APS, is a misleading term as well. Not all patients have lupus. While aPL have been demonstrated in up to one-third of the patients with lupus, less than 10% have the clinical syndrome of APS. Also, in the laboratory, LAs cause prolongation of clotting tests, while the clinical consequence is thrombosis rather than bleeding.

APS may exist in isolation without any definable associated disease (primary APS) or occur in association with SLE or another autoimmune rheumatic disease (secondary APS). As many as 5% of healthy individuals may show transient aPL antibodies giving rise to the thought that a "second hit" is required to incite the pro-thrombotic aPL (Fig. 18.2). This takes the form of risk factors like age, hypertension (HT), diabetes mellitus (DM), obesity, smoking, pregnancy, surgery, etc. which should be sought and addressed while treating APS.

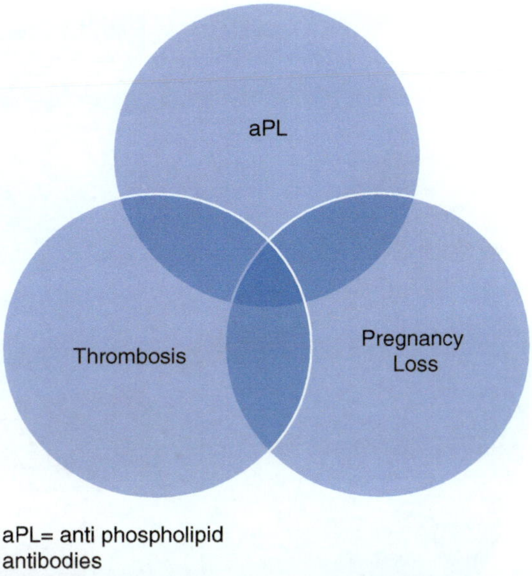

Fig. 18.1 Cardinal features of antiphospholipid syndrome

18.2 Clinical Recognition

The clinical manifestations of APS can be quite protean (Fig. 18.3). A clinician should suspect APS in the following situations:

- Thrombosis at a relatively early age (males <55 years, females <65 years), thrombosis in the absence of known risk factors, or recurrent episodes. This may take the form of deep vein thrombosis (DVT), pulmonary embo-

R. Handa, *Clinical Rheumatology*, https://doi.org/10.1007/978-981-33-4885-1_18

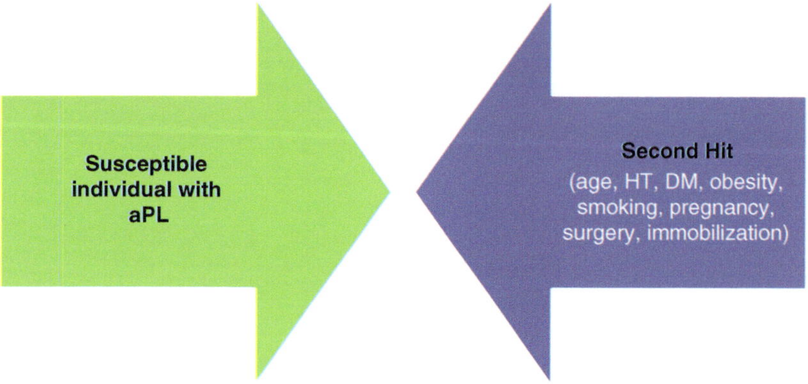

Fig. 18.2 Second hit in APS

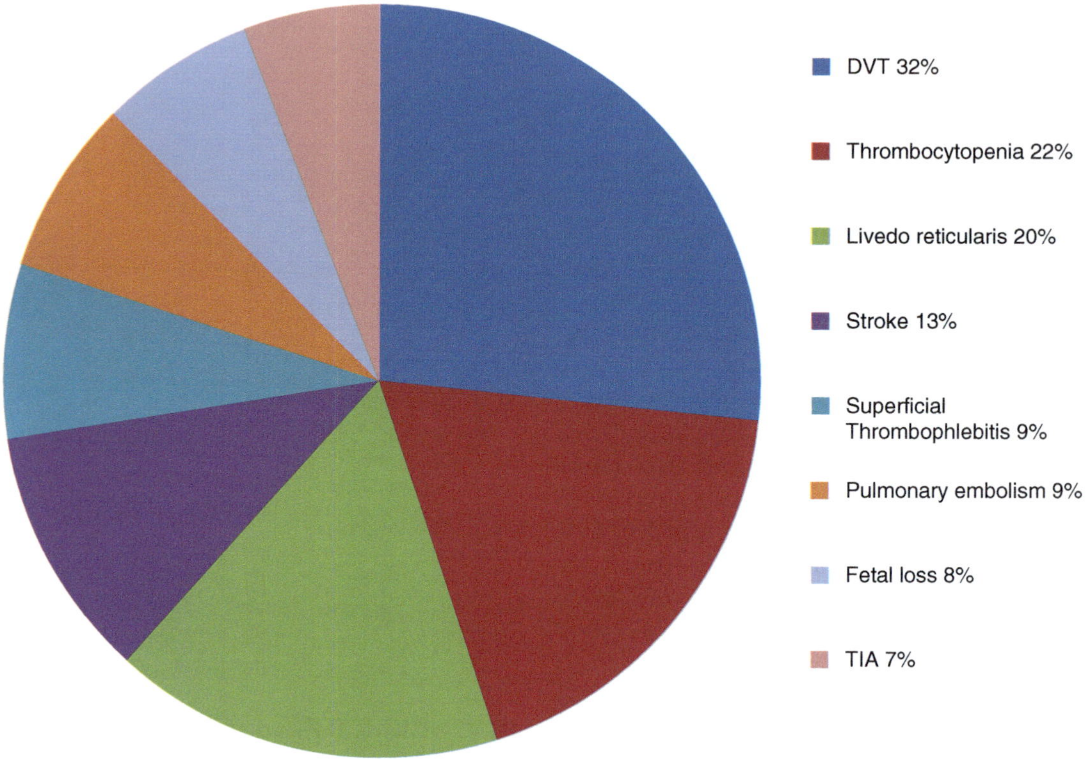

Fig. 18.3 Clinical features of APS in a large series of 1000 patients (820 female, 180 male) (Cervera et al. 2002)

lism (PE), myocardial infarction (MI), transient ischemic attack (TIA), stroke, digital gangrene, etc. (Figs. 18.4, 18.5, 18.6 and 18.7).

- Pregnancy loss (especially late trimester or recurrent) or premature birth.
- Cardiac valvular vegetations.
- Thrombocytopenia or hemolytic anemia.
- Nonthrombotic neurologic symptoms like migraine, chorea, seizures, Guillain–Barré syndrome, or transverse myelitis.
- Unexplained adrenal insufficiency.
- Unexplained osteonecrosis of bone.
- Unexplained nephropathy.

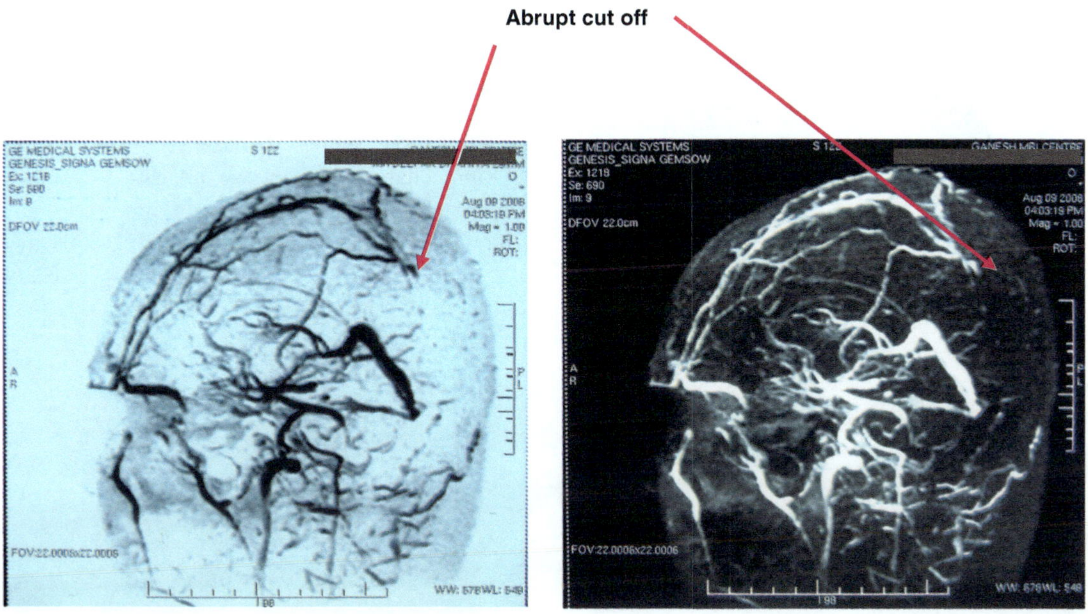

Fig. 18.4 Cerebral venous sinus thrombosis in APS

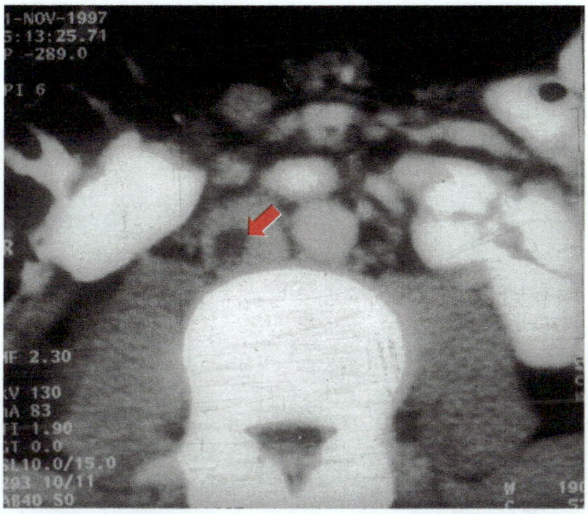

Fig. 18.5 Inferior vena cava thrombosis in APS

- Unexplained pulmonary hypertension.
- Livedo reticularis (Fig. 18.8)—appreciated with difficulty in dark-skinned individuals.

Patients can have vascular thrombosis without pregnancy complications or obstetric manifestations alone or a combination. The co-occurrence of both thrombosis and miscarriages is rare and affects only 2.5–5% of APS pregnancies.

The revised classification criteria for APS put forward in 2006 require at least one clinical and one laboratory criterion (Table 18.1). The clinical criteria comprise vascular thrombosis and pregnancy morbidity. Vascular thrombosis is defined as one or more clinical episodes of arterial, venous, or small-vessel thrombosis in any tissue or organ confirmed by findings from imaging studies, Doppler studies, or histopathology. Pregnancy losses are typically late pregnancy beyond 10 weeks of gestation. Since early pregnancy losses are not uncommon in the general population, APS screening is recommended only if there are three or more consecutive first-trimester abortions (Fig. 18.9). The other setting is one or more premature births of a morphologically healthy neonate at or before 34 weeks' gestation because of severe pre-eclampsia or eclampsia or severe placental insufficiency.

The laboratory criteria require demonstration of aPL with two caveats: levels have to be medium to high, and positivity has to be persistent—demonstrable on a minimum of two occasions at least 12 weeks apart. This is because low level, transient aPL positivity can be triggered by infections like malaria, hepatitis, HIV and by

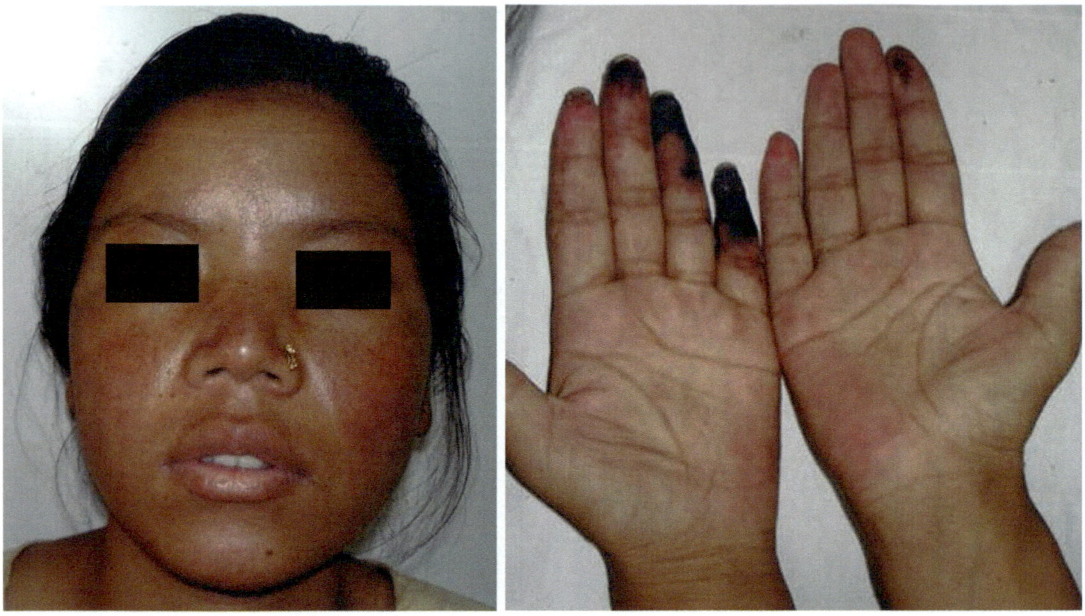

Fig. 18.6 Digital gangrene in a young girl with SLE and APS

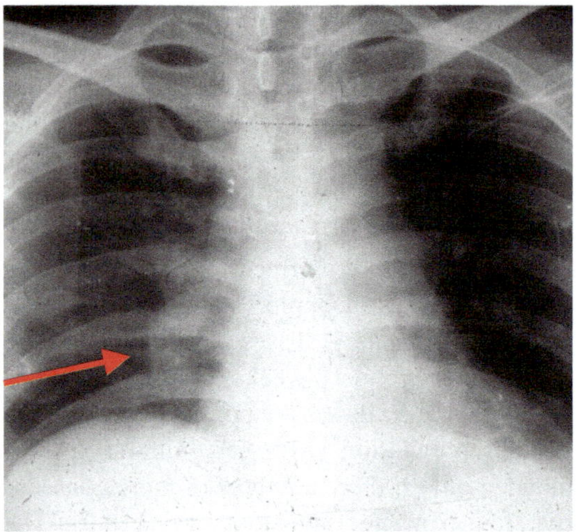

Fig. 18.7 Pulmonary thromboembolism in APS (Note the dilated right descending pulmonary artery with abrupt cut-off)

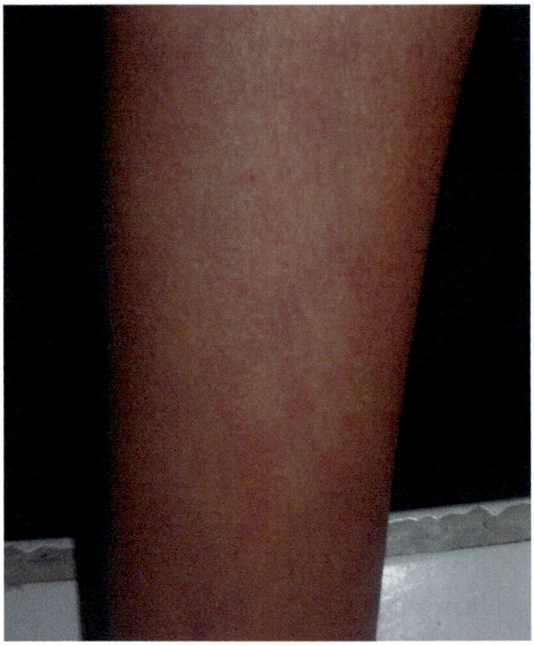

Fig. 18.8 Livedo reticularis on forearm in APS

drugs like procainamide, quinidine, propranolol, hydralazine, phenytoin, etc. APS patients may exhibit a false-positive test result for syphilis because serologic tests for syphilis employ cardiolipin as the dominant antigen.

The aPL antibodies are divided into two categories: criteria and noncriteria (Table 18.2). The former are included in the 2006 criteria and comprise medium to high levels of IgG or IgM anticardiolipin (aCL) or anti-beta-2 glycoprotein I (β-2 GPI) and lupus anticoagulant (LA). It is to be noted that IgA acL and IgA β-2 GPI are not included. Patients can have acL, β-2 GPI, LA in all combinations (single-positive, double-positive, or triple-positive).

A variety of clotting assays like activated partial thromboplastin time (aPTT), kaolin clotting time, and dilute Russell viper venom time (DRVVT) are used to detect LA. The test is done in three stages:

1. Screening tests—prolongation of clotting assay
2. Mixing studies—failure to correct with platelet-poor pooled plasma
3. Neutralization—by addition of phospholipids

Table 18.1 Antiphospholipid syndrome—Sydney Classification Criteria 2006

Clinical criteria
Vascular thrombosis: venous, arterial, or small vessel
Pregnancy morbidity: – three or more consecutive miscarriages (<10 weeks) – one or more fetal deaths (>10 weeks) – one or more premature births (<34 weeks) due to severe preeclampsia or eclampsia or placental insufficiency
Laboratory criteria (on two or more occasions, 12 weeks or more apart)
Anticardiolipin antibody: IgG and/or IgM (medium/high titer; >40 MPL/GPL)
Lupus anticoagulant
Anti-β 2 glycoprotein-I antibody: IgG and/or IgM (medium/high titer; >40 MPL/GPL)

Miyakis S, Lockshin MD, Atsumi T, Branch DW, Brey RL, Cervera R, et al. International consensus statement on an update of the classification criteria for definite anti phospholipid syndrome (APS). J Thromb Haemost 2006;4:295–306

In clotting factor deficiency, the addition of normal plasma corrects the prolonged clotting time. The shortening of the clotting time after the addition of phospholipid is often defined as a ratio (clotting time before the addition of phospholipid to clotting time after the addition of phospholipid). LA is suggested by a ratio greater than 1.3.

The differential diagnosis of APS includes other causes of hypercoagulable state (malignancy, oral pills, hormone replacement therapy, homocysteinemia, antithrombin III deficiency, protein C or S deficiency, factor V Leiden mutation, etc.), atherosclerotic vascular disease, systemic vasculitides, and cholesterol emboli syndrome.

Catastrophic APS (CAPS) is a subset seen in less than 1% of APS patients and is typified by widespread thrombotic disease and multi-organ failure. In CAPS, the thromboses typically involve multiple small blood vessels in various organs rather than a large vessel DVT or stroke. The criteria for CAPS require a history of APS and/or antiphospholipid antibodies (aPL); three or more new organ thromboses

Table 18.2 Antibodies in antiphospholipid syndrome

Criteria	Non-criteria
• LA • acL: IgG and IgM • β2 GP1: IgG and IgM)	• Antiprothrombin ab. • Anti-annexin V ab. • Anti-phosphatidylserine ab. • Antiphosphatidylinositol ab. • Domain specific abs. (D1)

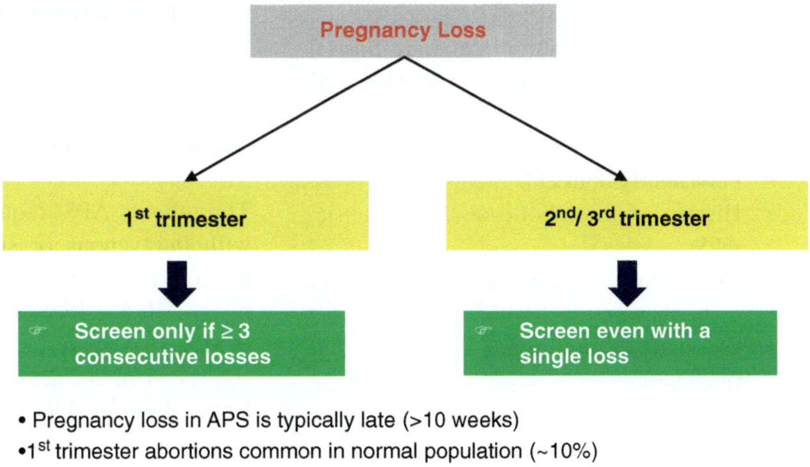

Fig. 18.9 Screening for APS in pregnancy

within a week; biopsy confirmation of a microthrombus and exclusion of other causes of multiple organ thromboses or microthromboses. The differential diagnosis includes disseminated intravascular coagulation (DIC) and thrombotic microangiopathies. The mortality rate in CAPS is very high (~50%).

Patients are risk-stratified according to the number and type of antibodies present. LA confers the strongest risk for thrombosis. The IgG subtype of aPL correlates most strongly with thrombotic events than IgM or IgA. "Triple-positive" patients (LA, anti-β-2 GPI antibodies, aCL antibodies) are at the highest risk for thrombosis or abnormal pregnancy. Scoring systems like the Global Antiphospholipid Syndrome Score (GAPSS) are available.

18.3 Management

It is important to seek and neutralize other risk factors for thrombosis like cigarette smoking, HT, diabetes mellitus, hyperlipidemia, obesity, oral pills, immobilization, etc. Statins are employed for dyslipidemia. The associated autoimmune disease should be treated on its own merit. Hydroxychloroquine is widely used, especially if there is underlying SLE. Prophylaxis is required during surgery or hospitalization. The profile of patients at high and low risk of thrombosis is outlined in Boxes 18.1 and 18.2.

Box 18.1 Patients at high risk of thrombosis

- Multiple aPL positivity (double or triple)
- Lupus anticoagulant
- Persistently high aPL titers
- History of thrombotic and/or obstetric APS
- Coexistence of other autoimmune rheumatic diseases such as SLE
- Presence of traditional cardiovascular risk factors.

Box 18.2 Patients at low risk of thrombosis

- Isolated aCL at low to medium titers, especially if transient
- Isolated anti-β-2 GPI at low to medium titers, especially if transient

18.3.1 Primary Thromboprophylaxis

This refers to the treatment of patients who demonstrate aPL without any clinical thrombotic event. Low-dose aspirin (75–100 mg daily) is employed. However, primary prevention is a controversial area, and current European League Against Rheumatism (EULAR) recommendations (summarized below) leave it to the treating physician's judgment in many circumstances. Primary prevention may be considered in the following situations:

1. In asymptomatic aPL carriers with a high-risk aPL profile with or without traditional risk factors.
2. In patients with SLE and no history of thrombosis or pregnancy complications:
   (A) With a high-risk aPL profile, prophylactic treatment is recommended.
   (B) With a low-risk aPL profile, prophylactic treatment may be considered.
3. In nonpregnant women with a history of obstetric APS only (with or without SLE), prophylactic treatment with low-dose aspirin after an adequate risk/benefit evaluation is recommended.

18.3.2 Treatment of Thrombotic APS

Thrombotic APS requires full anticoagulation with intravenous or subcutaneous heparin followed by warfarin (or other vitamin K antagonists—VKA). Low molecular weight heparin (LMWH) is preferred to unfractionated heparin (UFH). With unfractionated heparin, the prophylactic dose is 5000 units subcutaneous every

12 h. The therapeutic dose is 20–24,000 units intravenous per day. With LMWH using enoxaparin as an example, prophylactic enoxaparin dose is 20 or 40 mg subcutaneous every 24 h. The therapeutic dose of enoxaparin is 1 mg/KBW subcutaneous every 12 h or 1.5 mg/KBW subcutaneous every 24 h.

Activated partial thromboplastin time (APTT) is used to monitor UFH. For LMWH, APTT cannot be used. Anti-factor Xa levels are used (therapeutic range 0.2–0.6 units/ml). International normalized ratio (INR) is used to monitor oral anticoagulants. For venous thrombosis, the target INR is 2.0–3.0. For arterial thrombosis, the target INR is 3.0–4.0. A combination of warfarin and aspirin is used for severe or refractory cases. The intensity of treatment has to be individualized according to the patient's risk of bleeding and recurrent thrombosis. The treatment duration is generally lifelong in unprovoked venous thrombosis, recurrent thrombosis, and arterial thrombosis. In patients with provoked first venous thrombosis, cautious cessation of treatment can be considered after treatment has been given for a duration recommended for patients without APS according to international guidelines. Even in such patients, longer anticoagulation may be required in patients with high-risk aPL profile or other risk factors for recurrence.

Direct Oral Anticoagulants (DOACs) are employed in several thrombotic conditions. DOAC advantages include fixed dose, early onset of action obviating need for initial bridging with LMWH, fewer drug interactions, lack of need for routine anticoagulant monitoring, and no interactions with food. However, in APS, the use of DOACs has been mired in controversy following the TRAPS (Rivaroxaban in Thrombotic Antiphospholipid Syndrome) RCT. The use of rivaroxaban in high-risk patients with APS was associated with an increased rate of thromboembolic events compared with warfarin, thus showing no benefit and excess risk leading to premature trial termination. The European Medicines Agency (EMA) recommends against the use of DOACs, especially in patients who have APS with triple positivity for aPL.

18.3.3 Treatment of Obstetric APS

These patients may be divided into four clinical categories:

(a) Women with high-risk aPL profile but no clinical issues
(b) Obstetric APS alone
(c) Obstetric + Thrombotic APS
(d) Refractory patients

Pregnant women with a high-risk aPL profile but no history of thrombosis or pregnancy complications (with or without SLE) are treated with low-dose aspirin (LDA) 75–100 mg daily. Obstetric APS alone is treated with LDA and heparin at "prophylactic" dosage throughout pregnancy and 6 weeks postpartum. Therapy is withheld at the time of delivery and is resumed after delivery. In the case of obstetric and thrombotic APS, treatment entails LDA and heparin at "therapeutic dosage." In refractory cases, the heparin is increased to "therapeutic" dose with the addition of HCQ or low-dose prednisolone or IVIG singly or in combination.

Warfarin is contraindicated in pregnancy but is compatible with breastfeeding. Corticosteroids are not advised in primary APS because their use is associated with increased maternal morbidity and fetal prematurity. Using these treatment strategies, the success rate ranges from 70 to 80%. As many as 20–30% of pregnancies continue to have adverse outcomes.

18.3.4 Treatment of Catastrophic APS

Precipitating factors include infections, surgical stress, and discontinuation of anticoagulants.

CAPS is best managed in specialized centers using a combination of glucocorticoids, heparin, and plasma exchange or IVIG. Infections need appropriate antibiotics. Agents tried in refractory CAPS include B cell depletion therapies (rituximab) or complement inhibition therapies (eculizumab). The mortality despite treatment is high.

18.4 Conclusions

APS has a broad range of thrombotic, non-thrombotic, and obstetric clinical manifestations. The diagnosis has to be serologically supported by aPL antibodies. Given the commonality of low titer aPL in a variety of conditions and the vast clinical spectrum of APS, overdiagnosis and underdiagnosis are common. All tests should be interpreted in light of the clinical picture. The treatment of obstetric APS differs from thrombotic APS. VKAs are the mainstay of anticoagulation. DOACs are not recommended according to the current state of knowledge.

Suggested Reading

Andreoli L, Bertsias GK, Agmon-Levin N, Brown S, Cervera R, Costedoat-Chalumeau N, et al. EULAR recommendations for women's health and the management of family planning, assisted reproduction, pregnancy and menopause in patients with systemic lupus erythematosus and/or antiphospholipid syndrome. Ann Rheum Dis. 2017;76:476–85.

Cervera R, Piette JC, Font J, Khamashta MA, Shoenfeld Y, Camps MT, et al. Antiphospholipid syndrome: clinical and immunologic manifestations and patterns of disease expression in a cohort of 1,000 patients. Arthritis Rheum. 2002;46:1019–27.

Tektonidou MG, Andreoli L, Limper M, Amoura Z, Cervera R, Costedoat-Chalumeau N, et al. EULAR recommendations for the management of antiphospholipid syndrome in adults. Ann Rheum Dis. 2019;78:1296–13.

19 Inflammatory Muscle Diseases

19.1 Introduction

Inflammatory muscle diseases, also known as idiopathic inflammatory myositis (IIM) or inflammatory myopathies, are a heterogeneous group of rare, chronic, autoimmune conditions afflicting primarily the proximal muscles. The different conditions comprising this group include dermatomyositis (DM), polymyositis, necrotizing autoimmune myositis, inclusion-body myositis (IBM), and overlap myositis.

Symptoms reflect proximal muscle weakness. The onset is insidious. Acute onset is distinctly uncommon. Patients report difficulty getting up from a squatting position, arising from a chair, climbing stairs, combing, and tasks like removing or placing objects on an overhead shelf. Ocular muscles are spared. The weakness of neck extensors may lead to a head drop. Respiratory muscle weakness and dysphagia may come up. Muscle pains (myalgias) are mild and occur in no more than one-third to one-half of the patients. Table 19.1 lists causes of proximal muscle weakness.

The extra-muscular manifestations of IIM include constitutional features like fever and malaise, skin rashes of several types, arthralgias, Raynaud's phenomenon, interstitial lung disease (ILD), and rarely cardiac arrhythmias or left ventricular dysfunction.

Laboratory investigations characteristically show elevated muscle enzymes with myositis-specific antibodies (MSA) in some patients. Muscle biopsy is the current gold standard for diagnosis. Corticosteroids and other immunomodulators are useful in some of these conditions.

Table 19.1 Differential diagnosis of proximal muscle weakness

Idiopathic inflammatory myositis
Inherited myopathies (muscular dystrophies, mitochondrial myopathies)
Myasthenia gravis
Guillain–Barre syndrome
Endocrine causes: Hypothyroidism, hyperthyroidism, diabetes
Rhabdomyolysis
Vitamin D deficiency
Drugs: antimalarials (chloroquine much more than hydroxychloroquine), corticosteroids, zidovudine, statins, D-penicillamine, amiodarone
Others: Hypokalemia, glycogen storage diseases, pyomyositis, trichinella, etc.

19.2 Dermatomyositis

Dermatomyositis is seen in both children and adults (women more than men). The skin manifestations may precede or accompany muscle weakness. The characteristic dermatologic features include heliotrope (bluish purple) rash around the eyes, which may be associated with edema, Gottron's rash on the knuckles, facial erythema, periungual erythema, mechanic's hands (scaly, fissured hyperkeratotic, nonpruritic

R. Handa, *Clinical Rheumatology*, https://doi.org/10.1007/978-981-33-4885-1_19

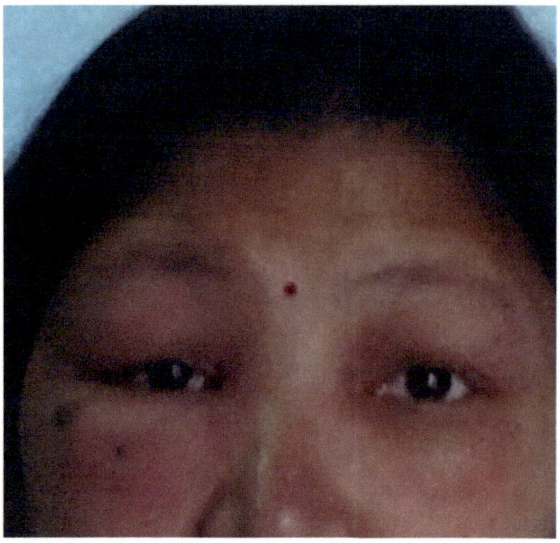

Fig. 19.1 Heliotrope rash in dermatomyositis

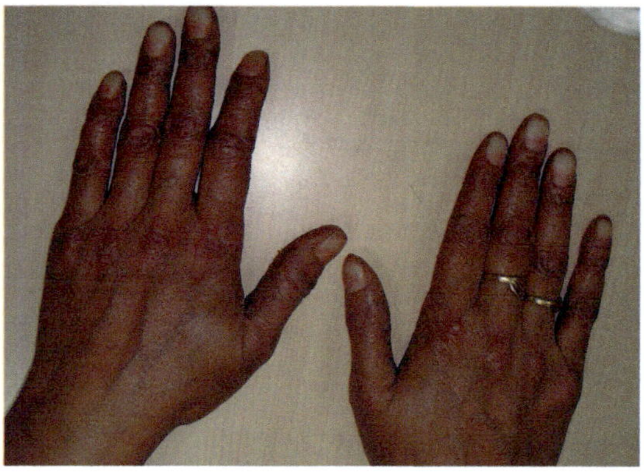

Fig. 19.2 Gottron's papules

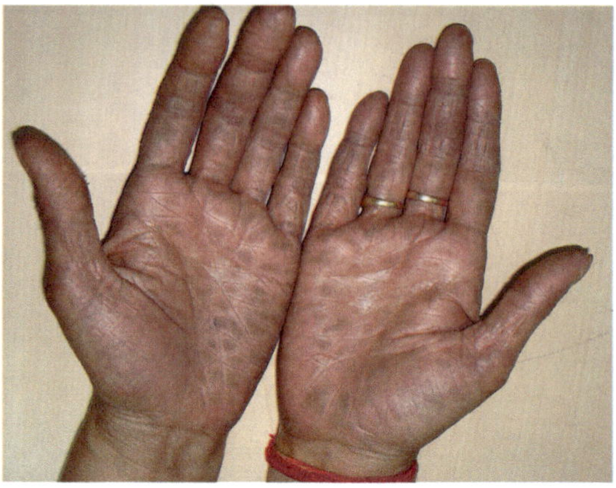

Fig. 19.3 Mechanic's hands

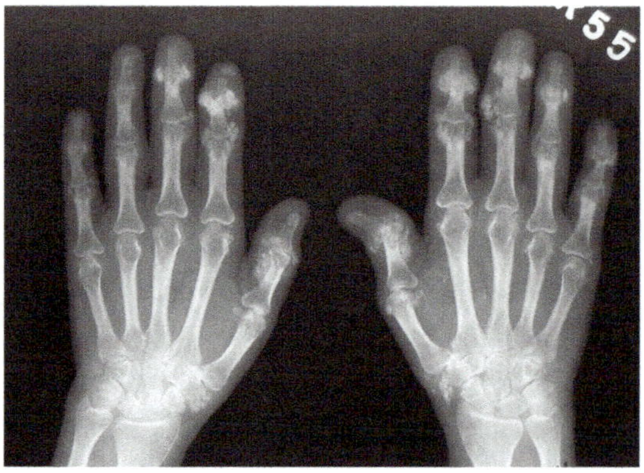

Fig. 19.4 Calcification in overlap myositis (scleroderma + myositis)

lesions on hands), calcinosis, etc. (Figs. 19.1, 19.2, 19.3 and 19.4). The facial rash can cross the labial fold (a feature used to differentiate it from the lupus rash which does not cross the nasolabial fold) (Fig. 19.5). Descriptors used in the literature for photo distributed erythematous rash vary according to the location of the rash: "V-sign" for the rash on the face, neck, and anterior chest; "shawl sign" for back and shoulders; "holster sign" for rash over the lateral hip; and "sleeve sign" for the rash on the lateral aspect of the upper arm. The rash is photosensitive. Both hypopigmentation and hyperpigmentation can be seen (poikiloderma).

Gottron's papules are erythematous, papular, scaly lesions over the knuckles while "inverse" Gottron's papules refer to papular lesions on the palms. Gottron's sign refers to erythematous macules and patches overlying the knuckles, elbows, and/or knees. Some authors prefer to use the term Gottron's papules for papular lesions and Gottron's sign for the flat macular rash. Others use the term Gottron's sign for lesions at sites except for the hands, namely knees, elbows, and ankles, preferring to use Gottron's papules for lesions on the knuckles.

The skin lesions are associated with muscle weakness. Some patients have only skin changes without muscle weakness (amyopathic dermatomyositis), while others have no skin changes

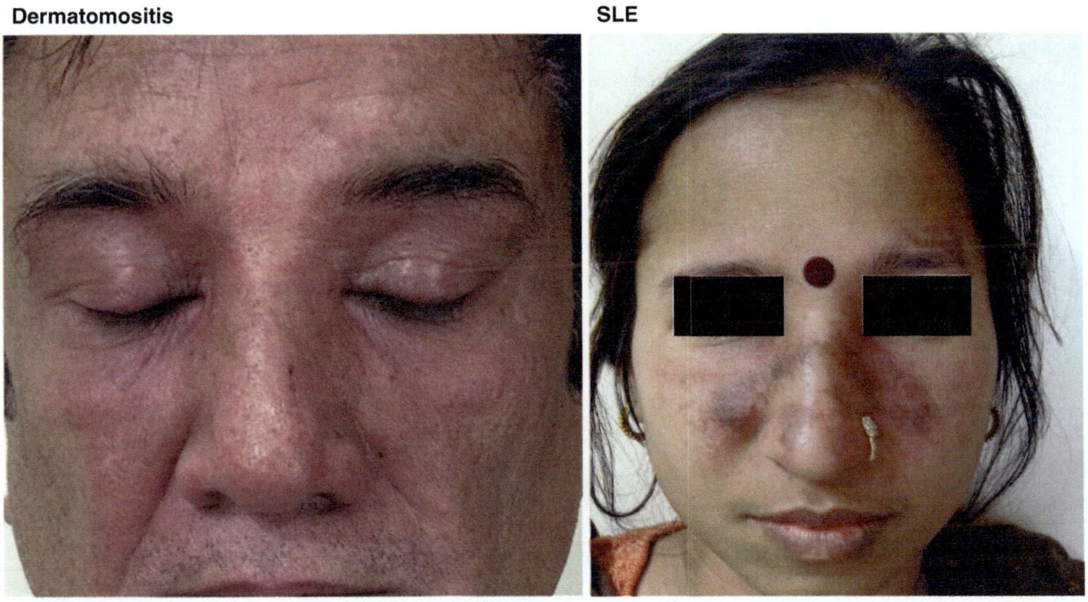

Fig. 19.5 Dermatomyositis rash crossing the nasolabial fold (cf. SLE where nasolabial folds are spared)

(adermatopathic dermatomyositis or dermatomyositis sine dermatitis), a condition that can be diagnosed only on muscle biopsy showing classical features of DM in the absence of cutaneous lesions.

Malignancy may be seen in up to 25% of patients with DM; the risk is much higher compared to polymyositis. Most malignancies are uncovered in the first year of disease onset but can appear anytime within 3–5 years. Cancers associated with DM include ovarian cancer, breast cancer, lung cancer, colorectal cancer, and non-Hodgkin's lymphoma. There is no consensus on the extent of screening needed for malignancy. A thorough clinical examination, chest X-ray, and ultrasound abdomen and pelvis are routinely carried out. Additional tests include mammography and pelvic exam with pap smear in case of women, prostate-specific antigen (PSA) in men, colonoscopy for patients >50 years, CT scan of chest, pelvis, and abdomen, PET-CT, and blood tumor markers depending on the index of suspicion, resource availability and patient concerns. After the first 5 years, screening procedures should follow the usual age- and gender-appropriate recommendations for all people.

19.3 Polymyositis

Polymyositis is the rarest of IIM and is considered a diagnosis of exclusion. Women are more affected than men. Unlike DM, it is virtually never seen in children. Patients have muscle weakness without rash. It is believed that many patients labeled as PM in the past were actually having inclusion-body myositis, necrotizing autoimmune myositis, or muscle dystrophy. Features that draw attention toward an alternate diagnosis in a patient with suspected DM/PM are listed in Box 19.1.

19.4 Necrotizing Autoimmune Myositis

Necrotizing autoimmune myositis (NAM), seen primarily in adults, can account for up to one-fifth of the inflammatory myopathies. The onset can be acute or subacute and result in profound weakness with very high CPK levels. NAM can be idiopathic or follow viral infections. Other causes include statin use, malignancy, or connective tissue diseases (CTDs), especially systemic

Box 19.1 Clinical clues pointing toward alternate diagnosis in a patient with suspected DM/PM

- Prominent muscle pains
- Asymmetric involvement
- Distal > Proximal weakness
- Intermittent symptoms
- Marked muscle atrophy especially in the beginning
- Family history suggestive of muscle disease
- Paresthesias, areflexia, or other features suggesting neuropathy
- Muscle fatigability (where muscle weakness develops as exercise proceeds). Rule out myasthenia gravis
- Presence of myotonia (slow relaxation that follows a normal muscle contraction)

Suspect IBM with distal weakness, muscle atrophy, and asymmetric involvement. The absence of skin rash does not exclude DM (adermatopathic DM).

sclerosis. The characteristic autoantibody is the anti-signal recognition particle (SRP) autoantibody. Statin-associated NAM is associated with autoantibodies against HMGCR (3-hydroxy-3-methyl-glutaryl-coenzyme A reductase) and interestingly does not improve despite the withdrawal of the statin.

19.5 Sporadic Inclusion-Body Myositis

Sporadic inclusion-body myositis (sIBM) is the commonest idiopathic inflammatory myositis in patients over 50 years and is more common in males (male:female::3:1). The disease has to be differentiated from familial IBM (IBM affecting two or more siblings in the same family) and hereditary inclusion-body myopathies (hIBM). The hIBM is a group that includes several autosomal recessive and autosomal dominant muscle disorders with earlier age of onset, the rarity of inflammatory features, and negative MHC class I expression. The "M" in hIBM stands for "myopathy" instead of "myositis."

Sporadic IBM is characterized by slowly progressive muscle weakness and atrophy, which at times may be asymmetrical. Clinical pointers toward diagnosis include early involvement of distal muscles, especially finger flexors and foot extensors. Patients report difficulty in buttoning or holding objects. Muscle atrophy is noticed early with selective atrophy of the quadriceps and forearm muscles. Frequent tripping and falls occur due to quadriceps weakness. Facial weakness is common and dysphagia is seen in 50% of cases. Axial muscle weakness may result in "bent spine syndrome," also known as camptocormia. This condition involves severe forward flexion of the thoracolumbar spine, which typically increases during walking or standing but completely disappears in the supine position. It is to be noted that sIBM is one of the causes and not the only cause of camptocormia.

19.6 Overlap Myositis

It is the largest subset of IIM, accounting for nearly half of all patients. It is characterized by clinical features of myositis overlapping with other CTDs like lupus, scleroderma, or Sjogren's syndrome. These include Raynaud's phenomenon, inflammatory arthritis, gastroesophageal reflux, or lupus features (butterfly rash to be distinguished from the photosensitive facial rash Fig. 19.5). The most well-described form of overlap myositis is the anti-synthetase syndrome, a term applied to the constellation of myositis, ILD, and inflammatory symmetrical polyarthritis of the small joints of the hands and feet. Other characteristic features include mechanic's hands, Raynaud's phenomenon, and fever, along with anti-synthetase antibodies to aminoacyl-transfer ribonucleic acid (tRNA) synthetase enzymes. The serological spectrum of overlap myositis includes several new autoantibodies.

19.7 Investigations

Muscle enzymes are used to diagnose muscle inflammation. These include creatinine kinase (CK), alanine aminotransferase (ALT), aspartate aminotransferase (AST), aldolase, and lactate dehydrogenase (LDH). Not all muscle enzymes need to be elevated in a given patient at the same time. Several conditions other than IIM may give rise to CK elevation (Table 19.2). CK is widely used not only for diagnosis but also for monitoring response to treatment with several caveats (Table 19.3).

The magnitude of CK rise varies in different conditions. Highest levels (more than 50 times the upper limit of normal (ULN) are seen in NAM. sIBM exhibits the lowest CK levels (less than ten times ULN). Intermediate levels up to 50 times ULN can be seen in DM and PM.

Table 19.2 Causes of CK elevation

Inflammatory myositis
Myocardial injury
Muscle dystrophies
Drugs
Rhabdomyolysis
Hypothyroidism
Malignant hyperthermia
Exercise
Infectious myopathies
Others: Alcohol, periodic paralysis, macro-CK, etc.
Idiopathic

Table 19.3 Caveats in the interpretation of CK

Elevated CK has several reasons, of which IIM is one.
Some patients with IIM may have normal CK but an elevation in other enzymes.
Rarely, patients with clinical muscle weakness, abnormal EMG, and positive muscle biopsy may have normal CK.
Amyopathic DM can have florid skin features with no muscle weakness and normal CK.
The biochemical response may not parallel clinical response to treatment. CK elevation may persist in the absence of muscle weakness.
CK normalization on treatment may take 3–4 months.
Recurrence of muscle weakness while on treatment with corticosteroids with normal CK should arouse suspicion of steroid myopathy.
Asymptomatic CK elevation without disease is occasionally seen. Reasons could be strenuous exercise, black ethnicity, macro-CK, and idiopathic.

Macro-CK refers to CK with an increased molecular weight that is cleared slowly from the circulation, leading to increased levels

EMG (electromyography) characteristically shows low voltage polyphasic potentials with fibrillation in acute phases. It is helpful in differentiation from neuropathies. However, the changes are not pathognomonic and are subject to variable interpretation. EMG should spare one lower limb to allow biopsy specimens from that side.

Skeletal muscle imaging using MRI is increasingly used in clinical practice to confirm muscle inflammation, pinpoint biopsy site, and sometimes monitor treatment. This is especially important in children with juvenile dermatomyositis and may help avoid an invasive muscle biopsy. To obviate the interference of fat signals, T2-weighted images with fat suppression or short tau inversion recovery (STIR) sequences are employed. Muscle edema is picked up as hyperintense (white) signals on T2-weighted and STIR images. Features of damage like fatty infiltration of muscle and muscle atrophy in chronic disease are better depicted on T1-weighted images. DM patients may show the involvement of connective tissue septa and muscle fascia.

Muscle biopsy is the current gold standard for diagnosis. The usual sites sampled are quadriceps or deltoid on the side where EMG has not been done. Open biopsy scores over closed needle biopsy because of the larger sample provided and because the orientation of muscle fibers is better preserved. Biopsy from grossly atrophic muscles and calf muscles are likely to have a low yield. The sample collection is important. Apart from formalin, cryo processing of the fresh specimen is required for immunohistochemistry and biochemical testing. Electron microscopy is needed in some situations.

Histologic features of IIM include muscle fiber necrosis, degeneration, regeneration, and inflammatory cell infiltration. In DM, the cellular infiltrate is predominantly perifascicular (located at the periphery of the fascicles or interfascicular septae) and perivascular. Microinfarcts may be seen. Skin biopsy reveals interface dermatitis (inflammation at the dermal–epidermal junction). PM is characterized by the cellular infiltrate predominantly within the fascicle with increased numbers of cytotoxic CD8+ T cells, which invade nonnecrotic healthy-looking muscle fibers expressing MHC Class I antigen. Vacuoles are absent. NAM shows an abundance of necrotic fibers invaded by macrophages. Vacuoles are absent, and complement deposits may be seen on capillaries. The biopsy in sIBM resembles PM. Healthy-looking, nonnecrotic fibers are invaded by macrophages and cytotoxic CD8+ T cells. Immunostaining reveals upregulation of MHC I (normal muscle fibers do not express this). In addition to inflammation, myofiber degeneration, regeneration, and necrosis may be seen. Other features include the variability of fiber size with scattered atrophic fibers. Sarcoplasmic rimmed vacuoles best picked up on Gomori-trichrome stain are a distinguishing feature. Intracellular amyloid deposits may be seen on Congo red staining. Electron microscopy reveals nuclear and cytoplasmic inclusions that consist of tubulofilaments. As many as 30% of patients with a clinical diagnosis of sIBM may not show vacuoles or amyloid deposits, leading to erroneous labeling of polymyositis. Muscle biopsies in anti-synthetase syndrome reveal changes of perifascicular atrophy akin to DM with an increase in the number of perifascicular necrotic fibers.

Antinuclear antibodies are seen in nearly three-fourths of the patients of DM by immunofluorescence. Autoantibodies in IIM are of two types: (1) Myositis-associated autoantibodies (MAA) and (2) Myositis-specific autoantibodies (MSA).

The MAA are not unique to IIM and can be seen in other CTDs as well. These include anti-Ro, anti-U1RNP, and anti-PM-Scl. The presence of anti-Ro52 without anti-Ro60 is more common in IIM (cf. Sjogren's syndrome, where both anti-Ro 52 and 60 may be seen in nearly the same frequency). Anti-Ro52 is more common in patients with anti-synthetase syndrome than other types of myositis.

MSAs are present in 30–60% of patients with IIM. They are directed against nuclear RNAs or cytoplasmic antigens and may point toward a specific phenotype. MSA includes antibodies to aminoacyl-transfer (t)RNA synthetases (anti-synthetase antibodies), antibodies to SRP, and antibodies to Mi-2. The most common anti-synthetase antibody is anti-Jo1, present in 20% of patients with IIM. The other anti-synthetases include PL-7, PL-12, EJ, KS, OJ, Ha, Zo, etc. and occur in fewer patients (<5%). Anti-synthetase antibodies are associated with myositis, mechanic's hand, interstitial lung disease (ILD), Raynaud's phenomenon, and arthritis.

NAM exhibits anti-SRP antibodies and anti-HMGCR antibodies. Anti-SRP antibodies are not exclusively seen in NAM. They may also occasionally be seen in other IIM. They denote aggressive refractory disease.

Antibodies to Mi-2 are found in 15–30% of DM patients and associated with a favorable prognosis. Anti-melanoma differentiation-associated gene 5 (MDA5) antibodies are associated with rapidly progressive ILD, severe skin rash, cutaneous ulceration involving Gottron's papules and Gottron's sign, and hypomyopathic or amyopathic dermatomyositis. Anti-MDA-5 antibodies are associated with poor survival. Antibody against cytosolic 5′nucleotidase 1A (anti-cN1A) may be seen in some patients of sIBM. A variety of other MSAs are being described in what is a rapidly changing field. Future classifications of IIM may subset patients based on autoantibody profiling.

19.8 Treatment of IIM

The non-IBM myositis (DM, PM, overlap myositis, and NAM) are treated along similar lines. Corticosteroids are the mainstay of treatment. The typical starting dose is prednisolone of 0.5–1 mg/KBW daily orally. Where scleroderma is a part of the overlap myositis, doses of steroids are kept low in order to avoid precipitation of scleroderma renal crisis. In severe cases with rapidly progressive ILD, dysphagia, or respiratory muscle involvement, daily intravenous methylprednisolone pulses of 500 mg to 1 g/day for 3–5 days are employed. Prednisolone is gradually tapered after 4–6 weeks depending on clinical response. The CK may lag behind clinical improvement. A vigil for corticosteroid adverse effects like deranged glycemic control, impaired bone health, etc. is maintained and appropriate measures adopted. The speed of tapering is governed by the clinical response and not the calendar. Treatment decisions often have to be individualized.

Most rheumatologists add a steroid-sparing agent from the very beginning. Methotrexate (15–25 mg/week orally or subcutaneously) is widely used. Other drugs include azathioprine (2–3 mg/kg/day) or mycophenolate mofetil (2–3 g/day divided into two doses). Cyclosporin and tacrolimus are sometimes used. Cyclophosphamide pulses are occasionally used for poorly responsive ILD. Agents employed for resistant cases include intravenous immunoglobulin (IVIG) (2 g/kg over 3–5 days) and rituximab (two doses of 1 g given by intravenous infusion 2 weeks apart).

Hydroxychloroquine is used for skin disease but does not help the muscle weakness. Photoprotection, topical glucocorticoids, or calcineurin inhibitors are employed for cutaneous manifestations. The treatment of calcinosis is frustrating. Diltiazem is used with rather poor results. Surgical excision may be needed in some patients.

Muscle-strengthening exercises and rehabilitation consults are rewarding. The usual duration of treatment is 1 year after remission. Many clinicians prefer to discontinue steroids before stopping methotrexate or azathioprine or mycophenolate. Relapses need retreatment with steroids.

The treatment of sporadic inclusion-body myositis is largely supportive because no pharmacological therapy is effective. Corticosteroids, azathioprine, methotrexate do not help.

19.9 Conclusions

IIM comprises five different entities: dermatomyositis, polymyositis, necrotizing autoimmune myositis, sporadic inclusion-body myositis, and overlap myositis. The clinical presentations, autoantibodies, and histopathologic features are quite variable. Treatment principles for all except sIBM are similar and involve steroids along with steroid-sparing strategies. There is no definitive treatment for sIBM.

Suggested Reading

Chinoy H, Lilleker JB. Pitfalls in the diagnosis of myositis. Best Pract Res Clin Rheumatol. 2020;34:101486.

Greenberg SA. Inclusion body myositis: clinical features and pathogenesis. Nat Rev Rheumatol. 2019;15:257–72.

Mariampillai K, Granger B, Amelin D, Guiguet M, Hachulla E, Maurier F, et al. Development of a new classification system for idiopathic inflammatory myopathies based on clinical manifestations and myositis-specific autoantibodies. JAMA Neurol. 2018;75:1528–37.

McHugh NJ, Tansley SL. Autoantibodies in myositis. Nat Rev Rheumatol. 2018;14:290–302.

Witt LJ, Curran JJ, Strek ME. The diagnosis and treatment of antisynthetase syndrome. Clin Pulm Med. 2016;23:218–26.

20 Vasculitis

20.1 Introduction

The vasculitides are a vast and heterogeneous group of clinical syndromes characterized by inflammation of blood vessels. They are classified based on the size of the blood vessels affected. The nomenclature and classification of vasculitides remain a matter of debate. The Chapel Hill Consensus Conference (CHCC) nomenclature system is widely used to define the various entities (Table 20.1). The manifestations are protean and diverse. Antineutrophil cytoplasmic antibody (ANCA) is a useful serologic marker of the ANCA-associated vasculitides—namely Wegener's granulomatosis (WG), microscopic polyangiitis (MPA), or Churg–Strauss Syndrome (CSS). There is a growing movement to shed eponyms. Wegener's Granulomatosis is now known as Granulomatosis with polyangiitis (GPA), while Churg–Strauss Syndrome is now known as eosinophilic granulomatosis with polyangiitis (EGPA). However, the older terminology continues to be widely used.

Table 20.1 International Chapel Hill Consensus Conference on the nomenclature of vasculitides (CHCC 2012)

Large vessel vasculitis
1. Takayasu's arteritis 2. Giant cell arteritis (temporal arteritis)
Medium vessel vasculitis
1. Polyarteritis nodosa (PAN) 2. Kawasaki disease
Small vessel vasculitis
1. Microscopic polyangiitis (MPA) 2. Wegener's granulomatosis (WG) or granulomatosis with polyangiitis (GPA) 3. Allergic granulomatosis (Churg–Strauss Syndrome—CSS) or eosinophilic granulomatosis with polyangiitis (EGPA)
4. Immune complex vasculitis
5. Anti-glomerular basement membrane (GBM) disease
6. Cryoglobulinemic vasculitis
7. IgA vasculitis (Henoch–Schonlein vasculitis)
8. Hypocomplementemic urticarial vasculitis (HUV) (anti-C1q vasculitis)
Variable vessel vasculitis
1. Behcet syndrome 2. Cogan's syndrome
Single organ vasculitis
Vasculitis associated with systemic disease
Vasculitis associated with probable etiology

WG (GPA), CSS (EGPA), and MPA are grouped under ANCA-associated vasculitides

20.2 Clinical Approach

Vasculitis should be suspected whenever a physician confronts unexplained systemic illness with fever, anorexia, and weight loss; multiorgan involvement without any apparent cause; skin lesions, especially palpable purpura or skin necrosis, with prominent systemic features; unexplained renal failure; FUO (fever of unknown origin); mononeuritis multiplex; arthralgias and arthritis with fever; unexplained hemoptysis; pulmonary–renal syndrome, etc. (Fig. 20.1). Some patients present with eye inflammation, notably

R. Handa, *Clinical Rheumatology*, https://doi.org/10.1007/978-981-33-4885-1_20

scleritis (Fig. 20.2). Despite the myriads of presentations, pattern recognition enables a clinician to identify particular types. For example, ear nose throat (ENT) symptoms like nasal stuffiness, epistaxis, or excessive crusting may be the presenting features of GPA—Wegener's. Limb claudication, pulse inequality or absence, jaw claudication, or new-onset hypertension may be seen in Takayasu's arteritis. Headache, jaw claudication, scalp tenderness, and visual disturbances in an elderly patient are suggestive of temporal arteritis.

Laboratory tests reveal high erythrocyte sedimentation rate (ESR), elevated C reactive protein (CRP), and leukocytosis reflecting acute phase response. Proteinuria and an active urinary sediment point toward kidney involvement. Additional tests are governed by the type of vasculitis suspected. These may include autoantibodies, complement levels, nerve conduction studies, imaging investigations like chest radiograph, ultrasound abdomen, computerized tomography (CT) or magnetic resonance imaging (MRI) scans or Positron emission tomography (PET)-CT scan, CT or MR angiography, and biopsies for tissue diagnosis.

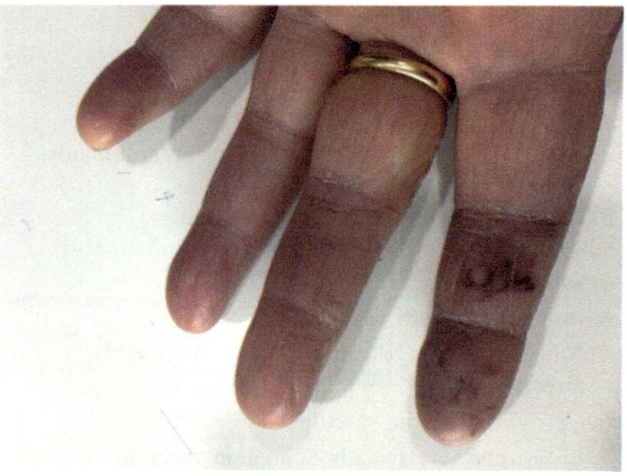

Fig. 20.1 Vasculitic skin rash in GPA

ANCA should not be used as a screening test. The current recommendations advocate the use of high-quality immunoassays as the preferred first method for ANCA detection. A second PR3-MPO-ANCA or immunofluorescence (IIF) can be considered for negative results in patients with a high clinical suspicion (to increase sensitivity) or in case of low antibody levels (to increase specificity).

Ideally, the diagnosis of vasculitis should be confirmed by histopathology, which continues to be the gold standard for diagnosing vasculitis. This may not be possible in many cases like Takayasu's arteritis, polyarteritis nodosa (PAN), etc. Blind biopsies are discouraged as yield is low. Tissues that can be sampled include skin in case of purpuric lesions or skin ulcers, temporal artery biopsy in suspected temporal arteritis, kidney biopsy in patients with active urine sediment, sural nerve biopsy, muscle biopsy, lung biopsy, or upper airway biopsy as dictated by the clinical requirement. Superficial biopsies of the skin may be inconclusive. Demonstration of medium vasculitis requires adequate skin and subcutaneous tissue, usually by excisional biopsy.

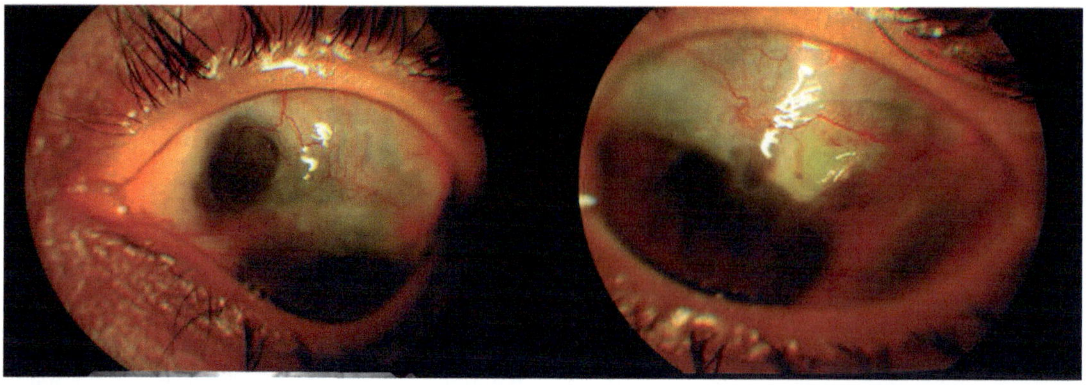

Fig. 20.2 Scleritis in GPA

Immunofluorescence is required to get additional information. Biopsy samples in ANCA-associated vasculitis do not show complement or immune complex deposits (pauci-immune) [cf. lupus nephritis which shows a full house pattern]. Henoch–Schonlein purpura (HSP) requires staining for IgA.

The bedside approach to vasculitis is considerably simplified if one takes into account that patients with vasculitis can present as one of the following three syndromes:

1. Systemic necrotizing vasculitis
2. Cutaneous vasculitis syndromes
3. Systemic vasculitis of large vessels

This syndromic approach facilitates treatment decisions even if a patient cannot be categorized into any definite entity since many vasculitides share common, overlapping clinical features. The systemic necrotizing vasculitides (SNV) are characterized by ischemia of the tissues supplied by the affected blood vessels. The different entities included in this group include GPA, EGPA, MPA, and PAN. These vasculitides, except for PAN, are associated with ANCA. The SNV differ from the predominantly cutaneous vasculitis syndromes like HSP and the large vessel vasculitides like Takayasu's arteritis and temporal arteritis in their clinical presentation. The clinical features of SNV include prominent constitutional symptoms like fever, night sweats, weight loss, and anorexia. Mononeuritis multiplex, renal involvement, gastrointestinal bleeding, musculoskeletal symptoms, pulmonary involvement, and vasculitic skin lesions are typical. The laboratory workup in SNV reveals leukocytosis, raised ESR, anemia, polyclonal gammopathy, high eosinophil count (in EGPA), and ANCA (except PAN). Untreated, these diseases are usually fatal.

In contrast to the SNV, the cutaneous vasculitis syndromes like HSP, etc. present with palpable purpura. Less common modes of presentation include urticaria, subcutaneous nodules, ulcers, necrotic lesions, livedo reticularis, etc. Constitutional symptoms are uncommon, and internal organ involvement, seen in only half the cases, is rarely life-threatening.

Large vessel vasculitides like Takayasu and temporal arteritis differ from SNV in that skin, lung, renal parenchymal, and gastrointestinal involvement are uncommon. Rapid progression, unlike SNV, is not usually seen.

Many a time, it is not possible to accurately classify the vasculitis. In such instances, delineation of the organs involved helps guide treatment.

20.3 Disease Activity and Damage Assessment in Vasculitis

The vasculitides are characterized by remission and relapses. Some patients exhibit chronically active disease. The intensity of treatment is based on the concept of disease activity, which refers to the current state of inflammation and reflects the need for treatment at that point in time. The Birmingham Vasculitis Activity Score (BVAS) is a validated tool for assessing disease activity in patients with many different forms of vasculitis. In contrast to disease activity that is reversible, damage refers to irreversible sequelae of the disease. In the face of damage, treatment escalation can be counterproductive. Validated instruments to measure disease activity, damage, and function are now available, a detailed discussion of which is beyond the scope of this chapter.

The differentiation of disease activity from damage is based on physical examination, laboratory investigations, imaging, and physician judgment. Disease activity has to be differentiated from infection so very common in patients on immunosuppressives. Periods on increased activity (flares) may supervene on chronic damage making distinction difficult.

20.4 Pseudovasculitis Syndromes/Mimics

Several conditions may mimic vasculitis. These include purpura fulminans, bacterial endocarditis, atrial myxoma, thoracic outlet syndromes, and cholesterol emboli syndrome.

20.5 Granulomatosis with Polyangiitis (GPA)-Wegener's Granulomatosis

Wegener's granulomatosis is a systemic necrotizing vasculitis of small and medium vessels that typically involves the upper and lower respiratory tracts and the kidneys. Cases without renal involvement are termed "Limited Wegener's granulomatosis." There is no sex predilection. The etiology is unknown. Most patients present with upper respiratory tract symptoms like purulent or bloody nasal discharge, paranasal sinus drainage or pain, nasal mucosal ulcerations, nasal stuffiness, or ear discharge. It is not uncommon for the patients to first present to the ear, nose, and throat (ENT) surgeon. In the first go, these symptoms are not linked to systemic disease, leading to a delay in diagnosis. The patients may develop saddle nose deformity (Fig. 20.3). The other causes of saddle nose deformity include leprosy, syphilis, and relapsing polychondritis. Palatal perforation may occur. Constitutional symptoms, arthralgias, and weight loss are common.

Lung involvement may be asymptomatic or manifest as cough, shortness of breath, or hemoptysis. The chest X-rays may show infiltrates, nodules, cavitary lesions, or any combination of these lesions (Fig. 20.4). Pleural effusion, pneumothorax, and hydropneumothorax are rare. The radiologic picture may be indistinguishable from pulmonary tuberculosis (PTB). Many patients receive an initial diagnosis of pulmonary tuberculosis and antitubercular treatment. The presence of active urine sediment, a sputum smear consistently negative for acid-fast bacilli, and prominent ENT symptoms should alert the physician to the presence of GPA. Careful examination of the urine is an inexpensive and rewarding investigation in this setting. Renal disease in GPA is most often asymptomatic. Urinalysis reveals proteinuria, hematuria, and RBC casts (active sediment). Eye involvement may take the form of proptosis, conjunctivitis, scleritis, episcleritis, uveitis, or optic nerve vasculitis. Nasolacrimal duct obstruction may be seen. Other organs affected include the skin, heart, GI tract, and the nervous system. Oral lesions occur in less than 10% of GPA patients but can be quite striking (Figs. 20.5 and 20.6).

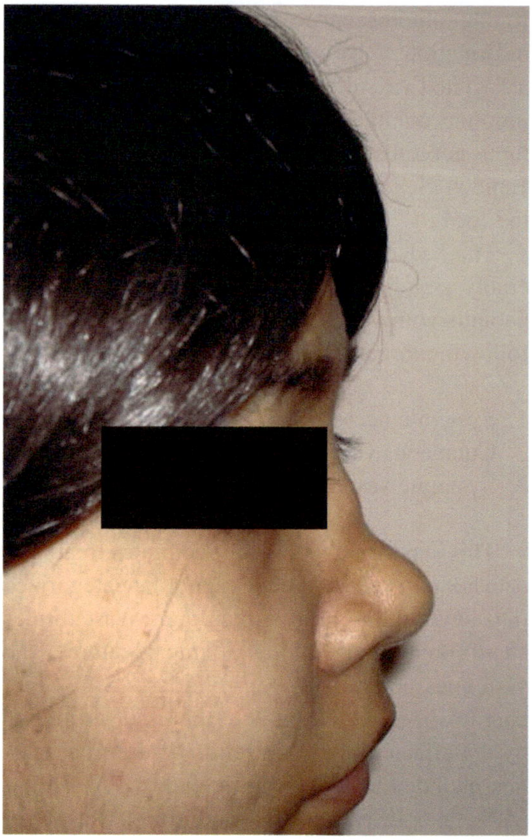

Fig. 20.3 Saddle nose deformity in GPA

PR-3 ANCA is positive in 85–90% of patients with active WG and 40% of patients in remission. The ANCA levels may not correlate with disease activity. The histopathologic hallmark of WG is necrotizing vasculitis of small arteries and veins with granuloma formation that may be intravascular or extravascular. The other granulomatous vasculitides include Takayasu's disease, Temporal arteritis, and CSS. Of these, the first two do not involve the lungs. Tissue biopsy from the upper airways (sinuses or nasopharynx) in WG usually reveals inflammation, necrosis, or granulomatous changes. Often, vasculitis is not present. The diagnostic yield of biopsy from the upper airways is maximum from paranasal sinuses, followed in decreasing order by the nose

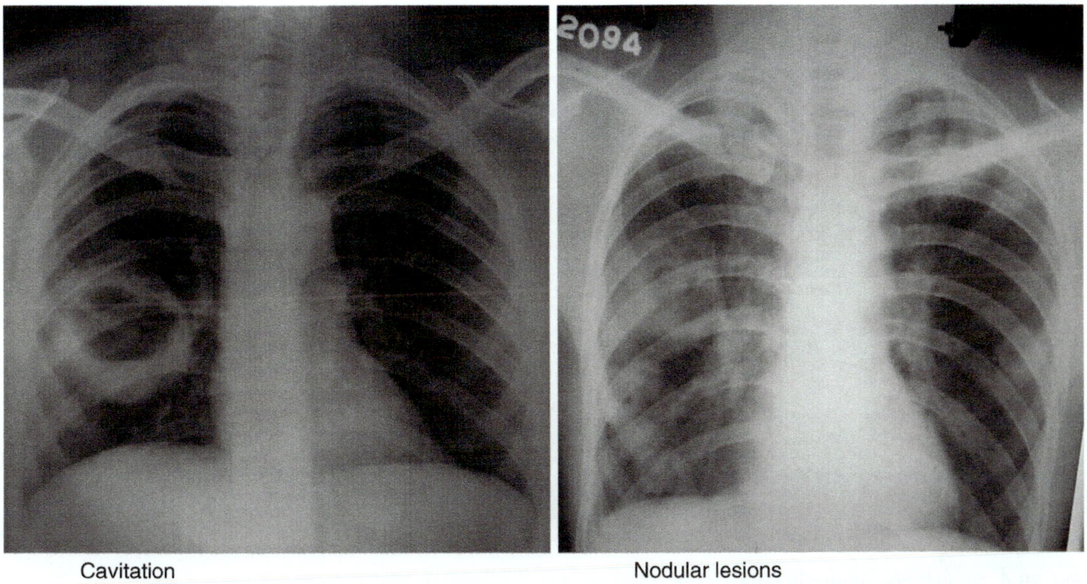

Fig. 20.4 Chest radiographs in GPA

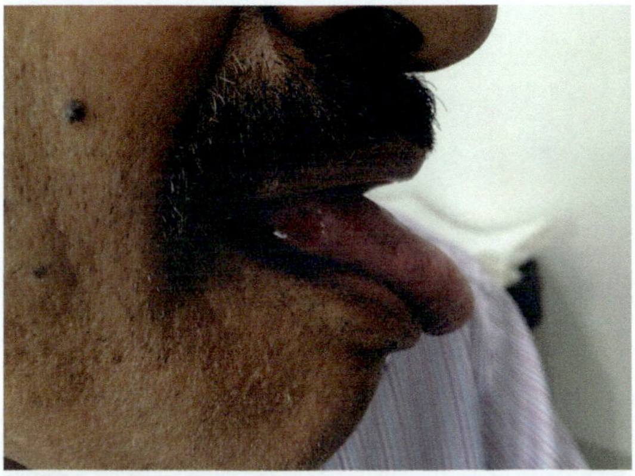

Fig. 20.5 Tongue ulcer in GPA

and the subglottic region, probably a reflection of the amount of tissue obtained by each procedure. Lung biopsies usually reveal both granuloma and vasculitis, while granulomas are rarely seen in a renal biopsy. The characteristic feature of a kidney biopsy is focal, segmental necrotizing glomerulonephritis. It is important to note that on immunofluorescence (IF) microscopy, immune deposits are not seen in GPA ("paucimmune" disease) in sharp contrast to systemic lupus erythematosus where IF reveals complement and immunoglobulin deposits. Skin biopsies usually show leukocytoclastic vasculitis.

Long-term morbidity is related to renal insufficiency, hearing impairment, tracheal stenosis, saddle nose deformity, chronic sinusitis, and side effects due to long-term use of prednisolone and cyclophosphamide. Factors contributing to mortality include renal disease, pulmonary disease, infections, and malignancy.

20.6 Microscopic Polyangiitis (MPA)

Microscopic polyangiitis (MPA) is one of the vasculitides previously included in the polyarteritis nodosa (PAN) group. The Chapel Hill Consensus Conference has clarified these issues significantly. Likely, many of the patients of PAN in the older literature were actually MPA. Urinalysis is a simple yet invaluable investigation in differentiating classical PAN from MPA. The urine sediment is active in MPA in contrast to the inactive sediment in PAN. Renal involvement is the central feature of MPA and takes the form of rapidly progressive glomerulonephritis (RPGN). Lung involvement takes the

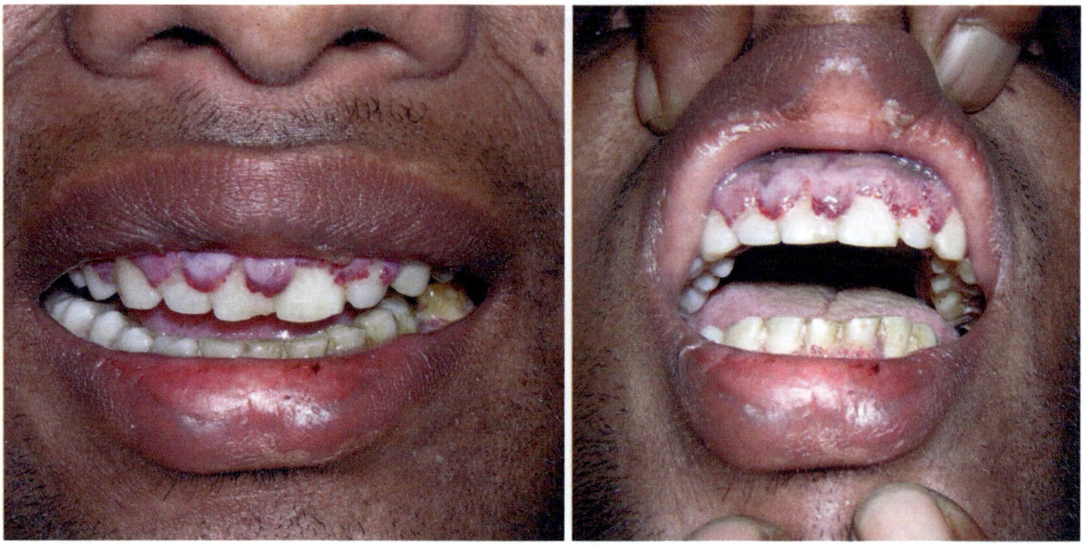

Fig. 20.6 Strawberry gingiva in GPA

form of diffuse alveolar hemorrhage (Fig. 20.7). A diagnosis of MPA is usually considered when necrotizing focal segmental glomerulonephritis and/or lung hemorrhage are present. Other clinical features include arthralgias, pain abdomen, gastrointestinal bleeding, and peripheral neuropathy. Nearly 90% of patients are ANCA positive with >95% MPO positivity.

20.7 Eosinophilic Granulomatosis with Polyangiitis (EGPA)-Churg–Strauss Syndrome

Also known as Allergic angiitis and granulomatosis, this vasculitis is characterized by granulomatous inflammation of small and medium-sized vessels. Peripheral and tissue eosinophilia are frequent, and lung involvement is common.

The disease may follow three phases:

1. *Prodromal phase*: Characterized by atopy, nasal polyposis, and asthma. This may last for several years.
2. *Peripheral blood and tissue eosinophilia*: in which eosinophilia is a prominent feature.
3. *Systemic vasculitis*: which is heralded by fever, weight loss, and anorexia.

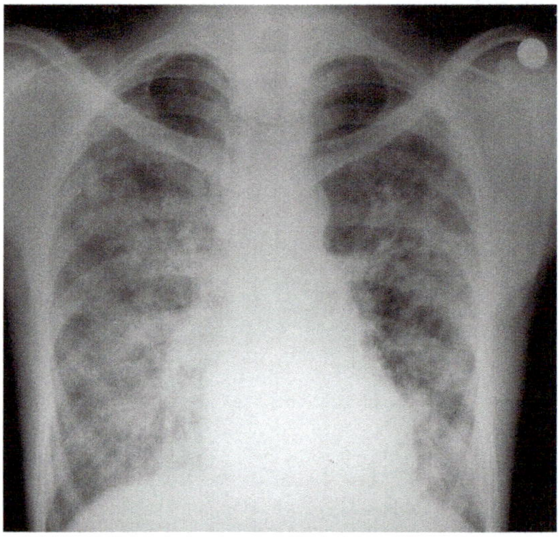

Fig. 20.7 Diffuse alveolar hemorrhage in microscopic polyangiitis

Asthma usually subsides when vasculitis emerges. However, it is essential to keep in mind that all three phases may appear simultaneously. Skin lesions, peripheral neuropathy, and renal disease are also seen. Approximately 50% of patients are ANCA positive with the majority (~80%) showing MPO positivity. Histopathology reveals necrotizing granulomatous eosinophilic vasculitis.

20.8 Treatment of ANCA-Associated Vasculitis (GPA, MPA, EGPA)

The treatment is divided into two phases:

(a) Induction of Remission
(b) Maintenance of Remission

Induction requires sharp curtailment of disease activity and is achieved by medium to high doses of steroids and an additional immunosuppressive. The maintenance phase sees the de-escalation of dosages—the focus shifts to continued disease control and relapse prevention alongside the minimization of drug toxicity. The treatment specifics vary according to the vasculitis type and the extent of organ involvement. The patients are divided into two broad categories: those with organ or life-threatening disease and those with a nonorgan or non-life-threatening disease (Table 20.2). These concepts help guide the intensity of therapy at a point in time but are not sacrosanct. Disease quiescent at a point of time may relapse and become active and organ threatening at another point of time. Therefore, constant vigil and regular monitoring are advised. Also, grumbling attacks of non-life-threatening diseases may result in substantial cumulative damage over time. Physician judgment plays a vital role in assessing the gravity of the situation.

Induction of remission in severe AAV is achieved by a combination of corticosteroids (1 mg/KBW of prednisolone daily) and cyclophosphamide or rituximab. Organ-threatening or life-threatening situations are tackled by intravenous methylprednisolone pulses of 500–1000 mg daily for 3–5 days at the start of treatment. The dose employed for pulse intravenous cyclophosphamide is 15 mg/KBW every 3–4 weeks while the oral dose of cyclophosphamide is 2 mg/KBW/day. Despite being effective, oral cyclophosphamide is infrequently used because of the higher cumulative dose delivered by oral administration and a growing tendency to limit exposure to cyclophosphamide given its long-term toxicity. Many rheumatologists use monthly cyclophosphamide pulses to induce remission and switch over to maintenance therapies after 6 months. Rituximab is employed as an alternative to cyclophosphamide in organ-threatening or life-threatening ANCA-associated vasculitis. The dose employed is 375 mg/m^2 of body surface area, once a week for four infusions. Biosimilars of rituximab are available in India. The choice between cyclophosphamide or rituximab is based on patient preference, cost considerations, and physician choice.

Table 20.2 Organ involvement in ANCA-associated vasculitis

Organ- or life-threatening disease	Nonorgan or non-life-threatening disease
• Pulmonary hemorrhage • Rapidly deteriorating renal function • Motor neuropathy • Cerebral vasculitis • Myocarditis, pericarditis • Gastrointestinal bleed due to vasculitis • Orbital pseudotumor	• Upper airway disease • Arthritis • Pulmonary nodules

Plasma exchange has also been popular as a part of induction treatment in AAV in patients with rapidly progressive glomerulonephritis and diffuse alveolar hemorrhage. It is also used in concomitant anti-GBM disease. The recent PEXIVAS trial published in 2020 reported that the use of plasma exchange did not result in a lower incidence of the primary composite outcome of end-stage kidney disease or death from any cause. The subgroup analysis in the PEXIVAS trial suggested a potential benefit of plasma exchange in patients with pulmonary hemorrhage. This influential trial has raised a question mark over the utility of plasma exchange in AAV.

For remission-induction of non-organ-threatening AAV, a combination of glucocorticoids and either methotrexate or mycophenolate mofetil (MMF) is used. The usual methotrexate dose employed is 15–25 mg/week, oral or parenteral. MMF is used in a dose of 2–3 g/day. However, in certain situations, methotrexate or mycophenolate should not be used (Box 20.1).

Box 20.1 Situations where methotrexate or mycophenolate should not be used for remission induction in ANCA-associated vasculitis

- Meningeal involvement
- Retro-orbital disease
- Cardiac involvement
- Mesenteric involvement
- Acute-onset mononeuritis multiplex
- Pulmonary hemorrhage of any severity

Trimethoprim–sulfamethoxazole (80 mg/400 mg) tablet daily is administered as prophylaxis against infection, especially pneumocystis. The double-strength tablet (160 mg/800 mg) may be used on alternate days.

After successful induction, steroids are slowly and steadily reduced if the disease is quiescent. Maintenance doses of 5–10 mg prednisolone daily are continued for 12–18 months depending on the situation. Maintenance therapy is generally started when the effect of induction therapy is wearing off. The TLC count should be >4000 cells/μl, and the ANC (absolute neutrophil count) >1500. With intravenous pulse cyclophosphamide, maintenance therapy is started after 2–4 weeks provided TLC and ANC are normal, as outlined above. The lag is not so much with oral cyclophosphamide, where maintenance treatment is started within days. With rituximab, it is prudent to wait 4–6 months after the last dose. Remission-maintenance therapy for AAV be continued for at least 24 months following induction of sustained remission. Some subsets where the risk for relapse is high like persistent PR3-ANCA positivity, pulmonary involvement, upper respiratory tract involvement require even more extended maintenance therapy for up to 36 months. Patients with multiple relapses (≥2 relapses) require indefinite treatment.

The agents used for maintenance therapy in AAV include rituximab, azathioprine (2 mg/KBW/day), methotrexate (15–25 mg/week), or mycophenolate mofetil (2–3 g/day). Some authorities recommend azathioprine or methotrexate maintenance in GPA or MPA who are MPO-ANCA positive because of the lower risk of relapse in these patients. Rituximab has emerged as a preferred treatment for maintenance after the publication of Maintenance of Remission using Rituximab in Systemic ANCA-associated Vasculitis (MAINRITSAN) trial. It is dosed as two 500 mg doses separated by 14 days at the start of maintenance therapy, followed by 500 mg again at months 6, 12, and 18. Some rheumatologists dose according to CD19-positive cells, which are depleted by rituximab. Redosing is carried out when B lymphocytes reconstitute.

Relapses are common in AAV. Predictors of relapse include a diagnosis of GPA (versus MPA), PR3-ANCA (versus MPO-ANCA), and history of relapses in the past. Relapsing disease in GPA or MPA requires reinduction with rituximab or cyclophosphamide. The timing of the relapse influences maintenance therapy in these patients. Patients who relapse during maintenance therapy with azathioprine or methotrexate, are shifted to rituximab for maintenance. Patients who relapse during maintenance therapy with rituximab are switched to azathioprine, methotrexate, or mycophenolate mofetil. When relapse occurs after discontinuation of maintenance, the drugs that were initially used for successful maintenance are retried, albeit with advice to continue indefinitely.

The disease severity in EGPA (Churg–Strauss) is assessed by the "five-factors score" (FFS) which looks at the presence or absence of five clinical factors: age >65 years; cardiac insufficiency; renal insufficiency; gastrointestinal involvement; and the absence of ENT manifestations (presence is associated with better prognosis). The treatment principles of EGPA are extrapolated from AAV trials. Prednisolone 0.5–1 mg/KBW/day is used to induce remission, followed by a slow taper. Cyclophosphamide is added in patients with severe disease (FFS ≥ 2). However, some patients with FFS of 1 with critical organ involvement may also benefit from cyclophosphamide. Agents used for maintenance include methotrexate, leflunomide, azathioprine, and MMF for 1–2 years. The role of rituximab is not as clearly defined as in AAV. HT and asthma are managed with appropriate drugs.

Mepolizumab, a humanized monoclonal antibody to IL-5, is used in patients with severe difficult to control asthma in a dose of 300 mg subcutaneously every 4 weeks.

20.9 Polyarteritis Nodosa

Classic polyarteritis nodosa (PAN or c-PAN) is characterized by necrotizing inflammatory lesions of medium-sized and small muscular arteries. The vasculitis leads to microaneurysms that may rupture with hemorrhage, thrombosis, and consequent organ ischemia. Hepatitis B virus (HBV) used to be an important cause of PAN in the earlier days, accounting for one-third of cases. With the widespread adoption of hepatitis B vaccination, the incidence of HBV-PAN is declining. This vasculitis most commonly affects the skin, joints, peripheral nerves, the gut, and the kidney. The lungs are typically spared. The clinical features include fever, weight loss, skin ulcerations or tender nodules, arthralgias, myalgias, livedo reticularis, testicular pain, mononeuritis multiplex, etc. (Figs. 20.8 and 20.9). ANCA is notably absent, and the urine sediment is bland (cf. MPA) (Table 20.3). Visceral angiograms, including the celiac axis, superior mesenteric artery, and renal arteries, may show aneurysms, stenotic lesions, or occlusions. The smaller lesions can only be picked up by conventional angiography, while computed tomography (CT) or magnetic resonance (MR) angiography can detect larger aneurysms and stenoses. Tissue diagnosis is possible from the skin, sural nerve, and skeletal muscle. Blind biopsies are not recommended.

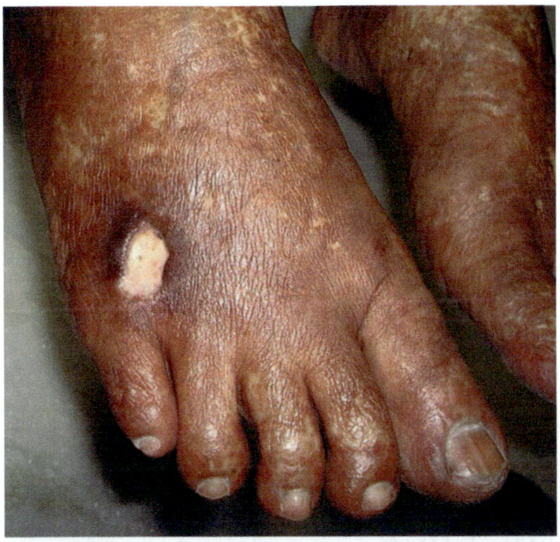

Fig. 20.8 Cutaneous PAN

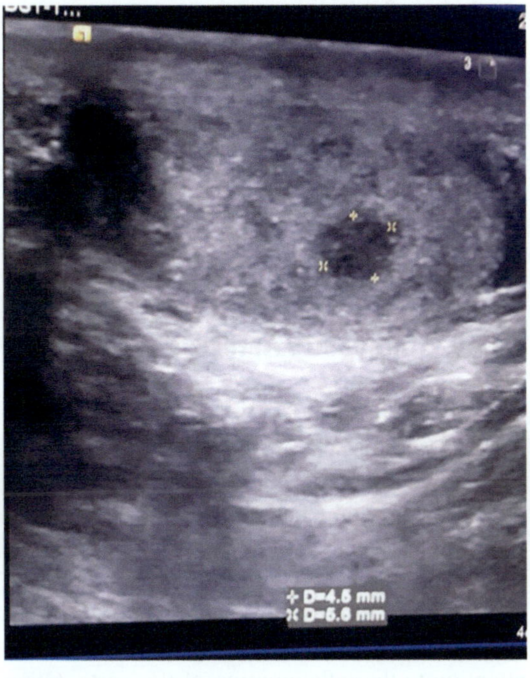

Fig. 20.9 Ultrasound showing testicular infarct in PAN

Patients with mild disease (absence of renal, GI, or neurologic involvement) are treated with steroids with or without azathioprine, methotrexate, or mycophenolate. This includes patients with cutaneous PAN, arthritis, and constitutional features. Patients unable to reduce steroids are offered steroid-sparing drugs early. Cyclophosphamide is employed in moderate to severe disease. Rituximab may be used in refractory disease, although large trial data is not available to guide treatment decisions. The treatment of PAN associated with hepatitis B or C (HBV or HCV) entails the use of antivirals primarily. Patients exhibiting severe vasculitic features are given short-term steroids and plasma exchange until antiviral therapy becomes effective. When vasculitis does not abate with these measures, additional immunosuppression may be considered.

Deficiency of adenosine deaminase 2 (DADA2) is a recently described monogenic

Table 20.3 Differences between polyarteritis nodosa (PAN) and microscopic polyangiitis (MPA)

	Classical PAN	MPA
Vessel size	Medium- and small-sized arteries	Small vessels (capillaries, venules, arterioles)
Frequency	Rare	Common
HbsAg	~30%	Not associated
Renal	Microaneurysms and/or multiple stenoses of renal arteries	Focal segmental necrotizing glomerulonephritis
Urine sediment	Normal	Mostly active
Lung involvement	Rare	Common
ANCA (anti-MPO)	Absent	>90%
Relapse rate	Lesser	More

autoinflammatory disease that can mimic PAN. DADA2 is caused by loss-of-function mutations in the ADA2 (formerly known as CECR1) gene located in the long arm of chromosome 22. Patients with DADA2 present with a wide variety of symptoms, including childhood-onset stroke, systemic inflammation, immunodeficiency, vasculopathy, and hematological defects. Many of these patients were earlier labeled as atypical PAN. TNF inhibitors constitute the mainstay of treatment of this rare syndrome.

20.10 Takayasu's Arteritis

Takayasu's arteritis (TA) is the commonest large vessel vasculitis seen in India. TA affects young people who present mainly with renovascular hypertension. Some patients are picked up in the pre-pulseless stage with nonspecific features like fever, arthralgias, myalgias, high ESR, etc. A computerized tomography (CT) scan of the chest or abdomen done as a workup for fever draws attention to the inflammation of the aorta. Other findings are absent/unequal pulses, blood pressure inequality, and vascular bruits. The clinical spectrum includes but is not limited to claudication, especially upper limb, carotidynia, aortic regurgitation, headaches, visual disturbances, TIAs (transient ischemic attacks), and strokes. Some patients have a monophasic and self-limited course while the majority have a relapsing and remitting course.

The diagnosis is confirmed by CT or MR angiography which are less invasive than conventional angiography, and are the preferred imaging modalities. Angiographic features include focal stenosis or occlusion, with secondary collaterals. Regions of multisegmental dilation alternating with regions of the normal-appearing arterial wall and fusiform aneurysms can occur.

Takayasu arteritis is angiographically divided into six types:

1. Type I—Branches of the aortic arch
2. Type IIa—Ascending aorta, aortic arch, and its branches
3. Type IIb—Type IIa region plus descending thoracic aorta
4. Type III—Thoracic descending aorta, abdominal aorta, renal arteries, or a combination
5. Type IV—Abdominal aorta, renal arteries, or both
6. Type V—Entire aorta and its branches

Disease activity assessment can be quite challenging in the absence of biomarkers. Clinical symptomatology, acute phase reactants (ESR and CRP), and vascular imaging are employed. PET-CT has also been employed as a marker of disease activity. Serial MR angiography is preferred to CT angiography to avoid radiation exposure.

The treatment revolves around the use of corticosteroids along with methotrexate or azathioprine as steroid-sparing agents. Women desirous of conceiving are offered azathioprine. Alternative steroid-sparing agents are MMF and leflunomide. The refractory disease requires biologics. Tocilizumab and TNF inhibitors are employed. Low dose aspirin (75 mg/day) is frequently used in patients with critical stenosis of carotid or vertebral arteries. Antihypertensives are used for hypertension. Endovascular intervention is used to treat stenotic lesions. Aneurysmal disease, severe aortic regurgitation, and aortic coarctation may require surgery. Surgical procedures are best avoided during the active phase of the disease.

20.11 Temporal Arteritis or Giant Cell Arteritis

Giant cell arteritis (GCA) is uncommon but not unknown in Indians. It is a disease of older people characterized by headache, polymyalgia rheumatica, and high ESR/CRP. About 50% of patients with GCA have PMR, while ~15% of individuals with PMR develop GCA. The temporal artery may be visibly dilated and tender. Jaw claudication is an important clue. It results from ischemia of the maxillary artery supplying the masseter muscles. Other features include visual disturbances, headache, neck pain, and scalp tenderness. Some patients have prominent constitutional features like fatigue, malaise, and fever. Vision loss is one of the most important complications in GCA with permanent visual impairment in nearly 20% of patients. Sometimes GCA may cause bilateral blindness. Vision loss in GCA is due to anterior ischemic optic neuropathy (AION) consequent to ischemia of the optic nerve head supplied by the posterior ciliary arteries.

Elevated ESR, CRP, and platelets are characteristic of GCA. Since the ESR is normal in ~10% of patients, a normal ESR does not rule out GCA. The levels of ESR may not correlate with disease severity. CRP has higher sensitivity and specificity than ESR and is relatively unaffected by age and gender.

Superficial temporal artery biopsy (TAB) is the criterion gold standard for diagnosing GCA. A positive TAB has 100% specificity but relatively low sensitivity, which ranges from 15% to 87%. "Skip lesions" may be seen. Therefore, an adequate sample size of 2–3 cm should be obtained. The histological changes on TAB remain positive for as long as 2 weeks after treatment is instituted. Therefore, treatment should not be delayed pending investigations.

Temporal artery ultrasound with or without axillary artery ultrasound is recommended as the imaging modality of choice in patients with suspected GCA. A noncompressible "halo" is highly suggestive of GCA. High-resolution MRI of cranial arteries can detect mural inflammation if ultrasound is not available, or the results are inconclusive.

Corticosteroids are the mainstay of treatment. Treatment is instituted with oral prednisolone 1 mg/KBW/day. For patients with threatened or established visual loss, methylprednisolone pulses 500–1000 mg intravenously daily for 3 days are recommended. GCA responds rather well to steroids, and tapering is started after the initial response. Relapses of disease activity are not uncommon when doses are lowered to less than 20 mg/day. These necessitate an escalation of dose and consideration of steroid-sparing strategies. ESR and CRP are used to track disease activity. Patients with a relapsing disease requiring prolonged or high-dose steroids are given tocilizumab or methotrexate. Subcutaneous tocilizumab has received FDA approval for GCA and may be more effective than methotrexate. The duration of treatment is variable. Attempts to stop steroids are made at the end of 1 year with variable results.

20.12 Henoch–Schonlein Purpura

This IgA vasculitis predominantly affects children and young adults. It is the most frequent vasculitis in childhood. The typical presentation includes palpable purpura, gastrointestinal tract involvement (GI), arthralgia, and glomerulonephritis (Fig. 20.10). Palpable purpura needs to be distinguished from nonpalpable purpura. This can easily be done at the bedside by running the hand over the skin. This distinction helps in the differential diagnosis (Table 20.4). GI involvement assumes the form of abdominal pain, melena, or bloody diarrhea. Arthralgias occur in

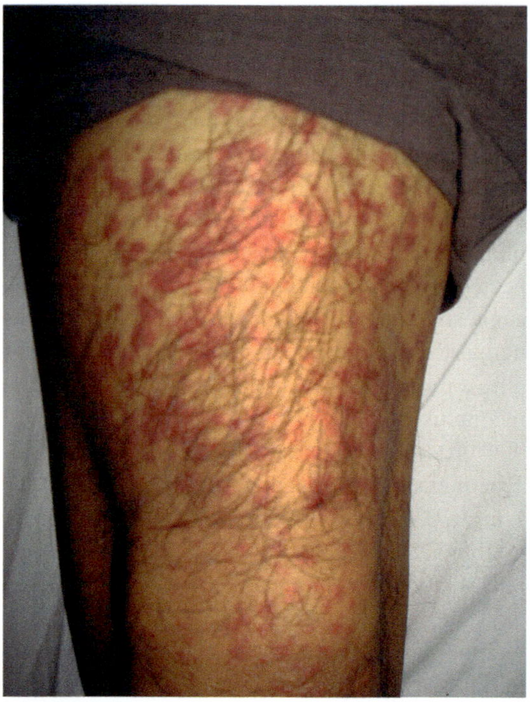

Fig. 20.10 Henoch Scholein Purpura

Table 20.4 Differential diagnosis of purpura

Nonpalpable	Palpable
• Senile • Corticosteroids • Thrombocytopenia	• Vasculitis • Meningococcemia/ gonococcemia • Rickettsial diseases

three-fourths of patients with HSP and are the presenting complaint in approximately one-fourth of the children. The large joints like the knees and ankles are the afflicted. Small joint involvement is unusual. Joint effusions are rare and deformities are unknown. Serum immunoglobulin A (IgA) levels are increased in about 50% of patients during the acute phase. Direct immunofluorescence of skin and kidney biopsies reveals IgA deposits.

In most instances, HSP is a self-limiting condition and does not require treatment. Some patients with severe bowel involvement and rapidly progressive renal failure need steroids and/or cytotoxic drug therapy. Children do better than adults. Less than 1% develop renal complications. Adults have a higher risk of developing significant renal disease.

The initial treatment involves adequate oral hydration and symptomatic treatment of joint and abdominal pain with NSAIDs. Naproxen is widely used in daily doses of 10–20 mg/kg/day. The usual adult dose is 250–500 mg twice daily. Patients not responding to NSAIDs are given steroids (oral prednisolone 1 mg/KBW/day). Sick patients may need intravenous steroids. The prophylactic use of steroids to prevent renal or GI complications is not recommended.

Patients with significant proteinuria (>1 g/day) and/or impaired renal function should be subjected to kidney biopsy. The presence of crescents is a poor prognostic sign. Patients with significant proteinuria, worsening renal function, or crescentic glomerulonephritis on biopsy are treated aggressively with intravenous (IV) methylprednisolone pulses daily for 3–5 days, followed by high-dose oral steroids. Stabilization is followed by a slow taper over 6 months. Angiotensin-converting enzyme (ACE) inhibitors or angiotensin receptor blockers (ARB) are employed to reduce proteinuria. Patients not responding to treatment with steroid alone and evidence of crescentic or proliferative glomerulonephritis are treated with cyclophosphamide or mycophenolate for 6–12 months. There are no large-scale trials to inform treatment decisions.

20.13 Conclusions

The vasculitides represent multisystem diseases with a course ranging from benign skin lesions to rapidly fatal diseases. Considerable overlap exists among the vasculitis syndromes. Often, definite classification into a particular type may not be possible. The physician's endeavor, in such cases, should be to define the extent of involvement and treat accordingly. The disease course is punctuated by remissions and relapses requiring long-term treatment. Drug toxicity, in the long run, becomes as much important as damage due to disease. Rituximab has emerged as an important treatment for induction and maintenance in AAV. In the absence of large, controlled clinical trials, many principles of AAV are extrapolated to other conditions.

Suggested Reading

Bossuyt X, Cohen Tervaert JW, Arimura Y, Blockmans D, Flores-Suárez LF, Guillevin L, et al. Position paper: Revised 2017 international consensus on testing of ANCAs in granulomatosis with polyangiitis and microscopic polyangiitis. Nat Rev Rheumatol. 2017;13:683–92.

Dejaco C, Ramiro S, Duftner C, Besson FL, Bley TA, Blockmans D, et al. EULAR recommendations for the use of imaging in large vessel vasculitis in clinical practice. Ann Rheum Dis. 2018;77:636–43.

Guillevin L, Pagnoux C, Karras A, Khouatra C, Aumaître O, Cohen P, et al. Rituximab versus azathioprine for maintenance in ANCA-associated vasculitis. N Engl J Med. 2014;371:1771–80.

Jennette JC, Falk RJ, Bacon PA, Basu N, Cid MC, Ferrario F, et al. 2012 revised International Chapel Hill Consensus Conference nomenclature of vasculitides. Arthritis Rheum. 2013;65:1.

Walsh M, Merkel PA, Peh CA, Szpirt WM, Puéchal X, Fujimoto S, et al. Plasma exchange and glucocorticoids in severe ANCA-associated vasculitis. N Engl J Med. 2020;382:622–31.

21 Osteoporosis

21.1 Introduction

Osteoporosis is a metabolic bone disease characterized by reduced bone mass and microarchitectural deterioration in bone tissue resulting in increased susceptibility to fragility fractures. Common sites for fragility fractures are the spine, hip, and wrist. The importance of osteoporosis can be gauged by the fact that a woman's lifetime risk of hip fracture equals the combined risk of breast, uterine, and ovarian cancers. The risk of dying from hip fracture equals mortality from breast cancer. Men, too, are at risk as they account for nearly 20–30% of all hip fractures that occur, and one-third of these men do not survive more than a year. The economic consequences of osteoporosis continue to mount as the life span of populations around the world increases. Ideally, osteoporosis should be diagnosed and treated much before the occurrence of complications like fractures.

21.2 Definition

The World Health Organisation (WHO) defines osteoporosis based on bone mass measurement compared to the peak bone mass in a young adult of the same race and sex (T-score). The difference between the patient's value and the norm is expressed in terms of standard deviations (SD) below the mean. Osteopenia is defined as bone mineral density (BMD) between −1 and 2.5 SD below the young adult reference mean. Osteoporosis is BMD −2.5 or more SD below the young adult reference mean. Established or severe osteoporosis is defined as T-score below −2.5 in the presence of one or more fragility fractures. From a clinical standpoint, it is pertinent to mention that the presence of one or more fragility fractures is sufficient to classify a patient as severe osteoporosis even if the BMD is normal.

In general, fracture risk approximately doubles for each −1 SD decrease in T-score. The International Society of Clinical Densitometry (ISCD) position statement while retaining the term "osteopenia" has suggested that "low bone mass" or "low bone density" be preferred. The WHO classification is derived from studies of white postmenopausal women and does not apply to children or premenopausal women. It may also be used for men older than 50 years. The Indian Council for Medical Research carried out a large multicenter study to generate an India-specific database which confirmed data from smaller, single-center studies and showed that Indians have lower BMD than Caucasians.

ISCD recommends the use of Z-scores in premenopausal women, men younger than 50 years, and children. Z-scores compare individual BMD measurements to age-matched reference populations. A Z-score lower than −2 is defined as "below the expected range for age." The diagnosis of osteoporosis in children, adolescents, and men below 50 should not be made on the basis of densitometric criteria alone. Fracture risk assessment is preferred in these groups. The posterior-anterior

R. Handa, *Clinical Rheumatology*, https://doi.org/10.1007/978-981-33-4885-1_21

(PA) spine and total body less head (TBLH) are the preferred skeletal sites for performing bone mineral content (BMC) and areal BMD measurements in most pediatric subjects. The hip is not a preferred measurement site in growing children due to variability in skeletal development.

21.3 Clinical Approach

Osteoporosis typically produces no symptoms. Often the first manifestation is a low impact fracture, defined as a fracture resulting from trauma equal to or less than a fall from standing height. Fractures commonly occur in the distal forearm, vertebrae, and hips, though any bone can be involved. Vertebral crush fractures lead to spinal deformities, kyphosis (Dowager's hump), loss of height, and a protuberant abdomen. Isolated involvement of the upper dorsal vertebrae should arouse suspicion of causes other than osteoporosis. Patients may complain of early satiety due to abdominal compression and breathlessness. Hip fractures are associated with excess mortality and are the most dreaded consequence of osteoporosis.

Baseline investigations in a patient with osteoporosis should include blood counts, renal and liver function tests, serum calcium, phosphorus, alkaline phosphatase, and urinary calcium excretion. In postmenopausal osteoporosis, these hematological and biochemical investigations are within normal limits and serve to rule out secondary causes.

The clinical approach revolves around four issues:

1. Who should be screened for osteoporosis?
2. What should be the screening modality?
3. When should one intervene?
4. How should one intervene?

21.3.1 Who Should Be Screened for Osteoporosis?

Resource constraints do not permit universal screening of all postmenopausal women in most countries. The ISCD recommends screening for osteoporosis in:

- Women aged 65 and older.
- Postmenopausal women under age 65 with risk factors: medical disorders like rheumatoid arthritis, patients on long-term corticosteroids (>3 months), current smoking, thinness (BMI < 21), parents with a history of fragility fracture and previous history of fragility fracture.
- Women during the menopausal transition with clinical risk factors for fracture, such as low body weight, prior fracture, or high-risk medication use.
- Men aged 70 and older.
- Men under age 70 with clinical risk factors for fracture.
- Adults with a fragility fracture.
- Adults with a disease or condition associated with low bone mass or bone loss.
- Adults taking medications associated with low bone mass or bone loss.
- Anyone being considered for pharmacologic therapy.
- Anyone being treated, to monitor treatment effect.
- Anyone not receiving therapy in whom evidence of bone loss would lead to treatment.
- Women discontinuing estrogen should be considered for bone density testing according to the indications listed above.

21.3.2 How Should Screening Be Done?

In the absence of tools to measure bone quality, bone mass has become the surrogate marker used to define osteoporosis. The current gold standard to measure BMD is DXA (dual-energy X-ray absorptiometry). The correct terminology, as approved by ICSD, is DXA, not DEXA. DXA can be used for the lumbar spine, proximal femur, forearm, and even for assessment of total body mineral composition. The radiation risk is negligible.

21.3.2.1 DXA (Dual-Energy X-Ray Absorptiometry)

DXA should ideally be performed at two sites: hip and spine (anteroposterior). The correlation of BMD at different sites is modest, and BMD at a specific site is the best predictor of fracture at that particular site. Osteophytes may interfere with BMD measurement in the AP view in the elderly. Lateral spine DXA, though less precise because accurate positioning is difficult, is less affected by degenerative spinal disease. The lumbar spine is the best site for monitoring response to treatment because of the greater quantity of trabecular bone that is more sensitive to the BMD changes that occur in response to drug treatment. Contraindications for bone densitometry include pregnancy, recent gastrointestinal contrast studies, and radionuclide tests. DXA results may be inaccurate in the presence of osteomalacia, osteoarthritis, vascular calcification, previous fracture, etc. Box 21.1 outlines some important practical points about DXA.

Peripheral DXA (pDXA) can measure BMD at peripheral sites like the heel, phalanges, and forearm. It is recommended that pDXA measurements should be interpreted with device-specific upper and lower thresholds.

DXA is also now utilized to pick up vertebral fractures. Vertebral Fracture Assessment (VFA) refers to densitometric spine imaging performed to detect vertebral fractures simultaneously with BMD measurement. This is important because the vertebral fracture is the most common osteoporotic fracture and often remains undetected. Apart from this, measurements of bone strength that can be obtained by DXA, with appropriate software, include hip structural analysis, trabecular bone scores (TBS), and finite element analysis. TBS is a DXA-derived measurement of bone strength that uses "gray-level texture measurements" from two-dimensional DXA scans of the lumbar spine to derive bone strength parameters.

Quantitative ultrasound (QUS) is an inexpensive modality of measuring BMD. It may provide some idea about bone quality. The parameters measured include speed of sound (SOS) and broadband ultrasound attenuation (BUA) at the calcaneus. Different systems yield different values which are not comparable. The current role of QUS is as a screening procedure. It cannot be used to diagnose osteoporosis or make treatment decisions. Low QUS is an independent risk factor for fracture in postmenopausal women over 65 years of age.

Box 21.1 Practical points about DXA

- DXA machines of different companies differ in calibration.
- An individual patient's bone density reading can differ by as much as 12% when different DXA machines are used. Whenever possible, follow-up measurements for a given patient should use the same scanning procedure and instrument as the original measurement.
- An increase in BMD of at least 3–4% is required as "the least significant difference" that exceeds the measurement error.
- Most treatments lead to an increase in BMD of 1–6% over 3 years. The small magnitude of change in response to treatment necessitates that repeat BMD measurements be spaced relatively far apart, usually 2 years or more.
- Although BMD is useful in guiding decisions to initiate treatment, subsequent changes in BMD do not fully explain reductions in fracture risk.
- Overreliance solely on BMD should be avoided. Fracture protection benefits may be realized even before BMD gains are detected.
- No change in BMD should not be taken to imply that therapy is not working because treatment may have prevented bone loss.

21.3.2.2 Osteoporosis Screening Intervals

Recommendations regarding rescreening are limited. Frequent BMD testing is unlikely to improve fracture prediction. Age and baseline BMD are

Table 21.1 When to repeat DXA?

Clinical setting	Frequency of DXA
Osteoporosis on treatment	Not earlier than 2 years
Osteopenia	2 years
Patients with normal BMD	3–5 years. Recent evidence also suggests that healthy women 67 years and older with normal bone mass may not need additional DXA testing for up to 10 years provided osteoporosis risk factors do not significantly change.

important factors which influence the interval for repeat bone density testing. Table 21.1 summarizes the current thinking.

21.3.2.3 Biochemical Markers of Bone Turnover

These provide an integrated assessment of global disease activity in contrast to DXA, which is regional. Several markers are available. The commonly utilized resorption marker is serum C-terminal telopeptide (S-CTX), and the formation marker is serum carboxy-terminal propeptide of type I collagen (PINP). The important points about biochemical markers of bone turnover (BTMs) are set out in Box 21.2. The urinary markers include CTX, N-telopeptide of type I collagen (NTX), free deoxypyridinoline, free pyridinoline, hydroxyproline, etc.

Box 21.2 Salient facts about biochemical markers of bone turnover

- Usually employed to monitor response to treatment or adherence.
- Do not help in the diagnosis of osteoporosis or the prediction of fracture risk.
- Bone resorption markers decrease relatively faster than bone formation markers.
- Potential advantage is the reduction of the need for repeated BMD measurements.
- Demonstrable fall in these markers may increase patient compliance.
- In general, a decrease of 30% after 3 months of treatment with antiresorptives is considered a treatment response.
- Bone formative agents like teriparatide increase markers of bone formation as well as bone resorption due to the physiological coupling of bone formation with resorption.
- Use in clinical practice limited by high in vivo and assay variability, poor predictive ability in individual patients, and lack of evidence-based thresholds for clinical decision-making.

21.4 Fracture Risk Assessment

Bone densitometry has several limitations apart from availability, cost, and lack of normative reference values. It does not capture bone quality. Therefore, for a clinician fracture risk assessment assumes greater importance than BMD alone. The University of Sheffield has come out with an algorithm for a 10-year absolute fracture risk called FRAX™. This can give a 10-year probability of fracture risk, even if BMD values are not available. Risk factors included in FRAX™ (www.shef.ac.uk/FRAX) are age, sex, glucocorticoid use, secondary osteoporosis, rheumatoid arthritis, family history, prior fragility fracture, low BMI, current smoking, alcohol consumption >3 units/day and femoral neck BMD. Falls were not included as their risk is unlikely to be modified by pharmaceutical intervention. The FRAX algorithms are suitable for men and women between 40 and 90 years. Four FRAX™ assessment models have been constructed: the 10-year probability of hip fracture, with and without BMD at the femoral neck, and the 10-year probability of other osteoporotic fractures, with and without BMD at the femoral neck. Other osteoporotic fractures include the forearm, clinical spine, and humerus. FRAX models are available for several countries, including India. However, treatment decisions have to be individualized based on the fracture risk and are not provided by FRAX™. Other screening tools for predicting fracture include the Osteoporosis Risk

Assessment Instrument (ORAI), Osteoporosis Self-assessment Tool (OST), Osteoporosis Index of Risk (OSIRIS), and Simple Calculated Risk Estimation Score (SCORE).

21.5 Management

Nonpharmacologic treatment involves regular exercise, prevention of falls, and avoidance of tobacco, and moderation of alcohol. The rationale for exercise is different in different age groups. In children and young adults, it helps build bone mass. In patients with osteoporosis, exercise helps maintain bone mass. In the elderly, exercise is important to ensure better neuromuscular coordination, cardiovascular conditioning, and fall prevention. Adequate calcium intake is a must for all postmenopausal women. Dairy products (milk, cheese, yogurt, etc.), nuts, spinach, lettuce, kale, chickpeas, sesame, tofu, sardines are dietary sources of calcium. Those with adequate dietary intake do not need tablets. The usual daily recommendation is 1200 mg daily, along with 800 international units of vitamin D. All calcium preparations in equivalent doses are alike. Calcium carbonate is given with food. In patients without kidney/liver disease, there is no additional advantage of alfacalcidol and calcitriol.

21.5.1 When to Intervene?

Pharmacologic treatment is recommended in:

1. Patients with a history of fragility fracture irrespective of the BMD
2. Osteoporosis defined by BMD T-score ≤ -2.5
3. Osteopenia with a high risk of fracture based on the calculation of the 10-year probability of fracture

21.5.2 How to Intervene- Which Drug for Whom?

The choice of the drug depends on availability, patient preference, safety, cost, physician familiarity, and administration ease. Bisphosphonates are drugs of the first choice because of low cost and long experience (Fig. 21.1). Bisphosphonates in clinical use include alendronate, risedronate, zoledronate, and ibandronate (Table 21.2).

Some patients complain of pains and aches (bone, joint, and/or muscle pain) after starting a bisphosphonate. These may emerge at the start of treatment or may emerge later. These symptoms mostly resolve on drug withdrawal except in rare cases where they may persist even after bisphosphonate discontinuation. Intravenous bisphosphonates may be associated with an acute-phase

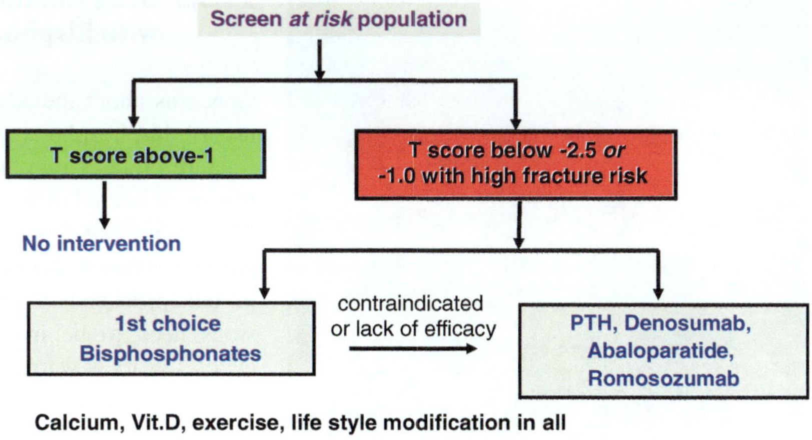

Fig. 21.1 Osteoporosis treatment algorithm

reaction in the first 24–48 h with low-grade fever, myalgias, and arthralgias. Paracetamol is used to alleviate these symptoms. In most patients, a recent fracture should not preclude the use of bisphosphonates, which can be initiated within 2–4 weeks. This may be delayed in patients who cannot sit upright.

Bisphosphonates are not recommended for use in patients with renal dysfunction (creatinine clearance <30). Rare complications of bisphosphonate therapy include osteonecrosis of the jaw (ONJ), atypical femoral fracture, and ocular inflammation. Risk factors for ONJ include cancer and anticancer therapy, dental extractions, dental implants, poorly fitting dentures, preexisting dental disease, smoking, diabetes, and corticosteroids. Good oral hygiene and regular dental care lower the risk of ONJ. Bisphosphonates are discontinued in patients who develop ONJ. There are no firm guidelines on stopping bisphosphonates before planned dental surgery. In general, patients on oral bisphosphonates for less than 4 years without clinical risk factors for developing ONJ may undergo dental extractions and implants without stopping bisphosphonates. For patients with risk factors like steroids or cancer and anticancer therapy, and prolonged use >4 years, bisphosphonates may be withheld 2 months before the dental procedure. Atypical femur fractures (Fig. 21.2) are a rare complication of chronic bisphosphonate therapy. The distinguishing features are listed in Box 21.3.

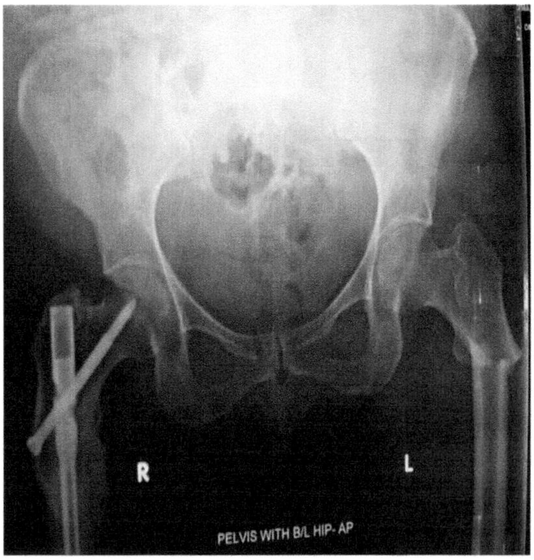

Fig. 21.2 Bisphosphonate induced fracture

Box 21.3 Characteristic features of bisphosphonate-induced atypical fractures

- Patients are younger than the typical femur fracture age group of >65 years.
- Bisphosphonate use longer than 5 years is seen in the majority of cases.
- Typically, minimal or no trauma.
- Frequently preceded by weeks to months of thigh pain.
- Bilateral in 47% of cases, in a similar location.
- Location is subtrochanteric or shaft (diaphyseal) part of the femur.
- Bone density is not severely decreased.
- X-rays show thick cortices, especially on the lateral side.

Ocular complications can rarely be seen with bisphosphonates. These include eye pain (1–2% of patients) or ocular inflammation (conjunctivitis, scleritis, episcleritis, uveitis, etc.) in 0.1–0.2% of patients.

21.5.3 Drug Holiday with Bisphosphonates

Concerns about the adverse effects of long-term use of bisphosphonates and the fact that antifracture efficacy may persist even after stopping treatment has led to the concept of "drug holiday." There is no trial data to determine the duration of a drug holiday and resumption strategy. One suggested approach is listed in Fig. 21.3. These decisions need to be individualized. Reassessment every 2 years is warranted. Progressive bone loss (≥5%) or the rise of bone turnover markers above the normal premenopausal range are sometimes used to aid decision-making. While repeating DXA, care should be taken to use the DXA scanner of the same model and make.

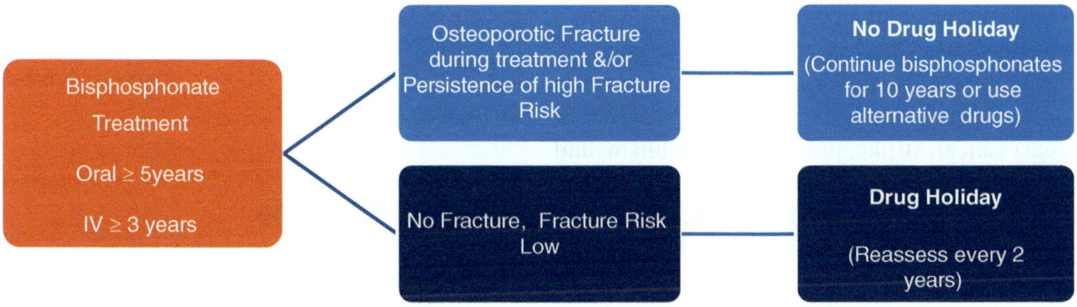

Fig. 21.3 Drug holiday with bisphosphonates

Table 21.2 Drugs used to treat osteoporosis (IV intravenous, SC subcutaneous)

Drug	Dose	Comments
Alendronate	Oral: 35–70 mg once a week	Benefit in vertebral, hip, and nonvertebral fractures. Do not use in chronic kidney disease (CKD; eGFR <30 ml/min), patients with esophageal disorders, patients unable to stay upright for at least 30–60 min
Risedronate	Oral: 35 mg once a week or 150 mg once a month	
Zoledronate	IV: 5 mg once a year for 3–5 years	
Ibandronate	Oral: 150 mg once monthly. IV: 3 mg every 3 months.	Reduction in hip fracture risk has not been established in randomized trials
Teriparatide	SC: 20 mcg once daily. Cumulative use for no more than 24 months in a lifetime	It is used for severe osteoporosis (T-score of ≤ -3.5 even in the absence of fractures, T-score of ≤ -2.5 plus a fragility fracture), patients with intolerance or contraindications to bisphosphonates
Denosumab	SC: 60 mg once in 6 months	Osteoporosis at high risk for fracture. It can be used in CKD. Rebound bone loss on stopping treatment.
Abaloparatide	SC: 80 mcg once daily. Cumulative use for no more than 24 months in a lifetime.	Abaloparatide has been approved in the USA, but registration was denied in Europe on the grounds of concerns about its effectiveness in reducing nonvertebral fractures, and increases in heart rate and palpitations.
Romosozumab	SC: 210 mg once monthly for 12 months	A monoclonal antibody that increases bone formation and decreases bone resorption. Sclerostin inhibitor. May increase the risk of myocardial infarction, stroke, and cardiovascular death. Do not initiate in patients who have had a myocardial infarction or stroke within the preceding year. No dosage adjustment in renal impairment.

21.5.4 Drugs other than Bisphosphonates

Teriparatide is recommended in patients with severe osteoporosis (T-score of ≤ -2.5 plus a fragility fracture) or patients who continue to fracture despite bisphosphonates. Second-line drugs used in select circumstances include denosumab, abaloparatide, and romosozumab (Table 21.2). Denosumab is a treatment option in patients with impaired renal function, patients intolerant or unresponsive to other therapies, or patients where adherence may be an issue. Combination treatment of teriparatide and denosumab has shown encouraging results in clinical trials. Bisphosphonates are not used in combination with anabolic agents. Abaloparatide is a synthetic 34 amino acid peptide analog of human parathyroid hormone-related peptide PTHrP(1-34). It is an osteoanabolic agent with 41% homology to hPTH(1-34) and 76% homology to hPTHrP(1-34). Romosozumab is a second-line drug that increases bone formation as well as reduces bone resorption. It is reserved for patients with multiple fragility fractures intolerant or refractory to other treatments.

Hormone replacement therapy (HRT) relieves menopausal symptoms and reduces hip and vertebral fracture risk but is seldom used for bone protection because of increased risk of breast cancer, stroke, pulmonary embolism, and coronary artery disease. Selective estrogen receptor modulators (SERMs) like raloxifene reduce the risk of breast cancer but increase the risk of deep vein thrombosis, pulmonary embolism, and hot flashes. There is no effect on heart disease or the endometrium. Raloxifene is much more widely used than bazedoxifene. The use of calcitonin has declined steeply because of the availability of more effective drugs and safety concerns. It has an analgesic effect in vertebral fracture. Safety concerns include increased risk of cancers like basal cell carcinoma, prostate carcinoma, liver cancer, etc. Some countries like Canada have withdrawn nasal calcitonin.

21.6 Conclusions

Physician awareness is important for the detection of osteoporosis before the first fracture. BMD determination by DXA is currently the gold standard for diagnosis. Bisphosphonates are the anchor drugs for the treatment of osteoporosis. Recent elucidation of pathophysiologic mechanisms has opened new vistas for novel therapies.

Suggested Reading

Eastell R, Rosen CJ, Black DM, Cheung AM, Murad MH, Shoback D. Pharmacological management of osteoporosis in postmenopausal women: an Endocrine Society Clinical Practice Guideline. J Clin Endocrinol Metab. 2019;104:1595–622.

Fink HA, MacDonald R, Forte ML, Rosebush CE, Ensrud KE, Schousboe JT, et al. Long-term drug therapy and drug discontinuations and holidays for osteoporosis fracture prevention: a systematic review. Ann Intern Med. 2019;171:37–50.

International Society for Clinical Densitometry Official Positions. 2019. https://www.iscd.org/official-positions/2019-iscd-official-positions-adult/

Saag KG, Petersen J, Brandi ML, Karaplis AC, Lorentzon M, Thomas T, et al. Romosozumab or alendronate for fracture prevention in women with osteoporosis. N Engl J Med. 2017;377:1417–27.

Shoback D, Rosen CJ, Black DM, Cheung AM, Murad MH, Eastell R. Pharmacological management of osteoporosis in postmenopausal women: an Endocrine Society Clinical Practice Guideline. J Clin Endocrinol Metab. 2020;105:dgaa048.

World Health Organisation. Assessment of fracture risk and its application to screening for postmenopausal osteoporosis: report of a WHO Study Group. WHO Technical Report Series 843. 1994;1–29.

22 Behcet's Syndrome

22.1 Introduction

Named after Hulusi Behcet, a Turkish dermatologist, this eponymous disease is characterized by a triad of recurrent oral aphthous ulcers, genital ulcers, and uveitis. Other clinical features include skin lesions, arthritis, gastrointestinal involvement, neurologic disease, and vascular disease. Mucocutaneous and ocular disease are more active in the early years, while the vascular and neurologic disease tends to come up later in the disease course. Patients may manifest one or several of these features. Incomplete forms are well known. The disease is common along the ancient silk route extending from east Asia to the Mediterranean. Behcet's syndrome or disease is a variable vessel vasculitis that has a propensity to involve arteries, veins, and capillaries of all sizes (large, medium, and small). There is no gender predilection in Behcet's syndrome (BS) in areas where it is common. However, some publications from North America and northern Europe mention women are affected more than men. The typical age group is young adults (20–40 years).

The classic pathologic lesion in BS is a necrotizing leukocytoclastic obliterative perivasculitis with lymphocytic infiltration. HLA-B51, one of the split antigens of HLA-B5, has been associated with BS in different ethnic groups. HLA-B5101 is the major suballele associated with BS. The prevalence varies, and its contribution to susceptibility is about 20%.

22.2 Clinical Recognition

In the absence of any pathognomic test, the diagnosis of BS is clinical. Recurrent (more than three episodes in 1 year) and painful mucocutaneous ulcers dominate the clinical picture. Oral ulcers are the presenting symptom in the overwhelming majority of patients. The other causes of oral ulcers are listed in Table 22.1. Clues that point toward a diagnosis of BS are outlined in Box 22.1. First to appear, oral ulcers are usually the last to regress in the disease course. The ulcers are painful, demonstrate well-defined borders with a white-yellow necrotic base, and may

Table 22.1 Differential diagnosis of oral aphthous ulcers

Aphthous stomatitis (canker sores)
Rheumatologic diseases/drugs
Systemic lupus erythematosus
Reactive arthritis
Methotrexate
Gastrointestinal diseases
Ulcerative colitis
Crohn's disease
Celiac disease
Infections
Herpes simplex virus (cold sore)
Human immunodeficiency virus
Dermatologic diseases
Pemphigoid
Pemphigus
Lichen planus
Stevens–Johnson syndrome
Deficiency Diseases
Vitamin B12, iron, and folic acid

R. Handa, *Clinical Rheumatology*, https://doi.org/10.1007/978-981-33-4885-1_22

Box 22.1 Clinical pointers toward Behcet's Syndrome in a patient with oral aphthous ulcers

- Concomitant genital ulcers especially scrotal or vulval
- Ocular inflammation especially panuveitis
- Deep vein thrombosis or superficial thrombophlebitis
- Neurologic disease
- Skin lesions like acne, pseudofolliculitis, erythema nodosum
- Arthritis

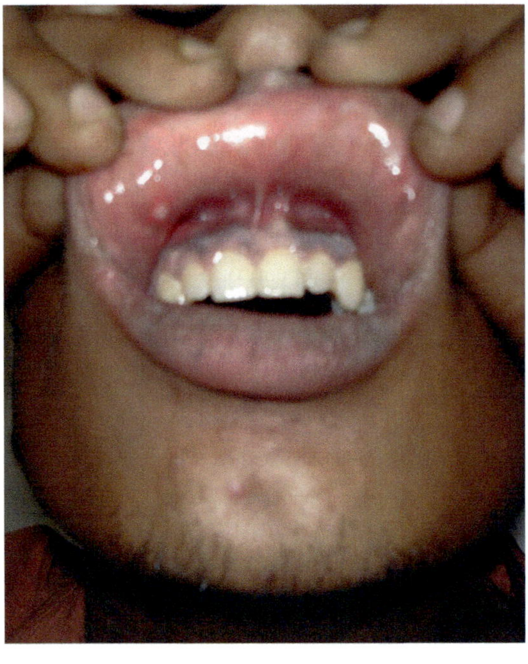

Fig. 22.1 Oral ulcer in Behcet's syndrome

demonstrate surrounding erythema (Fig. 22.1). Ulcers with a diameter of less than 1 cm are termed minor ulcers, and ulcers more than 1 cm in diameter are called major ulcers. Scarring is unusual. While individual ulcers resolve in 1–3 weeks, new lesions come up at other locations. The ulcers are commonly located on the tongue, inner portion of lips, buccal mucosa, and gingiva. The palate, tonsils, and pharynx are less common sites. The outer portions of the lips are spared (cf. Herpes simplex induced herpes labialis or cold sores, where lips are affected). Differentiation from the garden variety of aphthous stomatitis (canker sores) can be difficult. The ulcers tend to be more extensive in BS.

Genital ulcers are less common (~75% patients) than oral ulcers but are more specific. The lesions are painful and typically located on the scrotum in males and the vulva in females. The morphology resembles oral ulcers. However, recurrence is less, and scarring is more as compared to oral ulcers. Post ulcer scrotal scarring in a male patient should arouse suspicion of BS. Apart from the scrotum, ulcers may be sited on the penis (Fig. 22.2). Vaginal ulcers in women are less common and may be painless in contrast to the vulval lesions that are painful.

A variety of skin lesions constitute the dermatologic spectrum of BS. Seen in nearly 75% of patients; these include acneiform lesions, papulovesicular lesions, pustules (Fig. 22.3), pseudofolliculitis, erythema nodosum, pyoderma gangrenosum, superficial thrombophlebitis, purpura, and erythema multiforme. Pathergy (an erythematous papular or pustular response to a local skin injury) is seen in 50–60% of patients. It can come up at the venepuncture site from where blood samples have been taken. At the bedside, it is elicited by pricking the skin with a sterile 20-gauge needle and watching for a pustule or papule that appears in 24–48 h.

Ocular inflammation, encountered in 25–75% of patients, is an important contributor to the morbidity of BS. Males are more likely to get eye disease as compared to females. Uveitis is the predominant feature of ocular BS. Characteristically, it is a panuveitis and bilateral. Isolated anterior uveitis is uncommon. Though episodic, the inflammation may not resolve fully between episodes. Other inflammatory eye lesions include hypopyon (severe anterior uveitis with purulent material in the anterior chamber), posterior uveitis, neovascularization, retinal vasculitis, and optic neuritis. Rare features include conjunctivitis, scleritis, episcleritis, and sicca syndrome. Ocular Behcet's maybe the only sign of disease.

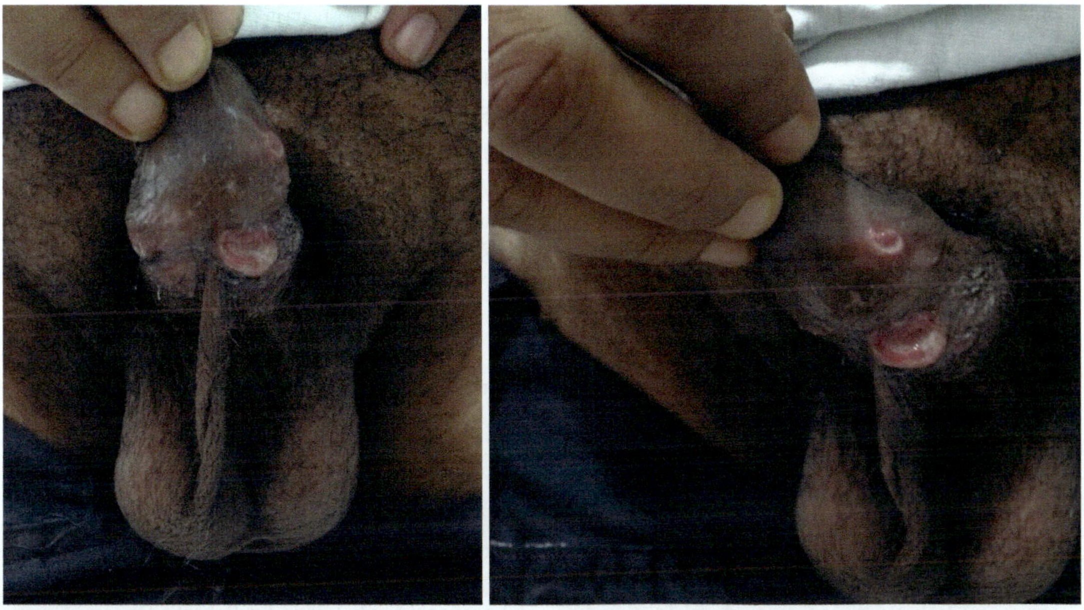

Fig. 22.2 Scrotal and penile lesions in Behcet's syndrome

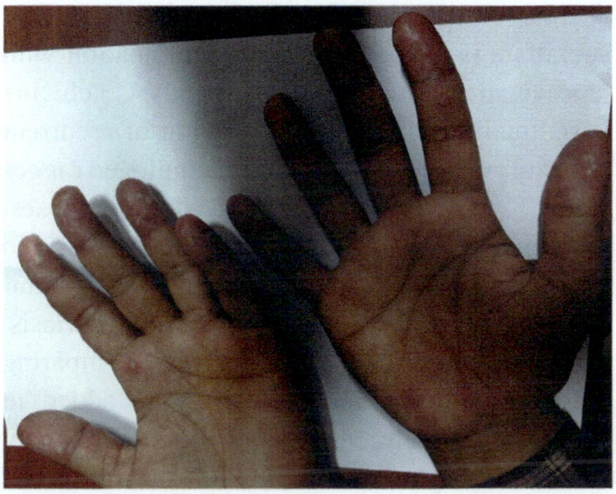

Fig. 22.3 Pustular lesions in Behcet's syndrome

Neurologic disease, like eye disease, is commoner in males and seen in 10% of patients. It assumes two forms: parenchymal or non-parenchymal. The spectrum of neuro-Behcet's is vast. Parenchymal lesions may be seen in the corticospinal tract, brainstem, periventricular white matter, spinal cord, and basal ganglia. Clinical features include encephalopathy, seizures, ischemic strokes, hemisensory loss, and mental changes such as psychosis and cognitive dysfunction. Peripheral neuropathy is rare. Cerebrospinal fluid (CSF) may show increased protein and increased cells. Magnetic resonance imaging (MRI) is the imaging modality of choice for the detection of neuro-Behcet's. Non-parenchymal disease includes cerebral venous thrombosis, intracranial hypertension (pseudotumor cerebri), acute meningitis, and stroke because of arterial thrombosis. Intracranial blood vessels may demonstrate dissection or aneurysms.

Joint involvement, seen in nearly one-half of the patients with BS, may manifest as a nonerosive, asymmetric, nondeforming arthritis of large joints like the knee, ankle, and wrist. Renal disease is rare and manifests with mild proteinuria. Amyloidosis can occur. Symptomatic cardiac disease is uncommon in BS. Acute myocardial infarction due to coronary artery vasculitis is rare. Gastrointestinal (GI) Behcet's presents with abdominal pain, diarrhea, and bleeding due to ulcers mimicking inflammatory bowel disease.

Vascular disease in BS assumes the form of venous thrombosis and arterial disease. Venous disease is more common than arterial involvement and maybe an early feature of BS. The spectrum comprises superficial thrombophlebitis (Fig. 22.4), deep vein thrombosis, superior and

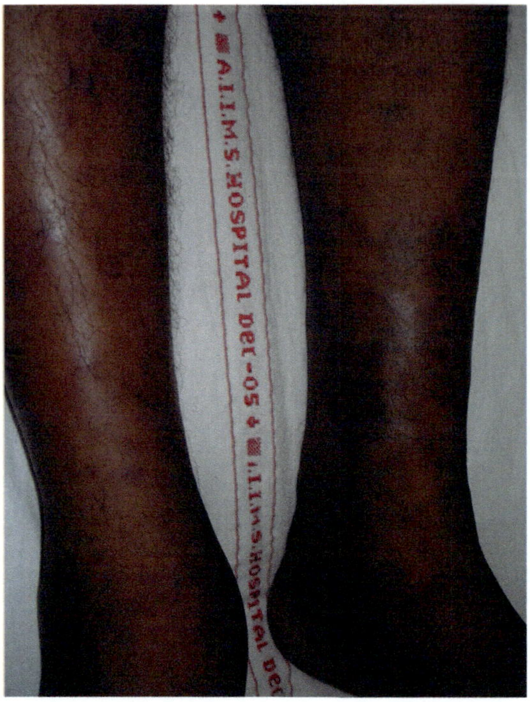

Fig. 22.4 Superficial thrombophlebitis in Behcet's syndrome

inferior vena cava occlusion, Budd–Chiari syndrome, and dural sinus thrombosis. The arteries involved include the carotid, pulmonary, aortic, iliac, femoral, and popliteal arteries. Pulmonary artery aneurysms are characteristic of BS, with hemoptysis being the most common presenting symptom. Other features include cough, dyspnea, fever, and pleuritic chest pain. Misdiagnosis, as pulmonary embolism, is not uncommon.

Several criteria set exist. The International Study Group (ISG) diagnostic criteria published in 1990 (Table 22.2) are widely used. The sensitivity and specificity approximates 95% and 100%, respectively.

Table 22.2 Diagnostic criteria for Behçet's syndrome

Recurrent oral ulceration	Aphthous (idiopathic) ulceration, observed by clinician or patient, with at least three episodes in any 12-month period
PLUS any two of:	
Recurrent genital ulceration	Aphthous ulceration or scarring, observed by clinician or patient
Eye lesions	Anterior or posterior uveitis, cells in vitreous in slit-lamp examination, or retinal vasculitis documented by ophthalmologist
Skin lesions	Erythema nodosum-like lesions observed by clinician or patient; papulopustular skin lesions or pseudofolliculitis with characteristic acneiform nodules observed by clinician
Pathergy test	Interpreted at 24–48 hours by clinician

International Study Group for Behcet's Disease. Criteria for diagnosis of Behcet's disease. Lancet 1990; 335:1078–80

22.3 Treatment

The treatment is governed by the organ involved and the severity of the disease within the affected organ system. Topical corticosteroids are employed for oral and genital ulcers. Topical anesthetics are added for symptom relief. Topical sucralfate is also employed in combination with or as an alternative to topical steroids. Colchicine is routinely used for the prevention of recurrent oral and genital ulcers. The dose employed ranges from 1 to 2 mg/day in two divided doses. Apremilast is used in patients not responding to colchicine—starting dose of 10 mg daily gradually escalated to 30 mg twice daily as in psoriasis. There is no head to head trial data comparing these two drugs. Corticosteroids are added in patients with refractory ulcers or multiple big ulcers, causing severe discomfort. The usual dose is 10 mg/day of prednisolone. The eventual dose and duration are governed by lesion severity. Azathioprine (2–3 mg/KBW/day) and tumor necrosis factor (TNF)-alpha inhibitors like infliximab or adalimumab are reserved for refractory disease. Thalidomide, an effective drug, is infrequently used for mucocutaneous BS because of the fear of neuropathy and teratogenicity. The usual dose is 100 mg/day. Bedtime use may help overcome the sedation associated with thalidomide.

The anterior uveitis of BS is generally treated with topical corticosteroids and mydriatics. Mydriatic eye drops relieve pain due to spasm of papillary muscles and prevent the formation of posterior synechiae. Patients with posterior uveitis and panuveitis are treated upfront with high-dose steroids (1 mg/KBW/day of prednisolone) in combination with azathioprine. Intravenous methylprednisolone pulses are employed for vision-threatening ocular disease. Azathioprine is usually started at 50 mg/day and titrated over 2–4 weeks to a target dose of 2–3 mg/KBW/day. Testing for thiopurine methyltransferase deficiency is recommended. The full effect of azathioprine may become apparent only after 3 months. TNF inhibitors are used in severe recalcitrant cases and refractory disease. Severe eye disease is defined by a sharp drop in visual acuity, retinal vasculitis, or macular involvement. Monoclonal antibodies are preferred over etanercept. There is greater data available with infliximab and adalimumab as compared to golimumab and certolizumab. The efficacy of infliximab and adalimumab is similar. The usual infliximab dose is 5 mg/KBW at 0, 2, 6 weeks, and every 8 weeks after that. Adalimumab is used in a loading dose of 80 mg given once subcutaneously, followed by 40 mg 1 week later, and 40 mg every 2 weeks thereafter. Alternative immunosuppressive agents include cyclosporine, cyclophosphamide, methotrexate, interferon-alpha, mycophenolate, and rituximab. Intravitreal steroid injections are used as adjuncts to systemic treatment.

Venous thrombosis in BS is thought to be due to vascular inflammation rather than a coagulation issue. The primary approach, therefore, involves control of systemic inflammation instead of anticoagulation. Treatment follows the principles of ocular inflammation—steroids in combination with another immunosuppressive agent. If venous thrombotic events occur, anticoagulants are added, like in any deep vein thrombosis. Arterial aneurysms of medium- and large-sized arteries require high-dose glucocorticoids and other immunosuppressives. Cyclophosphamide is often used. Some cases need surgical or interventional radiology treatments as a part of multispecialty care.

The cutaneous lesions are treated with colchicine, and low-dose steroids, if required. Erythema nodosum and pyoderma gangrenosum may require more aggressive treatment. Apart from nonsteroidal anti-inflammatory drugs (NSAIDs), agents useful for arthritis include colchicine, low-dose steroids, methotrexate, azathioprine, and TNF inhibitors. Significant neurologic parenchymal disease is treated with steroids and azathioprine. Other immunosuppressives for neuro-Behcet's include mycophenolate mofetil, methotrexate, and cyclophosphamide. GI ulcerations require systemic steroids (0.5–1 mg/KBW/day of prednisolone) plus azathioprine, with TNF inhibitors reserved for refractory cases. Sulfasalazine is also sometimes employed for GI disease.

The duration of treatment has to be individualized. Once disease activity has abated, the doses are reduced, and maintenance therapy continued for 18–24 months. Some patients require lifelong treatment.

22.4 Conclusions

Behcet's syndrome is an inflammatory condition characterized by oro-genital ulcers and a propensity to involve the eyes in addition to other organs. The disease follows a waxing and waning course with periods of quiescence followed by exacerbations. Treatment depends on the activity and severity of the organs involved. Ocular, neurologic, and large-vessel arterial or venous disease are important contributors to morbidity and mortality. An integrated multidisciplinary approach is necessary to ensure optimal care.

Suggested Reading

Davatchi F, Chams-Davatchi C, Shams H, Shahram F, Nadji A, Akhlaghi M, et al. Behcet's disease: epidemiology, clinical manifestations, and diagnosis. Expert Rev Clin Immunol. 2017;13:57–65.

Hatemi G, Christensen R, Bang D, Bodaghi B, Celik AF, Fortune F, et al. 2018 update of the EULAR recommendations for the management of Behçet's syndrome. Ann Rheum Dis. 2018;77:808–18.

Yazici H, Seyahi E, Hatemi G, Yazici Y. Behçet syndrome: a contemporary view. Nat Rev Rheumatol. 2018;14:107–119. [published correction appears in Nat Rev Rheumatol 2018 Jan 24;14 (2):119].

Soft Tissue Rheumatism and Regional Pain Syndromes

23

23.1 Introduction

Soft tissue rheumatism (STR) is ubiquitous in the community. It is an umbrella term incorporating musculoskeletal disorders that produce pain, swelling, and inflammation in the tissues and structures around a joint. While patients may attribute all pains "around" a joint to arthritis, STR refers to nonarticular pain. The joint per se is not affected. STR may be localized or generalized (Table 23.1). The salient STR entities around the different body regions are outlined in Tables 23.2, 23.3, 23.4, 23.5, 23.6 and 23.7.

These disorders are not associated with systemic signs and symptoms. Some may be self-limiting. In contrast to autoimmune rheumatic diseases like rheumatoid arthritis, vasculitis or lupus, multisystem involvement, and organ-/life-threatening disease are conspicuous by their absence. Despite being "non-serious" in that sense, the symptoms can be quite disconcerting and may adversely impact the quality of life.

Precipitating factors include repetitive strain, physical deconditioning, and occupational overuse. Nonsteroidal anti-inflammatory drugs (NSAIDs) and intralesional corticosteroid injections are invaluable in localized disorders. Generalized disorders like fibromyalgia syndrome (FMS) require a different approach. FMS is discussed separately in Chap. 24 and complex regional pain syndrome (CRPS) in Chap. 25.

Table 23.1 Classification of soft tissue rheumatism

Localized	Generalized
• Tendinitis • Bursitis • Enthesitis • Fasciitis • Epicondylitis • Nerve entrapment • Complex regional pain syndrome (CRPS) • Myofascial pain syndrome	• Fibromyalgia

23.2 Clinical Approach

The key to the diagnosis of STR lies in history and physical examination. For example, pain around the elbow may be due to tennis elbow, golfer's elbow, olecranon bursitis, or elbow arthritis. A careful physical examination can help differentiate between these causes. Arthritis pain tends to be more diffuse and deep-seated, is accompanied by joint swelling and tenderness, and pain increases both on active and passive movements. In STR, the pain is more localized and increases more on active than passive movements. The distinguishing characteristics are also discussed in Chap. 1.

Bone pains (as may be seen with leukemia, infection, osteomalacia, sickle cell anemia, etc.) are usually deep-seated, and tenderness can be elicited by pressing the bone. Growing pains are typically bilateral leg pains in children of 8–12 years and are a diagnosis of exclusion. Muscle

R. Handa, *Clinical Rheumatology*, https://doi.org/10.1007/978-981-33-4885-1_23

Table 23.2 Regional pain syndromes around the shoulder

Shoulder impingement syndrome (Swimmer's Shoulder)
Also known as subacromial impingement syndrome or painful arc syndrome, this is a broad and imprecise term that refers to a clinical condition in which there is difficulty in reaching overhead. Forward elevation of the arm from 60° to 120° may produce a painful arc of movement. Pain may be worse at night. Risk factors include activities like swimming, overhead sports like basketball, painting, lifting, etc. Often associated with supraspinatus tendinitis and rotator cuff injury.
Supraspinatus tendinitis
Patients complain of anterolateral shoulder pain worse at night when the patient rests on the affected side. Abduction is painful. This is often associated with shoulder impingement syndrome.
Rotator cuff syndrome
This is especially common in the elderly. The rotator cuff comprises four muscles—the supraspinatus, infraspinatus, teres minor, and subscapularis. The supraspinatus is commonly affected. Patients with partial tears have weakness in abduction and external rotation. Patients with full-thickness tears cannot initiate shoulder abduction from 0 to 20°.
Bicipital tendinitis
This presents as localized pain and tenderness in the area of the bicipital groove. The pain is aggravated by overhead movements, shoulder extension, and resisted supination or flexion of the forearm.
Adhesive capsulitis (Frozen shoulder)
This is common in diabetes. There is a painful restriction of all active and passive movements of the glenohumeral joint. Shoulder immobilization due to trauma or rotator cuff disease may contribute to the development of adhesive capsulitis. Adhesive capsulitis may be self-limiting with symptoms duration of 1–2 years. Three phases are described: painful inflammatory phase (2–9 months); adhesive phase (4–12 months) when the pain eases, but the shoulder remains frozen; recovery phase when shoulder mobility is regained.

Table 23.3 Regional pain syndromes around the elbow

Olecranon bursitis
Causes include repetitive mild trauma, rheumatoid arthritis, gout, and infection. Patients present with swelling, warmth, and pain over the olecranon process (Fig. 23.1).
Lateral epicondylitis (Tennis Elbow)
Lateral epicondylitis is the most commonly encountered elbow problem. It presents as pain around the lateral epicondyle. Examination reveals tenderness 1–2 cm distal to the lateral epicondyle. Lateral elbow pain can be produced by supination or wrist dorsiflexion against resistance.
Medial epicondylitis (Golfer's Elbow)
Medial epicondylitis presents with a medial elbow and proximal forearm pain that increases with wrist flexion and forearm pronation.

Table 23.4 Regional pain syndromes around the hand and wrist

de Quervain Tenosynovitis (DQT)
Named after Fritz de Quervain, a Swiss surgeon, this condition is characterized by pain at the radial side of the wrist and the base of the thumb during pinch grip, grasping, and lifting. Tendon swelling and tenderness are seen 1–2 cm proximal to the radial styloid (Fig. 23.2). Finklestein test is positive (pain is worsened when the patient positions his thumb inside a closed fist, and ulnar deviates the wrist).
Ganglia
Ganglia are unilocular or multilocular cysts overlying or attached to tendon sheaths and joint capsules (Fig. 23.3). Most ganglia are painless and spontaneous resolution is common.
Carpal tunnel syndrome (CTS)
CTS is due to compression of the median nerve within the carpal tunnel. Common causes include pregnancy, diabetes, hypothyroidism, and rheumatoid arthritis. The typical history is tingling of the first three digits worse at night. Tinel sign (sensation of tingling in the distribution of the nerve produced by tapping over the carpal tunnel) or Phalen sign (tingling caused by 90° wrist flexion) are employed but are insensitive. Electrodiagnostic studies are confirmatory.
Trigger finger
Stenosing digital tenosynovitis or trigger finger results from a nodular thickening or stenosis at the first annular pulley of the digit. The fingers catch or lock in a flexed position and require to be extended manually.
Dupuytren's contracture
This refers to fibroproliferative thickening and shortening of the aponeurotic fascia superficial to the flexor tendons and small muscles of the hand. It starts as a palmar nodule that eventually becomes cord-like and contracts resulting in a contracture of the fingers. Ring and little fingers are the ones most commonly affected, followed by the middle and index finger (Fig. 23.4).

pains, as are seen with statin use, overexertion, vitamin D deficiency, hypothyroidism, etc., tend to be diffuse and poorly localized. Muscle squeeze elicits pain. Contrary to popular perception, inflammatory muscle diseases like dermatomyositis and polymyositis do not cause prominent muscle pains. There can be a significant overlap in various conditions.

Myofascial pain syndrome (MPS) is a regional pain disorder characterized by trigger points within muscles. On palpation, the muscle may give the impression of a taut band with "hyperirritable spots." These points may be exquisitely painful on palpation, and the patient

Table 23.5 Regional pain syndromes around the hip

Piriformis syndrome
This results from compression or irritation of the sciatic nerve by the piriformis muscle. Patients complain of buttock pain, which may radiate down the posterior thigh and lower leg. The pain is aggravated by passive flexion, adduction, and internal rotation of the hip (FAIR test).
Trochanteric bursitis
Patients present with acute or chronic pain over the greater trochanter and the lateral thigh. It is mistaken for hip joint pain, which is characteristically felt in the groin and not laterally. The pain prevents patients from lying on the affected hip.
Iliopectineal (iliopsoas) bursitis
The bursa is located anterior to the hip joint and bursitis causes groin and anterior thigh pain. In order to relieve the pain, patients often position the affected hip in 20–30° flexion.
Ischial (ischiogluteal) bursitis (Weaver's Bottom)
This is caused by prolonged sitting on hard surfaces, especially in thin individuals. Pain radiates down the posterior thigh. Palpation with the hip flexed (this moves the gluteus maximus muscle off the ischial tuberosity) reveals point tenderness.

Table 23.6 Regional pain syndromes around the knee

Anserine bursitis
The bursa is located at the anteromedial portion of the proximal tibia. Anserine bursitis is common in osteoarthritis of the knees.
Iliotibial band syndrome
The presenting complaint is diffuse pain over the lateral aspect of the knee joint, especially after running or cycling. Examination reveals tenderness over the lateral condyle of the femur.
Runner's knee
This is a common term for any of the several conditions that cause pain around the knee cap. Causes include patellofemoral malalignment, chondromalacia patella, and iliotibial band syndrome.
Baker's cyst (Popliteal cyst)
Named after William Morrant Baker, an English surgeon, the eponym refers to a popliteal cyst that results from synovial outpouching into the popliteal fossa in patients with knee effusion (Fig. 23.5). The cyst may rupture and dissect down the calf causing calf pain, swelling, and redness that mimics deep venous thrombosis.
Prepatellar bursitis (Housemaid's Knee)
Colloquially termed Housemaid's Knee, this presents as swelling on the anterior patella (Fig. 23.6). Frequent kneeling for domestic chores is responsible. Other causes are gout and, rarely, infection.

Table 23.7 Regional pain syndromes around the ankle and foot

Posterior tibial tendinitis
A common cause of pain along the inside of the foot and ankle in overweight women over 50 years. May be associated with swelling around the medial malleolus. Most important cause of adult acquired flatfoot. May result in flat foot with valgus deformity.
Achilles tendinitis
It is a typical feature of spondarthritides and is also seen in athletes, ill-fitting footwear, and the elderly. Tenderness and pain occur proximal to the tendon insertion site and are aggravated by dorsiflexion of the foot. Tendon rupture can be detected by the Simmonds–Thompson test (absence of foot plantarflexion on calf compression when the patient lies prone).
Retrocalcaneal bursitis
Posterior heel pain is the presenting complaint. Some women exhibit a swelling (pump bump) due to high-heeled shoes or pumps. Tenderness in retrocalcaneal bursitis is at the sides of the distal Achilles tendon. It is also more proximal than tenderness in Achilles tendinitis, which is located more distally where the tendon inserts into the back of the heel. Both retrocalcaneal bursitis and Achilles tendinitis may coexist (Fig. 23.7). It is to be noted that the retrocalcaneal (subtendinous) bursa is anterior or deep to the tendon and is located between the Achilles tendon and the calcaneus. In contrast, the Achilles bursa is posterior or superficial to the Achilles tendon.
Plantar fasciitis
Plantar fascia extends from the calcaneus to the metatarsal region. Plantar heel pain that is especially prominent with the first few steps on awakening in the morning or after a period of sitting is characteristic. Pain may be aggravated on walking barefoot. There is point tenderness in the region of the medial calcaneal tuberosity. The pain often increases on passive dorsiflexion of the foot. Risk factors include prolonged standing and pes planus.
Tarsal tunnel syndrome
This is due to the posterior tibial nerve entrapment as it passes posterior and inferior to the medial malleolus. Patients complain of burning pain and numbness radiating from the medial malleolus to the plantar heel and sometimes to the distal sole and toes. Symptoms may be aggravated by foot dorsiflexion and eversion.
Morton neuroma
It is an entrapment neuropathy of the interdigital nerves. Common in women wearing high heels and tight-fitting shoes, the typical complaint is a burning pain with paresthesias between the metatarsals and surrounding digits.

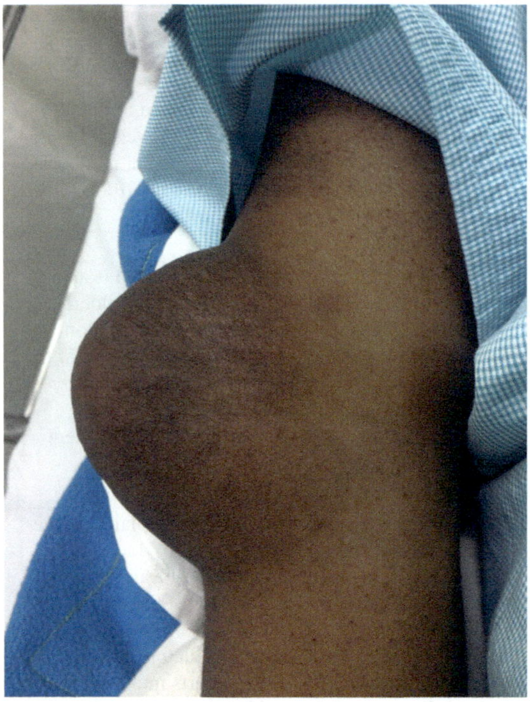

Fig. 23.1 Olecranon bursitis

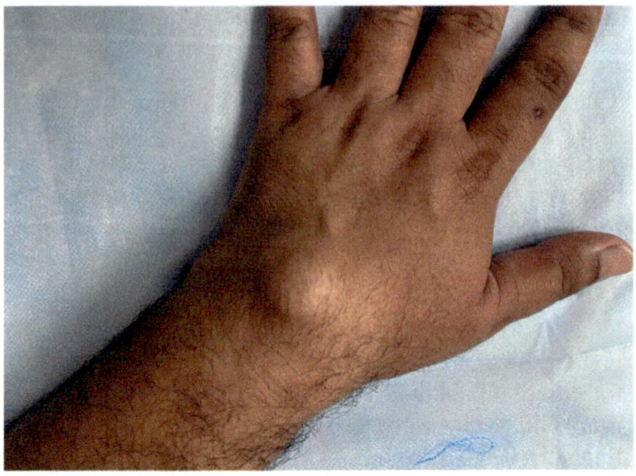

Fig. 23.3 Ganglion

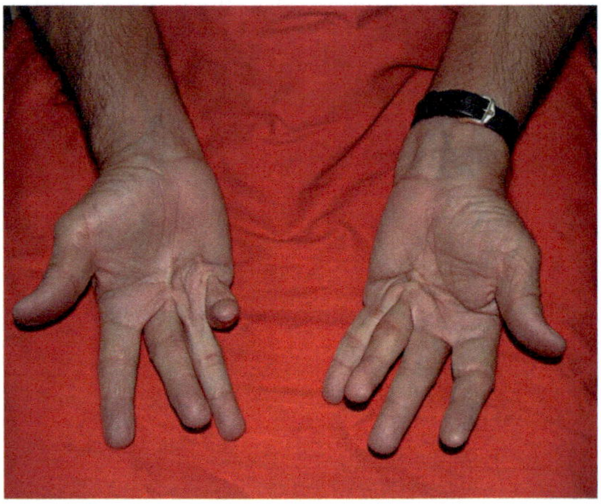

Fig. 23.4 Dupuytren's contracture

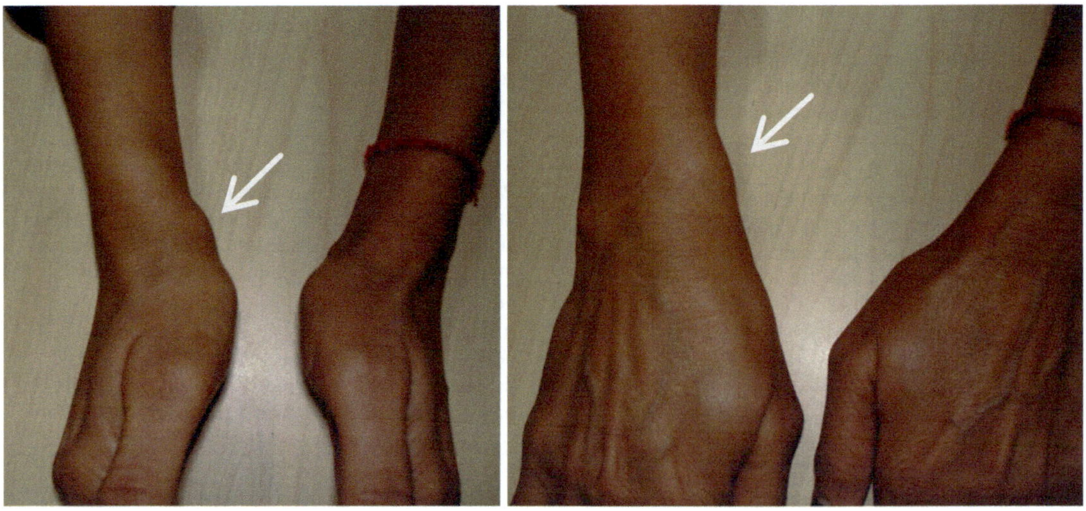

Fig. 23.2 de Quervain's tenosynovitis

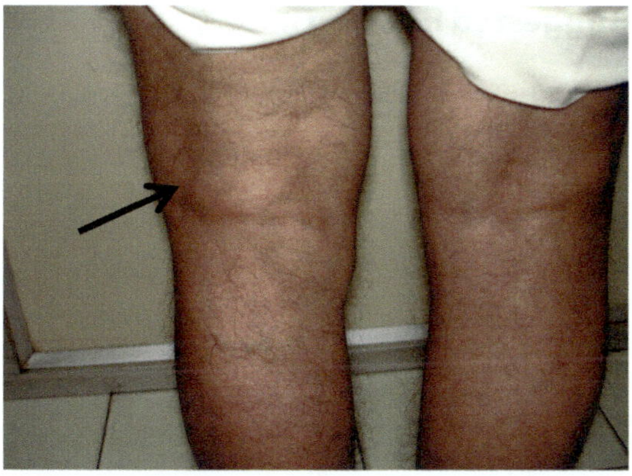

Fig. 23.5 Popliteal cyst

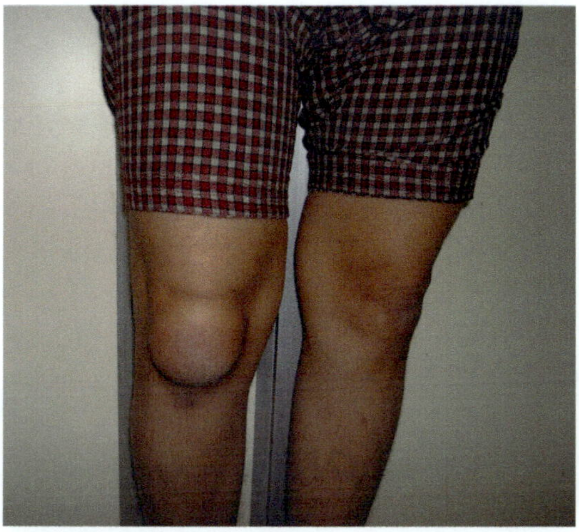

Fig. 23.6 Prepatellar bursitis

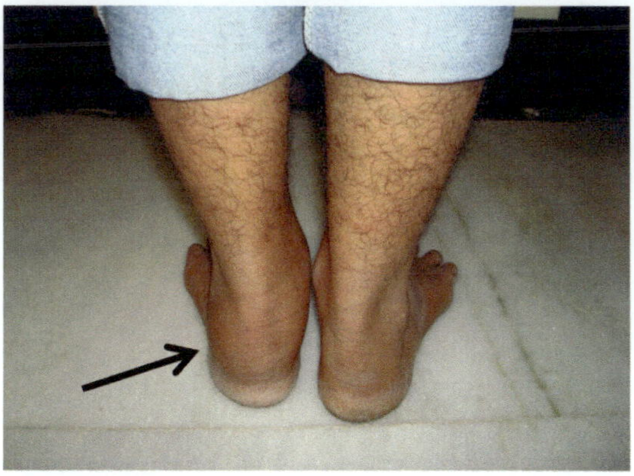

Fig. 23.7 Tendo achilles and retrocalcaneal bursitis

Table 23.8 Differentiation between fibromyalgia and myofascial pain

	Fibromyalgia	Myofascial pain
Pain	Generalized	Localized
Examination	Multiple tender points	Few trigger points
Fatigue, irritable bowel syndrome, non-refreshing sleep	Prominent	Less common

may jump up with pain—"jump sign." Referred pain in the "target zone" some distance away is not uncommon.

On the other hand, fibromyalgia is generalized soft tissue rheumatism with tender points (Table 23.8). Some experts question the difference between the two entities of MPS and FMS.

Laboratory investigations in STR are unremarkable and serve to rule out systemic disease. Imaging may buttress the clinical diagnosis but more often helps rule out sinister causes. For example, radiographs and magnetic resonance imaging (MRI) scans help rule out hip joint pathology in a patient with suspected trochanteric bursitis. In patients with an unequivocal diagnosis, imaging is not required.

23.3 Management

Treatment entails the removal of precipitating factors, exercises, and oral or topical NSAIDs. Local steroid injections are used in bursitis, tendinitis, carpal tunnel syndrome, or MPS.

Heat and cold applications are used in STR. The RICE regimen is employed for acute injuries: Rest, Ice, Compression of injured tissue, and Elevation. Heat is not indicated in acute conditions. It may help pain and muscle spasms in chronic injuries. Other modalities with variable evidence base include acupuncture, therapeutic ultrasound, low-level laser therapy, and botulinum toxin injections. The treatment of FMS has been dealt with separately.

23.4 Conclusions

STR is common in the community. The bedrock of diagnosis is history and physical examination. Accurate identification helps avoid unnecessary laboratory investigations and expensive imaging.

Suggested Reading

Hubbard MJ, Hildebrand BA, Battafarano MM, Battafarano DF. Common soft tissue musculoskeletal pain disorders. Prim Care. 2018;45:289–303.

Fibromyalgia 24

24.1 Introduction

Fibromyalgia syndrome (FMS) is a widely prevalent disorder more common in women and characterized by generalized musculoskeletal pain. Common accompaniments include fatigue, sleep disturbances, and multiple psychiatric symptoms. The etiopathogenesis is unknown. According to current thinking, FMS is a disorder of pain regulation and central sensitization.

24.2 Clinical Recognition

FMS may affect children and adults. The prevalence figures vary, but the striking feature is its commonality. Patients often complain of "hurting all over." The pain is chronic (>3 months) and widespread. It is also called multisite pain (MSP).

The pain is accompanied by other somatic symptoms, notably fatigue and sleep disturbances, as well as psychiatric and cognitive disturbances. The somatic symptomatology includes, but is not confined to, headaches, nonrefreshing sleep, abdominal pain, bloating, bowel irregularity, nausea, and paresthesias. Cognitive problems reported by patients include limited attention span, inability to concentrate, and forgetfulness—"fibro fog." Irritable bowel syndrome (IBS), migraine, anxiety, depression, bladder irritability, and restless leg syndrome commonly coexist. FMS may mimic or coexist with inflammatory rheumatic diseases like rheumatoid arthritis and lupus.

Despite impressive symptomatology, the physical examination is unremarkable except for diffuse soft tissue tenderness. The earlier criteria required the presence of tender points at specific locations. In contrast to rheumatoid arthritis, joint tenderness or swelling is not seen in FMS. Laboratory testing is normal, and acute phase reactants are not elevated. Unless clinically warranted, "autoimmune panels" are to be discouraged. FMS is a symptom-based clinical diagnosis.

24.3 Classification and Diagnostic Criteria for FMS

In the absence of pathognomonic laboratory or imaging findings, the diagnosis of FMS is symptom-based. Several classification criteria have been proposed. The initial 1990 American College of Rheumatology (ACR) classification criteria required symptoms of widespread pain, occurring both above and below the waist and affecting both the right and left sides of the body with the presence of at least 11 of 18 defined tender points. Over years of use, it became apparent that tender point examination was impossible to standardize. Also, these criteria neglected the multiple somatic symptoms in FMS.

R. Handa, *Clinical Rheumatology*, https://doi.org/10.1007/978-981-33-4885-1_24

The subsequent 2010 ACR preliminary diagnostic criteria for FMS do not require a tender point examination and provide a scale for the measurement of the severity of symptoms that are characteristic of FMS. A patient satisfies these diagnostic criteria if the following three conditions are met:

- Widespread pain index (WPI) >7 and symptom severity (SS) scale >5 or WPI 3–6 and SS scale >9.
- Symptoms have been present for at least 3 months.
- Absence of any other disorder that would explain the patient's symptoms.

The WPI is a measure of the number of painful body regions from a defined list of 19 areas. The SS score includes an estimate of the degree of fatigue, waking unrefreshed, cognitive symptoms, and somatic symptoms.

In 2016, the ACR criteria were further modified to stipulate that FMS patients have pain in 4 of 5 regions—termed multisite pain (MSP). This permitted better differentiation from regional pain syndromes.

AAPT criteria—In 2013, the Analgesic, Anesthetic, and Addiction Clinical Trial Translations Innovations Opportunities and Networks (ACTTION) public–private partnership with the US Food and Drug Administration (FDA) and American Pain Society (APS) initiated the ACTTION-APS Pain Taxonomy (AAPT) in an attempt to develop a diagnostic system that would be clinically useful and consistent across chronic pain disorders, including FMS. In 2019, the FMS working group suggested new AAPT diagnostic criteria for FMS:

- MSP defined as ≥6 pain sites out of a total of 9 possible sites (head, left arm, right arm, chest, abdomen, upper back, lower back/buttocks, left leg, right leg).
- Moderate to severe sleep problems or fatigue.
- Both these must have been present for at least 3 months.

According to the AAPT FMS diagnostic criteria, the presence of another pain disorder or related symptoms does not exclude the diagnosis of FMS.

24.4 Management

FMS treatment has to be individualized and multidisciplinary. Patient education and encouragement play a vital role in improving adherence. Nonpharmacologic measures are important. Regular physical activity, weight loss, and sleep hygiene should be advised to all patients. Walking, biking, swimming, tai chi, etc. are recommended based on patient preference. Drugs used include amitriptyline, duloxetine, milnacipran, or pregabalin. The general principle is to start low and go slow (gradual buildup of doses).

The initial amitriptyline dose is 10 mg at bedtime, going up to 25–75 mg/day. Duloxetine doses are 30–60 mg/day. Milnacipran is started at 12.5 mg daily, going up to 50 mg twice daily. Pregabalin may be used in patients with sleep disturbance. Initiation may be with low doses of 75–100 mg, going up to 300–450 mg/day. Gabapentin is started at 100 mg at bedtime, going up to 1200–2400 mg per day in divided doses. Opioids are generally not recommended. Patients refractory to monotherapy may benefit from combination treatment. Patients with persistent symptoms may benefit from referral to specialized facilities for cognitive behavioral therapy, relaxation techniques, biofeedback, and more complex behavioral treatments.

24.5 Conclusions

FMS is a common pain disorder that can be distressing for patients, frustrating for families, and challenging for physicians. The primary problem is altered pain processing. The diagnosis is clinical. Treatment involves a multimodal approach incorporating pharmacologic and nonpharmacologic measures.

Suggested Reading

1. Wolfe F, Smythe HA, Yunus MB, Bennett RM, Bombardier C, Goldenberg DL, et al. The American college of rheumatology 1990 criteria for the classification of fibromyalgia. Report of the multicenter criteria committee. Arthritis Rheum. 1990;33:160–72.
2. Wolfe F, Clauw DJ, Fitzcharles MA, Goldenberg DL, Katz RS, Mease P, et al. The American college of rheumatology preliminary diagnostic criteria for fibromyalgia and measurement of symptom severity. Arthritis Care Res (Hoboken). 2010;62:600–10.
3. Wolfe F, Clauw DJ, Fitzcharles MA, Goldenberg DL, Häuser W, Katz RL, et al. Revisions to the 2010/2011 fibromyalgia diagnostic criteria. Semin Arthritis Rheum. 2016;46:319–29.
4. Arnold LM, Bennett RM, Crofford LJ, Dean LE, Clauw DJ, Goldenberg DL, et al. AAPT diagnostic criteria for fibromyalgia. J Pain. 2019;20:611–28.

25 Complex Regional Pain Syndrome

25.1 Introduction

Complex Regional Pain Syndrome (CRPS) is a regional pain disorder that affects a distal extremity following a fracture, soft tissue injury, or surgery. No inciting event is discernible in 5–10% of patients. The pain is regional and not confined to the distribution of a specific nerve or dermatome. The onset of symptoms is days or weeks after the injury. Uncommonly, it may arise months after the noxious event. The presentation can be quite dramatic, with pain being disproportionate in time or degree to the inciting event's usual course. Unilateral involvement is characteristic (~95% cases). Women are affected more often, and the pain is frequently accompanied by abnormal sensory, motor, sudomotor, vasomotor, or trophic changes.

CRPS is subdivided into two types: CRPS-I and CRPS-II. Individuals without a nerve injury are classified as having CRPS-I (earlier termed as reflex sympathetic dystrophy syndrome—RSDS). CRPS-II (previously known as causalgia) refers to cases in which peripheral nerve injury is present.

Apart from RSDS, other terms used to describe CRPS include algodystrophy, causalgia, Sudeck atrophy, transient osteoporosis, and "shoulder-hand syndrome." The latter refers to upper extremity involvement following a stroke or myocardial infarction.

25.2 Clinical Recognition

The symptomatology includes pain, sensory changes, motor impairment, autonomic dysfunction, and trophic changes in the affected limb—with upper limbs being affected more than lower limbs.

Pain is the defining symptom of CRPS. Adjectives used to describe the pain include burning, stinging, lancinating, or tearing sensation felt deep inside the limb. Sensory abnormalities common in CRPS include, but are not limited to, hyperalgesia, allodynia, hypoesthesia, anesthesia dolorosa, and hyperpathia (Table 25.1). Of note, hyperalgesia is an increased response to a painful stimulus while hyperpathia, on the other hand, is an augmented response to any stimulus.

Table 25.1 Sensory abnormalities in CRPS

Condition	Descriptor
Hyperalgesia	Increased pain from a stimulus that usually provokes pain
Allodynia	Pain due to a stimulus that does not usually provoke pain
Hypoesthesia	Decrease in sensations like touch and temperature
Anesthesia dolorosa	Touch sensation is diminished or lost, but pain is intact—"painful numbness."
Hyperpathia	Abnormally painful reaction to a stimulus

R. Handa, *Clinical Rheumatology*, https://doi.org/10.1007/978-981-33-4885-1_25

Autonomic dysfunction manifests as sudomotor changes (abnormal sweating, sweating asymmetry), edema, and vasomotor instability leading to altered skin color and temperature (Figs. 25.1 and 25.2). The temperature may be reduced or increased giving rise to primarily cold CRPS, primarily warm CRPS, or secondarily cold CRPS. Over a period of time, atrophy of the soft tissues, muscles, and bones can occur. The Budapest criteria are employed to diagnose CRPS (Box 25.1).

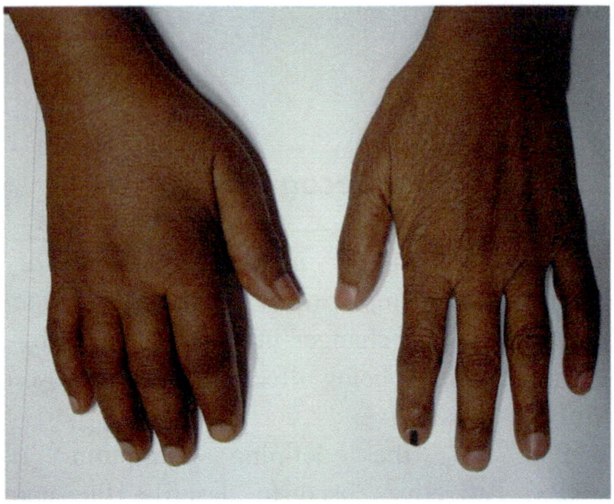

Fig. 25.1 Complex regional pain syndrome (Right Hand)

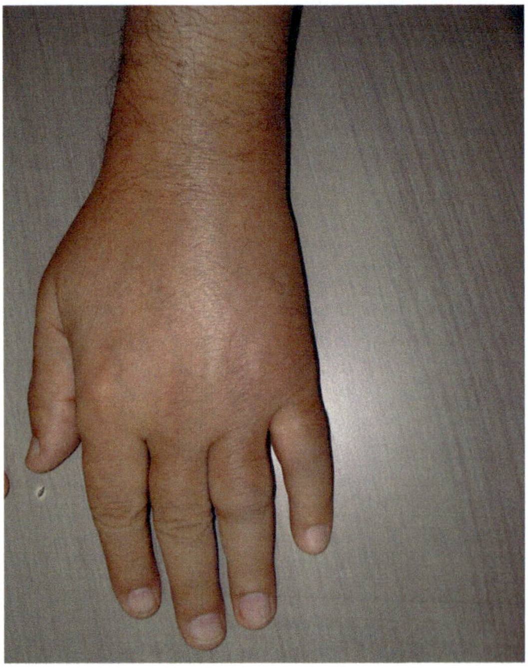

Fig. 25.2 Swelling and color change in complex regional pain syndrome

Box 25.1 Budapest Criteria for CRPS

A clinical diagnosis of CRPS can be made when the following criteria are met:

- Continuing pain that is disproportionate to any inciting event.
- At least one symptom reported in at least three of the following categories:
  - Sensory: Hyperesthesia or allodynia.
  - Vasomotor: Temperature asymmetry, skin color changes, skin color asymmetry.
  - Sudomotor/edema: Edema, sweating changes, or sweating asymmetry.
  - Motor/trophic: Decreased range of motion, motor dysfunction (e.g., weakness, tremor, dystonia), or trophic changes (e.g., hair, nail, skin).
- At least one sign at the time of evaluation in at least two of the following categories:
  - Sensory: Evidence of hyperalgesia (to pinprick), allodynia (to light touch, temperature sensation, deep somatic pressure, or joint movement).
  - Vasomotor: Evidence of temperature asymmetry (>1 °C), skin color changes, or asymmetry.
  - Sudomotor/edema: Evidence of edema, sweating changes, or sweating asymmetry.
  - Motor/trophic: Evidence of decreased range of motion, motor dysfunction (e.g., weakness, tremor, dystonia), or trophic changes (e.g., hair, nail, skin).
- No other diagnosis better explaining the signs and symptoms.

The differential diagnosis of CRPS includes conditions like infection of the skin, muscle, joint, or bone, peripheral vascular disease, compartment syndrome, thoracic outlet syndrome, atypical rheumatoid arthritis, Raynaud's phenomenon, etc.

There are no pathognomonic investigations. Radiographs in chronic stages of CRPS may reveal subperiosteal and trabecular bone resorption, localized bone demineralization, and/or osteoporosis. Three-phase bone scintigraphy is widely used. Herein, imaging is conducted at three time points: blood flow images (during injection), blood pool images (3–5 min after injection), and the delayed (skeletal phase) images 2–5 h after injection. The characteristic findings in CRPS are increased blood flow and blood pool activity due to hyperemia. Delayed images typically display increased periarticular uptake in the small and large joints of the affected limb (Fig. 25.3). These scintigraphic changes are more likely to be seen in the first year of disease and in adults. Pediatric patients may not exhibit these typical changes. Some patients exhibit atypical scintigraphic findings by way of decreased perfusion and decreased uptake. The sensitivity and specificity of the three-phase bone scan approach 90–95% and 80–85%, respectively, in early postfracture CRPS. A normal bone scan does not rule out CRPS.

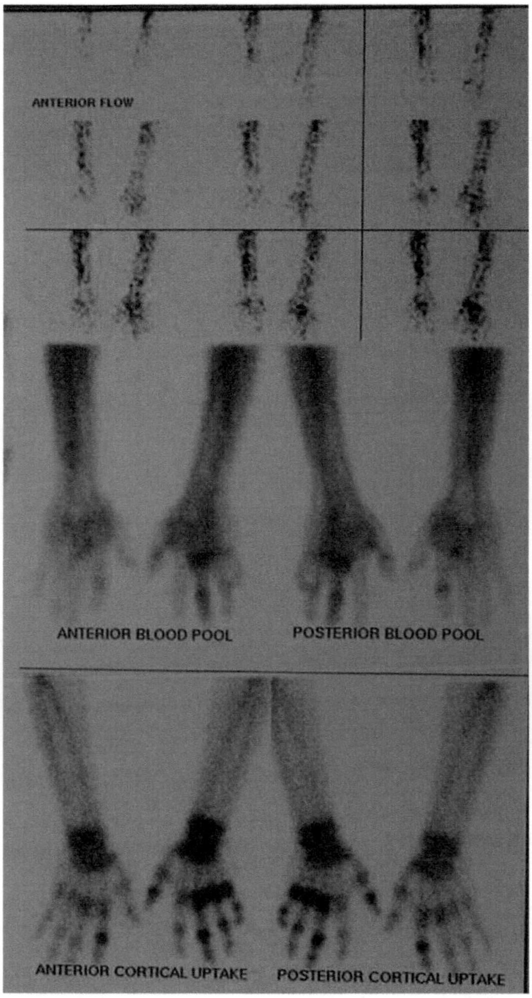

Fig. 25.3 Three phase bone scan in complex regional pain syndrome

25.3 Treatment

Nonsteroidal anti-inflammatory drugs (NSAIDs), amitriptyline, pregabalin, and gabapentin are used for symptom relief. Corticosteroids are widely used in early CRPS. The evidence base is small. Large, randomized, controlled trials are conspicuous by their absence. Oral steroids in the dose range of 20–40 mg daily for 4–12 weeks have been used with variable benefits. Follow-up data is lacking in most studies. Most authors believe that steroids have little/no efficacy in patients with symptoms for more than 6 months. Intranasal calcitonin and bisphosphonates have also been tried. Topical lidocaine and capsaicin, too, find mention as treatment modalities.

25.4 Conclusions

CRPS is a regional pain disorder affecting the extremities wherein the pain is disproportionate in time or degree to the usual course of the precipitating injury. Sensory changes, motor impairment, autonomic symptoms, and trophic changes are common accompaniments of the pain, which typically is not restricted to the anatomical territory of a nerve. NSAIDs, corticosteroids, amitriptyline, pregabalin, gabapentin, and bisphosphonates have been used to treat CRPS with variable results.

Suggested Reading

Harden RN, Bruehl S, Perez RS, Birklein F, Marinus J, Maihofner C, et al. Validation of proposed diagnostic criteria (the "Budapest Criteria") for complex regional pain syndrome. Pain. 2010;150:268–74.

Benign Joint Hypermobility Syndrome

26

26.1 Introduction

Benign Joint Hypermobility Syndrome (BJHS) is a connective tissue disorder characterized by chronic musculoskeletal pain due to hypermobility and greater than normal extensibility of the joints. It is the commonest entity amongst a group of conditions collectively termed "hereditary disorders of connective tissue"—HDCT. The diseases included in HDCT share common features of joint hypermobility, skin hyperextensibility, and tissue fragility and are listed in Fig. 26.1.

Joint hypermobility is extremely common in the general population. It may be limited to isolated joints or be more generalized. The prevalence is more in childhood and adolescence, in females, and Asians. Joint hypermobility without clinical symptomatology is not labeled as BJHS. The clinical label of BJHS requires joint hypermobility along with musculoskeletal symptoms like arthralgias, widespread pain, fatigue, dysautonomia, and gastrointestinal dysmotility. Joint hypermobility is assessed by Beighton's score while the diagnosis of BJHS is based on Brighton criteria.

Many experts believe that BJHS is a mild variant of Ehler–Danlos Syndrome (EDS). It closely resembles EDS type III (hypermobility type)—hEDS, which typically has joint pain, hypermobility, mild extra-articular involvement, and mild skin changes as its features. BJHS and hEDS are phenotypically very similar and difficult to separate clinically. Also, there is no genetic marker

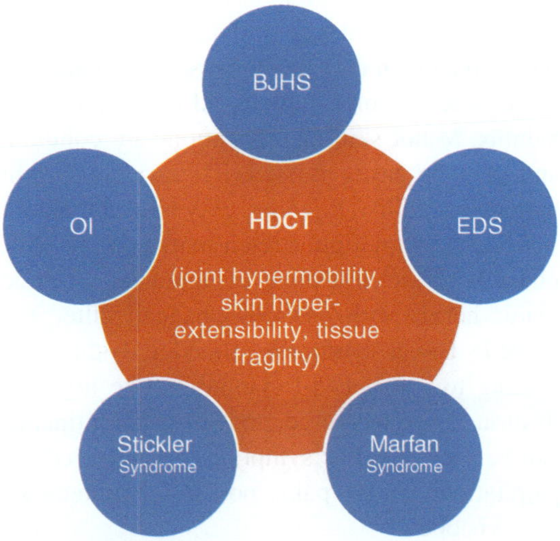

BJHS=Benign Joint Hypermobility Syndrome,
EDS= Ehler Danlos Syndrome,
OI=Osteogenesis Imperfecta

Fig. 26.1 Spectrum of Hereditary Disorders of Connective Tissue (HDCT)

for hEDS. An updated classification and terminology for EDS was published in 2017, which recognizes 13 subtypes of EDS. Stringent criteria were laid down to prevent hEDS from being lumped with BJHS. It has also been proposed that the term BJHS be replaced with the term "hypermobility spectrum disorder"—HSD—to describe those individuals with a hypermobility-related condition who do not fulfill the stringent criteria for hEDS or criteria for another HDCT. It needs emphasis that the term "spectrum" is used

R. Handa, *Clinical Rheumatology*, https://doi.org/10.1007/978-981-33-4885-1_26

to highlight the varied disease presentations in this group and not intended to convey a severity scale. Notwithstanding this, the term BJHS continues to enjoy widespread use.

26.2 Clinical Recognition

The musculoskeletal manifestations of BJHS include joint pains, frequent sprains, and ligament/tendon injuries, and recurrent joint subluxations or dislocations. These may either be spontaneous or result from minor trauma. Patellar displacements are common. Poor proprioception may lead to imbalance and falls. Fatigue with widespread pain may be the presenting feature in some patients. Some patients exhibit a Marfanoid habitus. Minor skin manifestations are common and may be easily missed. These include skin hyperextensibility, thinning, easy bruisability and scarring, and multiple stretch marks (striae atrophicae). Gastrointestinal complaints include hiatus hernia with gastroesophageal reflux and irritable bowel syndrome. Bladder dysfunction leading to a variety of symptoms like urgency, dysuria, frequency, urge, and stress incontinence can be seen. Cardiac symptoms encountered are palpitations, chest pain, postural hypotension, and syncope.

The diagnosis is entirely clinical. There are no confirmatory laboratory or imaging investigations. The Brighton 1998 criteria are employed, which rely upon the Beighton hypermobility score (Tables 26.1 and 26.2). Beighton score assesses hypermobility in the hands, elbows, lumbar spine, and knees. With the exception of the spine, the maneuvers (Fig. 26.2) are performed and scored bilaterally. Hypermobility is a score ≥ 4 out of a total score of 9. While the Beighton score is used to determine joint hypermobility, the Brighton criteria are employed to diagnose BJHS. The diagnosis requires two major criteria or one major and two minor criteria or four minor criteria. Two minor criteria suffice in the presence of an unequivocally affected first-degree relative.

Table 26.1 Beighton score for hypermobility

Maneuver	Right	Left
Passive apposition of the thumb to the volar aspect of the ipsilateral forearm	1	1
Passive hyperextension of fingers, demonstrated by passive dorsiflexion of the fifth metacarpophalangeal joint to at least 90 degrees	1	1
Hyperextension of the elbow to at least 10 degrees	1	1
Hyperextension of the knee to at least 10 degrees	1	1
Flexion of the spine with the placement of the palms flat on the floor without bending the knees	1	

Table 26.2 Brighton criteria for BJHS

Major criteria
1. Beighton score of 4/9 or greater (currently or historically)
2. Arthralgia for longer than 3 months in four or more joints
Minor criteria
1. A Beighton score of 1, 2, or 3/9 if age greater than 50 years
2. Arthralgia for longer than 3 months in one to three joints; back pain for 3 months or more; or spondylosis, spondylolysis, or spondylolisthesis. (the major criterion of arthralgia and this criterion are mutually exclusive).
3. Dislocation or subluxation in more than one joint, or in one joint on more than one occasion
4. Soft tissue rheumatism (e.g., epicondylitis, tenosynovitis, bursitis) in three or more locations
5. Marfanoid habitus
6. Abnormal skin (e.g., striae, hyperextensibility, thin skin, or papyraceous scarring)
7. Eye abnormalities, e.g., drooping eyelids, myopia, or anti-mongoloid slant (a downward slant of the palpebral fissure where the lateral canthus is lower than the medial canthus)
8. Varicose veins, hernia, or uterine/rectal prolapse

The first major and minor criteria (based upon the Beighton score) are mutually exclusive

While a few joints are assessed to determine the Beighton score, it is to be noted that this does not preclude assessment of other symptomatic joints like temporomandibular joints, shoulders, hips, etc. This is akin to the story of 28 joint count in rheumatoid arthritis (RA), which does not

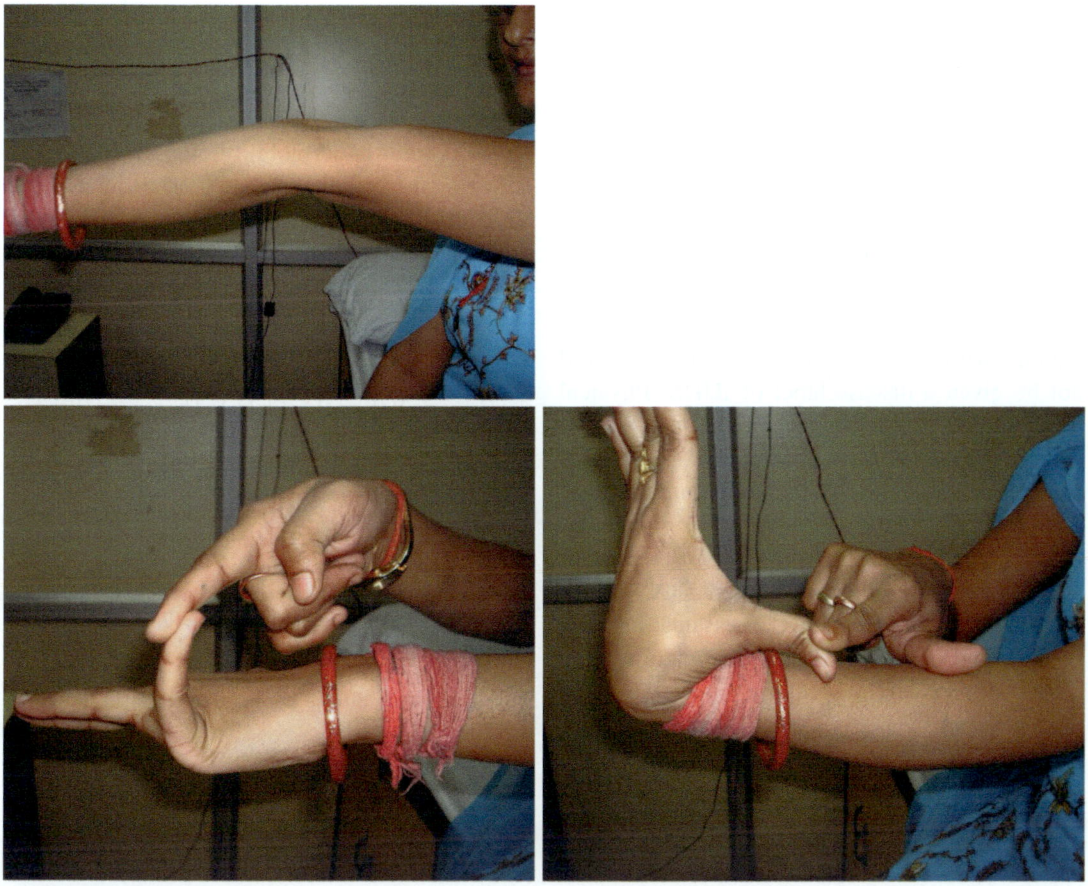

Fig. 26.2 Joint hypermobility

assess small joints of feet for brevity, despite feet being commonly affected in RA. Much in the same way, no hypermobility scoring system can include all joints. At the bedside, all symptomatic joints should be assessed despite not being part of the scoring system.

Patient-reported tools are also available. BJHS is suspected in patients who answer "yes" to two or more questions in a simple five-part questionnaire. This is not easy to administer in the vernacular:

1. Can you now (or could you ever) place your hands flat on the floor without bending your knees?
2. Can you now (or could you ever) bend your thumb to touch your forearm?
3. As a child did you amuse your friends by contorting your body into strange shapes OR could you do splits?
4. As a child or teenager, did your shoulder or kneecap dislocate on more than one occasion?
5. Do you consider yourself double-jointed?

The differential diagnosis of BJHS includes other conditions in the HDCT group. Since Marfanoid habitus is common in BJHS, distinction from Marfan syndrome can be challenging. Both have hypermobility in common. Features unique to Marfan syndrome like scoliosis, kyphosis, dilatation of the aortic root and aortic arch, aortic dissection, ectopia lentis, or dural ectasia, if present, may help in the differential diagnosis.

An ophthalmologic evaluation can be beneficial in addition to investigations like echocardiography and genetic testing for mutations in the fibrillin-1 (FBN1) gene. A consultation with a clinical geneticist may be required in difficult cases.

26.3 Management

Patient education and reassurance are important. Patients with isolated joint hypermobility should not be given a disease label of BJHS. Physical therapy, including exercises, splints, and adaptive devices are the mainstay of treatment. The goal is joint protection, improvement of joint stability and strength, and avoidance of joint injury. Chronic diffuse pain may require paracetamol or nonsteroidal anti-inflammatory drugs (NSAIDs). Some may benefit from antidepressants. Irritable bowel syndrome or bladder dysfunction may need appropriate specialty referral and management.

26.4 Conclusions

BJHS is the commonest disorder among the hereditary disorders of connective tissue. BJHS requires joint hypermobility plus musculoskeletal and other clinical features. The diagnosis is clinical. Physical therapy is the most important treatment available.

Suggested Reading

1. Grahame R, Bird HA, Child A. The revised (Brighton 1998) criteria for the diagnosis of Benign Joint Hypermobility Syndrome (BJHS). J Rheumatol. 2000;27:1777–9.
2. Bloom L, Byers P, Francomano C, Tinkle B, Malfait F; Steering committee of the international consortium on the Ehlers-Danlos syndromes. The international consortium on the Ehlers-Danlos syndromes. Am J Med Genet C Semin Med Genet. 2017;175:5–7.
3. Hakim AJ, Grahame RA. Simple questionnaire to detect hypermobility: an adjunct to the assessment of patients with diffuse musculoskeletal pain. Int J Clin Pract. 2003;57:163–6.

27 Tuberculous and Septic Arthritis

27.1 Introduction

Musculoskeletal (MSK) involvement is seen in 1–3% of all patients with tuberculosis (TB). It is primarily due to reactivation of a secondary focus that is seeded hematogenously during the primary illness. The commonest site of the primary lesion is the lung. Rarely, it could be the lymph nodes or other viscera. The primary lesion may be quiescent or active when MSK tuberculosis is diagnosed. Joints can also be affected by an adjacent focus of tuberculous osteomyelitis eroding through the articular surface. Unlike pyogenic infections, tuberculous joint infection is insidious with a slower rate of progression.

Septic arthritis is a destructive arthritis characterized by the rapid onset of severe joint pain, warmth, and tenderness. The usual patient profile is immunocompromised individuals like diabetics and transplant recipients or patients with prosthetic joints. It is uncommon in normal individuals. Septic arthritis is usually monomicrobial. *Staphylococcus aureus* (including methicillin-resistant *S. aureus*) is the commonest cause of septic arthritis in adults. Patients present with acute onset monoarthritis. The knee is the commonest joint affected.

27.2 Musculoskeletal Tuberculosis (MSK TB)

MSK TB is classified into four main types: (1) tuberculous spondylitis or Pott's spine; (2) TB of the diarthrodial joints; (3) bone TB or tuberculous osteomyelitis; and (4) miscellaneous involvement. Pott's spine constitutes ~50% of all MSK TB, followed by joint TB (~30–35% cases). Soft tissue TB is the least common type of MSK TB. Risk factors for MSK TB include poor socioeconomic status, chronic debilitating conditions like diabetes mellitus, malnutrition, chronic renal failure, cirrhosis of the liver, disseminated malignancy, and glucocorticoid therapy, dialysis, HIV infection, and preexisting joint diseases like rheumatoid arthritis. *Mycobacterium tuberculosis* is the most common cause of MSK TB worldwide. With the advent of the HIV pandemic, atypical mycobacteria esp. *M. kansasii* is increasingly seen. Such infections tend to affect synovial sheath more often than the osseous tissue.

R. Handa, *Clinical Rheumatology*, https://doi.org/10.1007/978-981-33-4885-1_27

27.2.1 Clinical Recognition of MSK TB

Tuberculous spondylitis commonly affects the lower thoracic and upper lumbar vertebrae. The involvement of the cervical and upper thoracic spine is less common. Patients complain of back pain with or without constitutional features. The infection starts at the anterior aspect of intervertebral joints and spreads behind the anterior ligament to involve the adjacent vertebral bodies. Subsequently, the infection involves the intervertebral disc space. Disc involvement occurs earlier in bacterial vertebral osteomyelitis as compared to TB. The characteristic features of spinal tuberculosis are vertebral body destruction, narrowing of intervertebral disk space, and paraspinal abscess. The intervertebral disc is usually spared in metastatic spinal lesions, and this is an important differentiating point from TB. Vertebral collapse may result in gibbus deformity and paraplegia due to cord compression.

Tuberculous joint involvement is usually monoarticular. Large weight-bearing joints like hip, knee, and shoulder are affected. Other joints that can be affected include sacroiliac, elbow, ankle, carpal, and tarsal joints. The involvement of small joints is uncommon but not unknown. Occasionally multiple joints may be affected. Prosthetic joints, too, may get infected with *M. tuberculosis*. These patients generally have a favorable outcome after standard antituberculous chemotherapy, even if the joint prosthesis is not removed. Initially, the infected joint exhibits synovial inflammation and swelling with restriction in the range of movement. Muscle spasm (splinting phenomenon) may contribute to this restricted movement. Plain X-rays exhibit increased joint space at this initial stage. Disease progression results in cartilage loss, lytic bone lesions, fibrous ankylosis of joint with reduced joint space, and degenerative changes. Cold abscesses and fistulae may form in untreated cases.

Bone involvement in TB affects the long bones (femur, tibia, and ulna). Short bones (e.g., phalanges—TB dactylitis) or small bones (carpals, tarsals) may also be affected especially in children. Soft tissue TB (bursitis, tenosynovitis, myositis, or fasciitis) is rare. Panniculitis is nonsuppurative inflammation in subcutaneous fat (panniculus). Two types are encountered in the setting of TB: erythema nodosum (EN), a form of septal panniculitis without vasculitis, and erythema induratum (EI), a lobular panniculitis associated with vasculitis of medium- or small-sized blood vessels. EI, also sometimes termed as "nodular vasculitis," may be seen on the calves while EN lesions are more on the shins (Fig. 27.1).

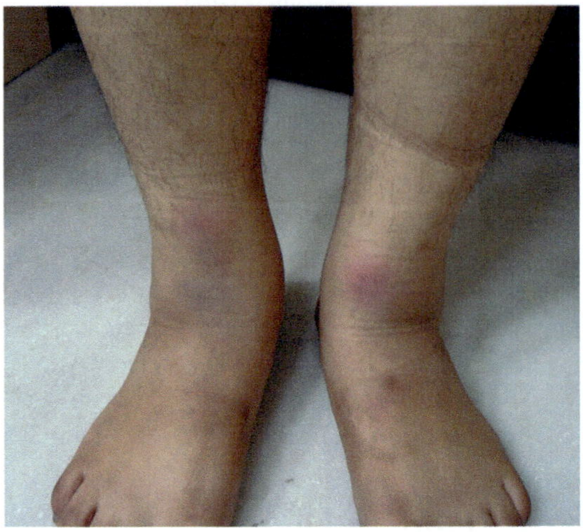

Fig. 27.1 Erythema nodosum in a patient with Lymph node TB

Poncet's disease or tubercular rheumatism is a nondestructive oligo- or polyarticular peripheral joint disease in the setting of active TB at a distant site. Mycobacteria are not demonstrable in the joint tissue, and no other cause of the joint disease can be established. It is thought to be a reactive (para-infectious) phenomenon and considered a diagnosis of exclusion. The disease subsides completely on antituberculous therapy without any complications.

27.2.2 Diagnosis of MSK TB

A high index of suspicion is required, especially in non-endemic areas. Synovial fluid findings are nonspecific and include raised protein, increased leukocyte count, and low levels of synovial fluid glucose. Radiographic evidence of pulmonary TB can be demonstrated in <50% of patients. Imaging findings are only "suggestive" and not diagnostic of MSK TB. Radiographic features of Pott's spine include involvement of >2 vertebral bodies, predominant involvement adjacent to endplates of vertebrae, intervertebral disc space narrowing, paravertebral abscess, bone fragments, and sub-ligamentous spread. MRI can pick up early lesions. "Phemister's triad" is considered typical of joint tuberculosis: (1) juxta-articular osteoporosis; (2) peripherally located osseous erosions; and (3) gradual narrowing of the joint space. Figure 27.2 reveals erosions in the shoulder joint.

The gold standard of MSK TB diagnosis is histopathological and/or microbiological confirmation of TB. Synovial fluid smear for AFB is positive in 20–40% of cases, while culture could yield a positive result in up to 80% cases. The yield of synovial biopsy approximates 90%. Xpert MTB/RIF, a commercially available diagnostic test for *M. tuberculosis* complex (MTB), that utilizes polymerase chain reaction (PCR) to test specimens for genetic material specific to MTB, and also detects a gene which confers resistance to rifampicin, *rpoB* is endorsed for the detection of pulmonary tuberculosis. A recent Cochrane review reported pooled Xpert sensitivity and specificity (defined by culture) of >80% and 82% in bone or joint fluid and tissue.

27.2.3 Treatment of MSK TB

The optimal duration of therapy for MSK TB is uncertain. Indian guidelines recommend that all patients with MSK TB should be treated with a 2-month intensive phase consisting of four drugs (isoniazid, rifampicin, pyrazinamide, and ethambutol), followed by a continuation phase lasting 10–16 months, consisting of three drugs (isoniazid, rifampicin, and ethambutol) depending on the site of disease and the patient's clinical course (i.e., the 2RHZE/10RHE regimen). The total treatment duration should be at least 12 months (extendable to 16–18 months on a case-by-case basis). While some patients with bone and joint TB require surgical intervention, most can achieve satisfactory recovery with medical treatment alone, especially if diagnosed and treated early in the disease course. Surgical aspects are beyond the purview of this chapter.

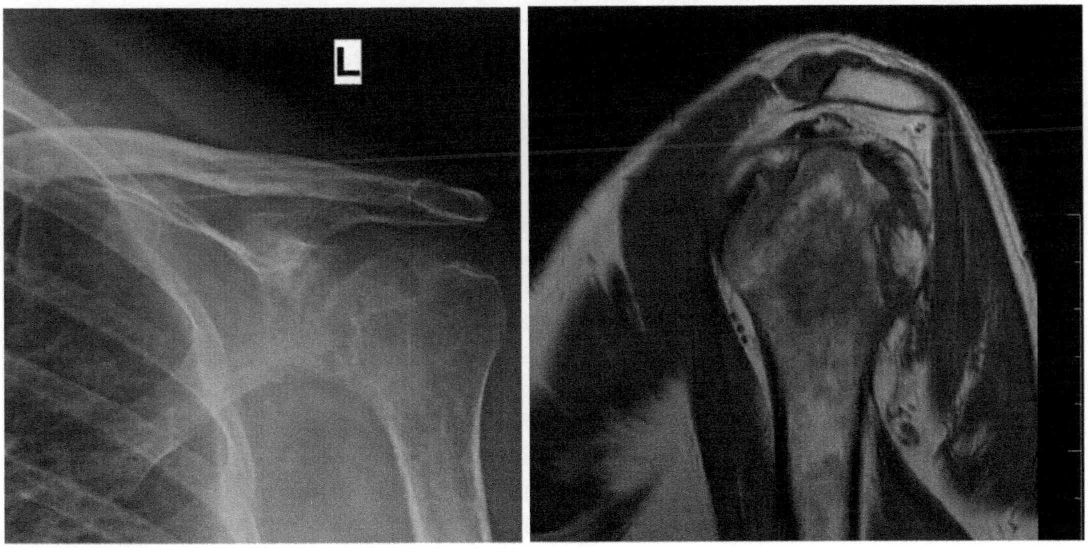

Fig. 27.2 Shoulder Joint TB. Courtesy: Dr. Sundeep Upadhyay

27.3 Septic Arthritis

The typical clinical presentation is a rapid onset of severe joint pain, warmth, and tenderness in a single joint. Large joints like the knee and hip are commonly involved. Polyarticular involvement is seen in 10–15% of patients. Elderly patients may not manifest fever or other signs of inflammation. *Staph. aureus* (including methicillin-resistant *Staph. aureus*) is the commonest organism followed by streptococcal species, Gram-negative organisms, and anaerobes. Gram-negative bacilli, including Pseudomonas, are seen in older patients and immunosuppressed patients. Gonococcal infections should be suspected in sexually active patients. The classical triad of disseminated gonococcal infection (DGI) comprises acute tenosynovitis, dermatitis, and arthritis. Tenosynovitis is most common over the dorsum of hands and wrists. In contrast, septic arthritis in DGI commonly affects the knee, ankle, wrist, and elbow in descending order of frequency. Maculopapular skin lesions are typical of DGI. Local genitourinary lesions are unusual in DGI.

The predisposing factors are age, preexisting joint disease like RA or OA, recent joint surgery or injection, intravenous drug use, diabetes, and other immunocompromised states. Polymicrobial septic arthritis is uncommon and usually follows penetrating trauma.

27.3.1 Clinical Approach

Joint aspiration is mandatory in patients with suspected septic arthritis. Since the mainstay of diagnosis is synovial fluid analysis, a definitive diagnosis can be made in the presence of positive synovial fluid Gram stain and/or culture. A presumptive diagnosis of septic arthritis is made when the synovial fluid is purulent and has a high leukocyte count, but synovial fluid cultures are negative. Gram stain is positive in 30–50% cases, while synovial fluid culture is positive in two-thirds of patients with nongonococcal bacterial arthritis. Negative synovial fluid cultures are the result of recent antibiotics or infection with a fastidious organism. Blood cultures may be positive in one-third to one-half of the cases. Plain radiographs, especially in the early stage, are normal. CT or MRI are helpful in the detection of bone and joint lesions and effusion.

27.3.2 Management of Septic Arthritis

Joint drainage is mandatory to drain the intraarticular pus. This can be achieved by large-bore needle aspiration or by arthroscopy. Surgical arthrotomy (open drainage) is usually required for septic hips/shoulders, if osteomyelitis coexists with septic arthritis and if the joint infection is not controlled by 5–7 days of needle/arthroscopic drainage.

Antibiotic selection depends on the results of Gram stain and culture. If the initial Gram stain of synovial fluid demonstrates Gram-positive cocci, intravenous vancomycin is started 15 mg/kg/dose every 12 h. Patients where synovial fluid culture shows methicillin-susceptible *S. aureus* are treated with a beta-lactam agent such as cefazolin (2 g IV every 8 h) or oxacillin (2 g IV every 4 h) or flucloxacillin (2 g IV every 6 h). If culture grows methicillin-resistant *S. aureus* preferred antibiotics are vancomycin (1 g IV every 12 h) or linezolid (600 mg oral or IV twice daily) or clindamycin (600 mg oral or IV three times daily).

Gram-negative bacilli are treated with cephalosporins viz. ceftriaxone (2 g IV once daily) or cefotaxime (1–2 g IV every 8 h) or ceftazidime (1–2 g IV every 8 h) or cefepime (1–2 g IV every 8–12 h). If *Pseudomonas aeruginosa* is suspected a combination of a cephalosporin with ciprofloxacin or an aminoglycoside is used. If Gram stain and culture are unrevealing, vancomycin is used in immunocompetent patients and vancomycin plus a cephalosporin in immunocompromised patients and patients with underlying trauma.

Antibiotics need to be given for 2 weeks parenterally followed by 2–6 weeks of oral therapy depending on clinical response.

27.4 Conclusions

Joint infections can be due to TB or septic arthritis. Synovial fluid analysis is essential and helps guide treatment. Medical management constitutes the mainstay of the treatment of joint TB. Some patients do require orthopedic intervention. Septic arthritis requires joint drainage with adequate antibiotics.

Suggested Reading

1. Kohli M, Schiller I, Dendukuri N, et al. Xpert® MTB/RIF assay for extrapulmonary tuberculosis and rifampicin resistance. Cochrane Database Syst Rev. 2018 Aug 27;8:CD012768.
2. Ministry of Health and Family Welfare. Index-TB Guidelines: guidelines on extrapulmonary tuberculosis for India. Central TB Division: World Health Organization Country Office for India. 2016; Available from: http://www.icmr.nic.in/guidelines/TB/Index-TB%20Guidelines%20-%20green%20colour%202594164.pdf. Accessed 10 January 2020.
3. Sharma SK, Ryan H, Khaparde S, et al. Index-TB guidelines: Guidelines on extrapulmonary tuberculosis for India. Indian J Med Res. 2017;145:448–63.

28 Viral Arthritis

28.1 Introduction

Viral arthritides are an important cause of acute polyarthritis, accounting for nearly 1% of such cases. The etiology varies according to the geographic location. Chikungunya, dengue, hepatitis B, and C, HIV, and parvovirus B19 are some well-known viral arthritides. The incidence of rubella arthritis has declined due to widespread vaccination. Arboviruses (ARthropod-BOrne viruses) are viruses transmitted by mosquitoes. Of these, Chikungunya belongs to the alphavirus genus of the Togaviridae family while dengue, Zika, and hepatitis C are part of the Flaviviridae family. In general, viral arthritides are self-limiting, and the treatment is symptomatic.

28.2 Chikungunya Arthritis

The chikungunya virus (CHIKV) was first identified in 1952–1953 during an outbreak in the Makonde plateau in the southern region of Tanzania bordering Mozambique. Etymologically, the word Chikungunya is derived from a Makonde word "that which bends up" describing the bent posture of persons with severe joint pains caused by this disease.

CHIKV is a single-stranded, positive-sense RNA virus with four genotypes based on E1 envelope glycoprotein sequence:

1. East Central South African (ECSA).
2. West African.
3. ECSA-diverged or Indian Ocean Lineage (IOL).
4. Asian lineage.

The two important vectors are *Aedes aegypti* and *Aedes albopictus* (Asian Tiger mosquito). The former is confined to tropical and subtropical regions, while *A. albopictus* has a wider distribution that includes temperate areas. CHIKV is spread by the bite of infected female Aedes mosquito. *Aedes aegypti* is a particularly efficient vector because it feeds preferentially on human blood, is capable of biting several people in a short period for one blood meal, is a daytime feeder, has a bite that is almost imperceptible, and is well adapted to life in urban settings.

Several factors have contributed to the spread of CHIV in nontropical areas (Fig. 28.1). An adaptive point mutation with substitution of alanine to valine at position 226 of the E1 envelope glycoprotein (E1-A226V) has enhanced both virus replication and transmission efficacy in *A.*

R. Handa, *Clinical Rheumatology*, https://doi.org/10.1007/978-981-33-4885-1_28

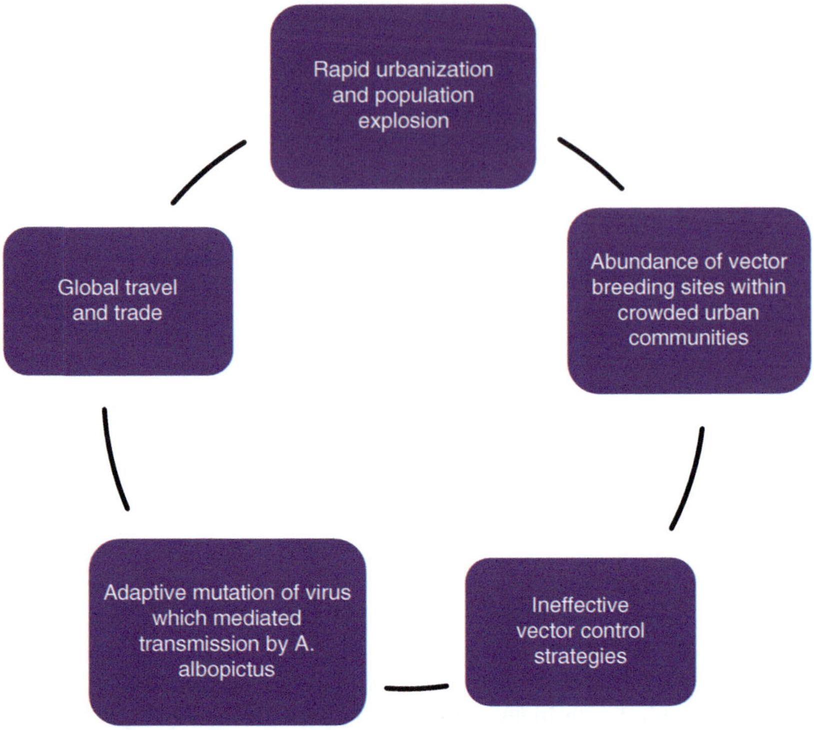

Fig. 28.1 Factors contributing to spread of Chikungunya

albopictus. It was responsible for >90% of viral sequences in the Indian Ocean outbreaks. It is to be noted that in Europe and the USA, the cases could be imported due to travel or autochthonous where *A. albopictus* serves as the vector.

28.2.1 Clinical Features of Chikungunya

Nearly 15% of infections are asymptomatic. The mean incubation period is 3 days. Patients report the abrupt onset of high fever (>39 °C) with severe arthralgias, myalgias, and an erythematous, maculopapular rash. The rash can be mild and localized or extensive, involving more than 90% of the skin. The rash and fever usually resolve within a few days. Less common features include conjunctivitis, uveitis, episcleritis, retinitis, encephalitis, myocarditis, hepatitis, and multi-organ failure. Hemorrhagic features are uncommon and should alert the clinician to an alternate diagnosis like dengue. The clinical course is arbitrarily divided by some authorities into three stages: acute stage (Day 1–Day 21); post-acute stage (from D21 to the end of the third month), and chronic stage (after 3 months). The post-acute stage and chronic stage are not observed in all patients.

28.2.2 Rheumatologic Spectrum of Chikungunya

In acute CHIKV infection, the joint pains are usually symmetric and involve large and small joints of both upper and lower limbs. The spine can be affected. The patients may bend up in pain and have difficulty in straightening. Periarticular edema may be seen around interphalangeal joints, wrists, and ankles (Fig. 28.2). Entheseal pains can occur.

While many patients may present with acute symptoms to rheumatologists, the bulk present to family physicians and general practitioners. The major rheumatologic impact is due to the propensity of musculoskeletal symptoms to persist in a substantial number of patients. A study of 150 patients followed up for 18 months in Kerala, India in 2011 reported that 14% of cases

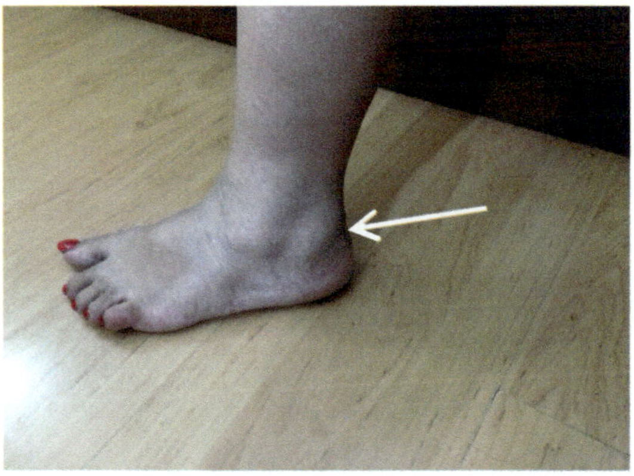

Fig. 28.2 Periarticular Swelling

showed persistence of arthralgia for 3–6 months, 54% for 6–12 months, and 22% for more than a year. The prevalence of post-CHIK chronic inflammatory rheumatism (CIR) has ranged from 27.27% in Indian studies to as high as 50.25% in French studies with a pooled prevalence of 40.22% in a recent meta-analysis. The spectrum of CHIK CIR is quite heterogeneous and includes arthralgias, arthritis, soft tissue symptoms like tendinitis, tenosynovitis, and plantar fasciitis, and a picture indistinguishable from rheumatoid arthritis (RA). As many as 14% of patients develop CHIK chronic arthritis. Deformities and erosive arthritis have been reported as sequelae of CHIKV.

Factors that may contribute to persistent symptoms include age > 45 years, severe or prolonged acute infection, high viral load (>10^9/mL) during the viremic phase, intense CHIKV immune response in the post-viremic phase (CHIKV specific IgG), and preexisting rheumatic disease. Current evidence suggests that it is a postinfectious inflammatory process rather than a persistent viral infection.

28.2.3 Diagnosis

The diagnosis is clinico-serologic. Complete blood counts reveal lymphopenia and thrombocytopenia. Blood chemistry may show transaminitis. Detection of CHIKV is possible during the phase of viremia (first week). Viral cultures are usually not available outside of a research setting. RT-PCR (Reverse transcriptase polymerase chain reaction) is commonly employed for viral RNA detection. Serodiagnosis relies on the detection of CHIKV IgM antibodies that appear by day 5 and may remain detectable for several months. Anti-CHIKV IgG antibodies appear nearly 2 weeks after symptom onset and remain elevated for months to years (Fig. 28.3).

28.2.4 Differential Diagnosis

Other tropical diseases like malaria, typhoid fever, leptospirosis, dengue, viral hemorrhagic fevers, and rickettsial diseases figure in the differential diagnosis of acute Chikungunya. The differential diagnosis of post-Chikungunya arthritis includes inflammatory arthritides like RA.

28.2.5 Treatment

Acute CHIKV infections are managed with supportive care. The World Health Organization (WHO) recommends adequate rest, hydration, paracetamol (acetaminophen)—up to 4 gm per day in divided doses. Aspirin should be avoided. Dengue should be ruled out before using nonsteroidal anti-inflammatory drugs (NSAIDs) because these drugs may aggravate the bleeding manifestations of dengue. All NSAIDs like ibuprofen, diclofenac, naproxen, indomethacin, or aceclofenac are equally effective, provided no contraindications exist. The available guidelines do not recommend corticosteroids in the acute phase (<3 weeks). In the sub-acute phase, low dose oral steroids (10 mg daily) may be added to NSAIDs for refractory joint pains or in situations where NSAIDs are contraindicated. Some authorities advise that the maximum dose of steroids should not exceed 0.5 mg/kg and for no more than 4 weeks. Some experts use intramuscular methylprednisolone injections (80 mg intramuscular weekly for 2–4 weeks). There is no trial data to back these recommendations, which need to be individualized against the common sense advice of restricting steroid use to the mini-

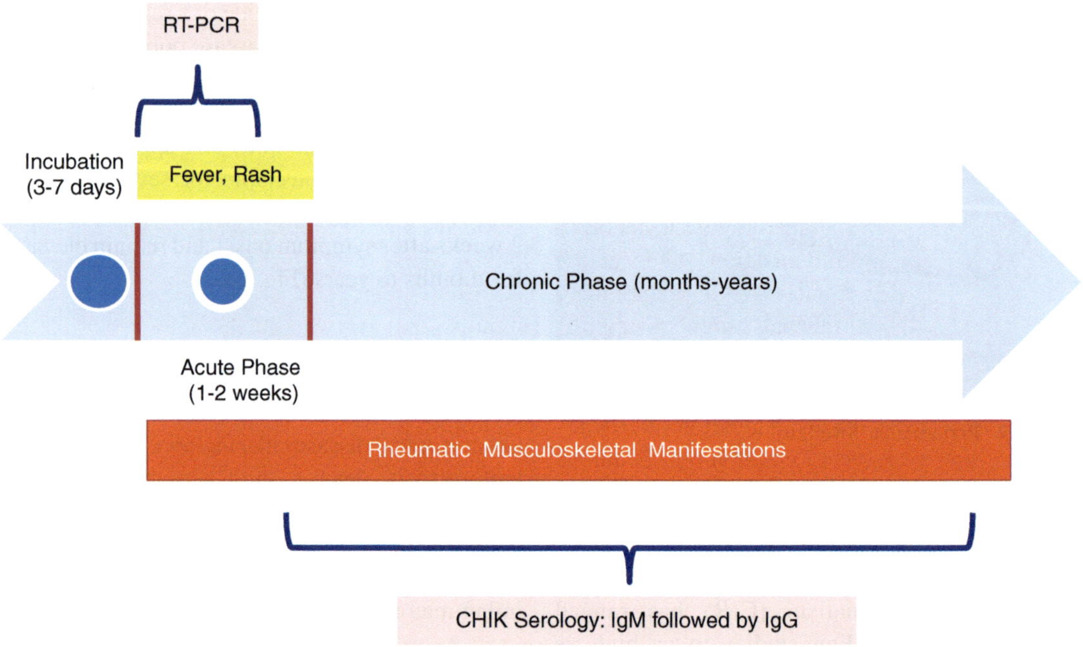

Fig. 28.3 Clinical course of Chikungunya infection and laboratory detection at different time points

Fig. 28.4 Chikungunya Treatment. *NSAIDs* Nonsteroidal antiinflammatory drugs, *DMARDs* Disease modifying antirheumatic drugs, *HCQ* Hydroxychloroquine, *SSZ* Sulfasalazine, *MTX* Methotrexate

	Acute stage	Post acute stage	Chronic stage
Physical treatment	+	+	+
Acetaminophen/NSAIDs	+	+	+
Corticosteroids	–	±	+
DMARDs (HCQ,SSZ,MTX)	–	±	+

mum possible. Codeine, tramadol, and pregabalin are sometimes employed in intractable pain.

Disease-modifying anti-rheumatic drugs (DMARDs), especially hydroxychloroquine, have been used for persistent synovitis (Fig. 28.4). Doses (5 mg/KBW/day) are similar to those used for RA. Other DMARDs include chloroquine, methotrexate, sulfasalazine, leflunomide and are used in a manner similar to RA. Some studies have used DMARD combinations. Occasional case reports detail the use of biologics such as tumor necrosis factor-α. No antivirals or vaccines have currently been approved for use in CHIK. Public health measures like vector control, personal protection, and community education and engagement are equally important.

28.3 Dengue Arthritis

Dengue virus (DENV) is a single-stranded, positive-sense RNA virus (family Flaviviridae) with four serotypes: DEN-1, DEN-2, DEN-3, and DEN-4. Each serotype has different genotypes with subtle antigenic differences that are not clinically relevant. Human infection with one serotype confers long-lived serotype-specific immunity, but only short-lived cross-immunity between serotypes. The vectors are *A. aegypti* and *A. albopictus*. Dengue is more widespread than CHIKV. Both infections are sometimes seen in the same patient. Unlike CHIK, almost 75% of DENV infections are asymptomatic. Children are more likely to be asymptomatic, and adults are more likely to be symptomatic.

Patients present with fever for 5–7 days (usually high fever). This may dissipate after 3–4 days and then recur—biphasic or "saddleback" fever pattern. Other features include severe headache, retro-orbital pain (behind eyes), back pain, joint pains, muscle or bone pains giving rise to the sobriquet of "break-bone fever." The rash may appear on day 3 or 4. Bleeding manifestations (e.g., nose or gum bleed, petechiae, easy bruising, vaginal bleeding, venepuncture site ooze) are seen in severe dengue.

Arthralgias are frequent in both DENV and CHIKV. However, arthritis occurs exclusively in Chikungunya. Joint effusion, restriction of joint movements, and deformities are characteristic of CHIK and virtually never seen in DEN. The joint examination is mostly unremarkable in dengue.

The diagnosis is made by RT-PCR during the viremic phase and later on by serology (IgM antibodies). Treatment is supportive. Acteaminophen (paracetamol) is used for symptom relief. NSAIDs are best avoided because of the fear of bleeding.

28.4 Other Viral Arthritides

Parvovirus B19 is a single-stranded DNA virus, and infections are often asymptomatic. Clinical features include erythema infectiosum (slapped cheek appearance), aplastic anemia, and acute arthritis. Children exhibit an asymmetric large-joint oligoarthritis of the knee while adults exhibit a picture like RA. A 9-year follow-up study from Christian Medical College, Vellore, India reported parvovirus B19 antibodies in 7 (14.8%) out the 47 patients with early inflammatory arthritis. The course is self-limited, and treatment is symptomatic. Hepatitis B, Hepatitis C, and HIV can have rheumatic symptoms that are well described in the literature.

28.5 Conclusions

Chikungunya is the most important arthritogenic arbovirus in India. The vectors are *Aedes aegypti* and *Aedes albopictus* mosquitoes. Global travel and trade, rapid urbanization, and lax vector control measures have led to the spread of Chikungunya to new areas. The propensity to develop persistent musculoskeletal symptoms brings this infectious disease in the ambit of rheumatologists. Novel approaches include repurposing standard DMARDs in combination with antiviral treatments.

Suggested Reading

1. Paixão ES, Rodrigues LC, Costa MDCN, Itaparica M, Barreto F, Gérardin P, et al. Chikungunya chronic disease: a systematic review and meta-analysis. Trans R Soc Trop Med Hyg. 2018;112:301–16.
2. Brito CAA, Marques CDL, Falcão MB, Cunha RVD, Simon F, Valadares LDA, et al. Update on the treatment of musculoskeletal manifestations in chikungunya fever: a guideline. Rev. Soc Bras Med Trop. 2020;53:e20190517.
3. Edington F, Varjão D, Melo P. Incidence of articular pain and arthritis after chikungunya fever in the Americas: a systematic review of the literature and meta-analysis. Joint Bone Spine. 2018;85:669–78.

Sarcoidosis: Rheumatological Considerations

29

29.1 Introduction

Sarcoidosis is a multisystem granulomatous disease of unknown etiology affecting patients between 20 and 60 years. It is not uncommon in India. More than 75% of patients present with lung involvement, while one-fourth of the patients present with extrathoracic features. Although all organs can be affected, the disease is incidentally picked up on chest radiographs in as many as 50% of patients. Common clinical features include bilateral hilar adenopathy (BHL), pulmonary reticular opacities, and skin, joint, or eye lesions. Differentiation from tuberculosis is difficult at times. The granulomas in sarcoidosis are typically noncaseating. This chapter focuses on aspects of sarcoidosis important for a rheumatologist.

29.2 Clinical Recognition

The usual presenting symptoms are cough, dyspnea, and constitutional features. Physical examination may be unremarkable. Clubbing is rare. Investigations reveal a variable rise in ESR and CRP. Patients with granulomatous liver disease may show a rise in serum alkaline phosphatase. Some patients show hypercalcemia and hypercalciuria. Serum angiotensin-converting enzyme (ACE) elevation is encountered in ~75% of patients with untreated sarcoidosis. The ACE levels do not mirror disease activity and have a limited role in monitoring the disease course. Apart from sarcoidosis, ACE can be elevated in other conditions like diabetes, asbestosis, silicosis, coccidioidomycosis, hyperthyroidism, leprosy, tuberculosis, Hodgkin's disease, lung cancer, hypersensitivity pneumonitis, etc.

Rheumatoid factor is positive in 15–20% of patients. Anti-citrullinated peptide antibodies have occasionally been reported in sarcoidosis (<5%). These patients may be erroneously labeled as RA based on serology. Rarely, sarcoidosis and RA may coexist. The tuberculin or Mantoux test is generally negative. The Kveim test (intradermal skin test using a suspension of sterilized splenic cells from patients with sarcoidosis) is seldom performed but always mentioned for historical reasons.

Lung involvement occurs in >90% of patients with sarcoidosis and is the presenting feature in nearly 75%. While 60–70% of patients demonstrate characteristic radiologic findings on chest X-rays, 25–30% of patients have atypical or nonspecific changes, and 5–10% have normal chest radiographs. Contrast-enhanced computerized tomography (CECT) is far more sensitive than X-rays in picking up mediastinal lymphadenopathy, while high-resolution CT (HRCT) is the modality of choice to detect interstitial lung disease.

BHL, the classic finding, is encountered in ~50% of cases (Fig. 29.1). Unilateral adenopathy is very uncommon (<5% cases). In sarcoidosis, hilar lymphadenopathy is frequently associated

R. Handa, *Clinical Rheumatology*, https://doi.org/10.1007/978-981-33-4885-1_29

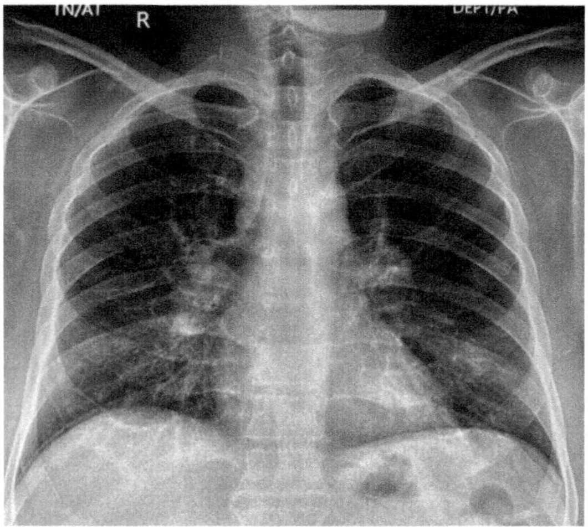

Fig. 29.1 Bilateral Hilar Lymphadenopathy

Table 29.1 Sarcoidosis—Radiographic stages

Stage I	Bilateral hilar adenopathy (BHL)
Stage II	BHL associated with a parenchymal abnormality
Stage III	Diffuse parenchymal disease without nodal enlargement
Stage IV	Pulmonary fibrosis

with mediastinal lymph node enlargement, especially the right paratracheal and subaortic nodes. However, isolated mediastinal lymphadenopathy without hilar involvement is rare and is more suggestive of lymphoma. The four well-known radiographic stages are enunciated in Table 29.1. These stages give an idea of anatomical lung involvement but do not reflect disease severity or activity. Spontaneous regression of hilar nodes over 1–2 years may occur in ~75% of patients. Stage II findings are seen in almost 25% of patients at presentation, of which as many as 50–60% may show spontaneous resolution. Patients generally complain of cough, dyspnea, and fever. A variety of radiographic patterns may be encountered: fine nodular, reticulonodular, nodules, coalescent opacities, etc. Advanced cases show fibrosis with distortion of the lung architecture and traction bronchiectasis. Cavitation is rare (<1% patients) and mandates exclusion of TB and fungal infections. Likewise, pleural effusion is rare (<5% cases). Dystrophic calcification of hilar or mediastinal lymph nodes is related to disease duration (3% cases after 5 years and ~ 20% after 10 years). Calcification may assume amorphous, punctate, popcornlike, or eggshell forms. HRCT reveals mid-to-upper zone predominance of lung parenchymal changes. These include areas of ground-glass attenuation, subpleural or perivascular nodules, and thickening of interlobular septa. The foci of ground-glass attenuation may represent active alveolitis. FDG-PET scan and Gallium-67 scans are occasionally employed. Of note, 18F-FDG PET may be positive in both malignancy and sarcoidosis.

Pulmonary function testing (PFT) is an important part of the workup. A full PFT should include spirometry, lung volumes, diffusion capacity for carbon monoxide (DLCO), and a 6-minute walk test (6MWT). PFTs obtained 3–6 monthly help assess respiratory impairment and are employed to monitor the course of the disease. The commonest PFT abnormality is a restrictive pattern (reduced vital capacity and total lung capacity) associated with reduced DLCO.

Nearly 25–30% of the patients present with extrapulmonary sarcoid. Common locations of extrapulmonary disease include the skin, eyes, musculoskeletal system, reticuloendothelial system, exocrine glands, heart, kidney, and central nervous system. Less than 10% of patients have an extrapulmonary disease without lung involvement, most commonly cutaneous sarcoidosis. Cutaneous involvement and ocular involvement are seen in ~25% of patients. A variety of skin lesions are described. Eye involvement includes uveitis, keratoconjunctivitis sicca, and adnexal (eyelid or conjunctival) granulomas. Cardiac sarcoidosis seen in 5% of cases can be asymptomatic or cause heart block, arrhythmias, heart failure, and even sudden death. Cardiac MRI is the recommended investigative modality in suspected cardiac sarcoidosis in addition to 24 h Holter monitoring and echocardiography. Peripheral lymphadenopathy is present in 40% of patients.

Musculoskeletal involvement occurs in ~10% of patients with sarcoidosis. This may take the form of acute arthritis—Lofgren syndrome or chronic arthritis. Rheumatologists may often be the first point of contact in Lofgren syndrome, a constellation of BHL, erythema nodosum

(Fig. 29.2), and polyarthritis. Apart from this classic triad, some patients show fever, anterior uveitis, and ankle periarthritis. Chronic sarcoid arthropathy assumes the form of nondeforming arthritis with granulomatous synovitis, Jaccoud's deformity of the hands, or dactylitis (Fig. 29.3). Salivary gland swelling may mimic Sjogren's.

The eponym Heerfordt–Waldenström syndrome (uveo-parotid fever) refers to a rare presentation of sarcoidosis characterized by the parotid gland enlargement, facial palsy, anterior uveitis, and fever.

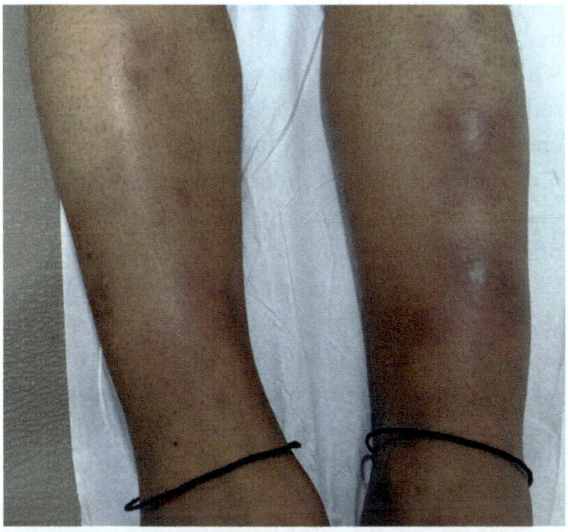

Fig. 29.2 Erythema nodosum in Sarcoidosis

Spontaneous resolution of the disease is fairly common. Progressive lung disease occurs in ~25% of patients. The prognosis of Lofgren's syndrome is good, with the vast majority resolving over a period of months.

29.3 Diagnosis

The diagnosis of sarcoidosis is clinico-radiologic combined with a histologic demonstration of noncaseating granulomas. Tissue diagnosis is recommended in most cases except in very typical situations like asymptomatic BHL and Lofgren syndrome. The choice of biopsy site depends on accessibility. Cutaneous lesions are easy to sample. It is pertinent to highlight that erythema nodosum biopsy in Lofgren's syndrome is not recommended as it shows panniculitis and not granulomas. Bronchoalveolar lavage is employed more to exclude infections and malignancy than confirm sarcoidosis. Endobronchial and transbronchial lung biopsy are commonly performed procedures with a yield

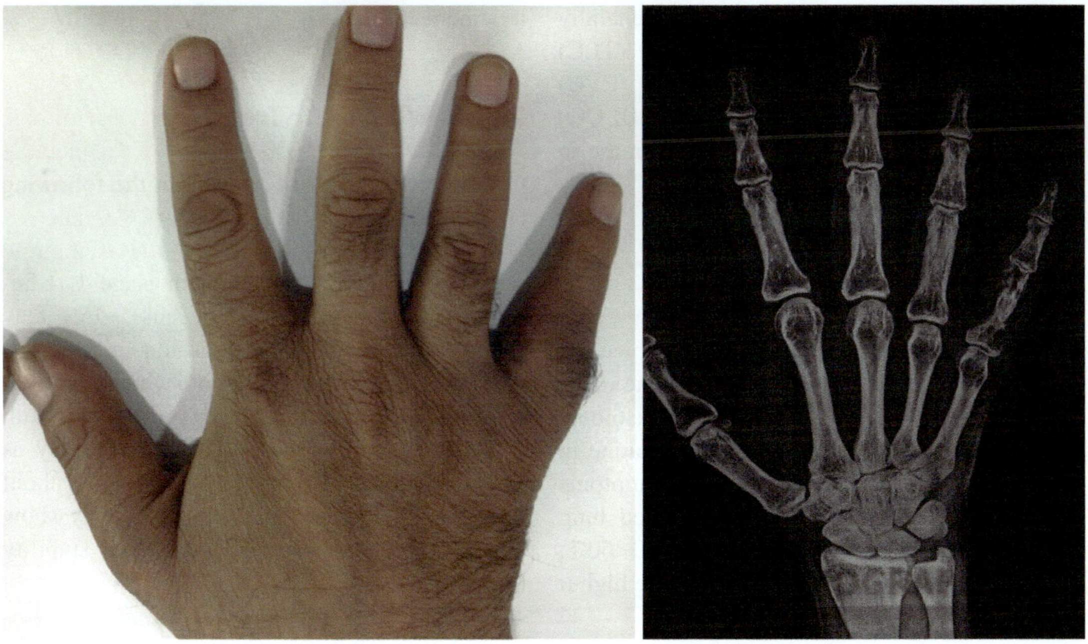

Fig. 29.3 Sarcoid dactylitis (5th finger)

of 50–75%. Endoscopic ultrasound-guided needle aspiration of intrathoracic lymph nodes via esophageal ultrasound (EUS) or endobronchial ultrasound (EBUS) has a diagnostic yield of 80–90%.

The important differential diagnoses include tuberculosis, fungal infections like histoplasmosis, blastomycosis, *Pneumocystis jirovecii*, and hypersensitivity pneumonitis. Rarely, TB and sarcoidosis can coexist.

29.4 Treatment

29.4.1 Who to Treat?

Many patients with pulmonary sarcoidosis do not require treatment because they have an asymptomatic, nonprogressive disease or undergo spontaneous remission. The decision to treat and how long to treat is not based on radiology alone but requires attention to clinical symptomatology and PFTs in addition. Serum ACE levels are not useful in following disease course. Indications of treatment include symptomatic patients with cough, shortness of breath, exercise intolerance, and chest pain. Patients with deteriorating PFTs and worsening radiology also need treatment. Significant impairment in pulmonary function is generally described as a fall in total lung capacity (TLC) ≥10%, decline in forced vital capacity (FVC) ≥15%, a reduction in diffusing capacity (DLCO) ≥20%, or pulse oximetry revealing a decrease in oxygen saturation ≥ 4% over 3–6 months.

29.4.2 How to Treat?

Oral corticosteroids are the drugs of choice for patients who are started on treatment. The usual daily dose is 0.25–0.5 mg/KBW of prednisolone. This works out to 15–30 mg of prednisolone in an average adult. Patients with severe symptoms at presentation or with severely impaired lung function (FVC<70%, FEV1<70%, DLCO<60%, and oxygen saturation <90%) may require higher doses of steroids and more aggressive treatment. The threshold for starting treatment is lower in hypercalcemia, ocular, neurologic, myocardial, or renal involvement because vision loss, fatal arrhythmias, or renal damage remain a distinct possibility. In such situations, even minor symptoms are not ignored.

After clinical improvement, the prednisolone dose is tapered slowly to 5–10 mg daily for ~1 year. Recurrence of symptoms is common (~60% patients). Therefore, treatment is continued for at least 6 months after remission. Patients with insufficient response to steroids or those requiring higher doses to keep disease activity in check are offered other immunosuppressives like methotrexate, azathioprine, or leflunomide. Some patients are not able to stop treatment because of ongoing symptoms.

Nonsteroidal anti-inflammatory drugs (NSAIDs) are employed to treat acute sarcoid arthropathy. Some people need low dose steroids for a short period. For major joint symptoms, hydroxychloroquine, colchicine, and methotrexate are widely used. In patients with suboptimal response to methotrexate, infliximab is used. Etanercept is not useful for pulmonary or ocular sarcoidosis. Adalimumab has been used in a few cases. Extra-articular disease also influences treatment choice.

29.4.3 Who not to Treat?

Corticosteroids are not advised in the following clinical settings:

(a) Asymptomatic patients with stage I radiographic changes (BHL) because ~75% may undergo spontaneous remission.
(b) Stage II or Stage III patients who are asymptomatic or minimally symptomatic with normal or near-normal PFTs. As many as 50% of patients with Stage II and about 30% of patients with Stage III may show radiologic resolution or sustained stability on follow-up.

29.5 Conclusions

Sarcoidosis can present in a variety of ways to several specialties. The diagnosis is clinico-radiologic and confirmed by the characteristic histology of noncaseating granulomas. Not all patients require treatment, and the mere diagnosis of sarcoidosis should not mean knee jerk institution of steroids in all patients. Follow-up requires clinical examination supplemented by PFTs and radiology.

Suggested Reading

Llanos O, Hamzeh N. Sarcoidosis. Med Clin North Am. 2019;103:527–34.

30 Emergencies in Rheumatology

30.1 Introduction

Urgencies and emergencies are common in the clinical practice of rheumatology. For purposes of convenience, rheumatological emergencies may be divided into three broad categories: primary rheumatological emergencies, medical emergencies in patients with systemic rheumatic disease, and iatrogenic emergencies (Table 30.1). Medical emergencies like infections, acute myocardial infarction, left ventricular failure (LVF), gastrointestinal (GI bleed), seizures, etc. in a systemic rheumatic disease are handled like in any other setting and are not discussed in this chapter. It is pertinent to point out that infections account for more than 50% of intensive care unit (ICU) admissions in patients with rheumatic diseases. The respiratory system is the commonest infection site. These infections may be related to disease-specific factors like compromised immunity, treatment-associated (immunosuppressant drugs), or unrelated.

Iatrogenic or drug-related problems are frequent in chronic rheumatic diseases. These include, but are not limited to, drug rash, gastrointestinal upset, cytopenias, kidney and liver injury, infections, etc. Nonsteroidal anti-inflammatory drugs (NSAIDs) can cause gastritis and gastrointestinal bleed, aggravation of asthma, worsening of blood pressure, transaminitis, and renal damage, amongst other drug-related adverse effects. Methotrexate, the anchor drug for rheumatoid arthritis (RA), is sometimes associated with severe nausea, vomiting, diarrhea, stomatitis, and bone marrow suppression. Inadvertent "daily" use instead of "weekly" dosing is usually the culprit, especially in elderly patients with multi-morbidities and several concomitant medications by multiple providers.

Table 30.1 Important rheumatological emergencies

(A) **Primary rheumatological emergencies**
1. Acute low back pain
2. Acute gout
3. Acute arthritis
(a) Arthritis arising de novo
(b) Acute exacerbation in a patient with chronic arthritis, e.g., rheumatoid flare
4. Lupus flare
5. Systemic necrotizing vasculitides
6. Scleroderma renal crisis
7. Catastrophic antiphospholipid syndrome
8. Erythema nodosum
9. Complex regional pain syndrome
(B) **Medical and iatrogenic emergencies in patients with systemic rheumatic disease**
1. Infections and sepsis
2. NSAID-induced gastrointestinal bleed
3. Acute left ventricular failure
4. Intracranial bleed
5. Accelerated hypertension
6. Tuberculous meningitis
7. Acute adrenal insufficiency due to sudden steroid withdrawal
8. Seizures
9. Cyclophosphamide-induced hemorrhagic cystitis
10. Drug (immunosuppressive)-induced bone marrow suppression, etc.

R. Handa, *Clinical Rheumatology*, https://doi.org/10.1007/978-981-33-4885-1_30

Sulfasalazine and leflunomide may cause a skin rash that necessitates emergency attention. Biologic use can be associated with infections. The adverse effects of corticosteroids are well known. It is not possible to catalog all the side effects of antirheumatic drugs in this chapter. However, it is prudent to rule in or rule out drug-related issues in patients with rheumatic diseases who present to the emergency room. One should carefully check not only about prescription drugs but also over the counter pills and alternative system treatments when going over the drug history in such patients. Prescription errors are occasionally the culprit.

The vast majority of primary rheumatologic emergencies are 'referred to' and 'handled by' orthopedic surgeons, despite the fact that surgical intervention is needed only in a small proportion of patients. In most instances, medical management suffices. Physician unfamiliarity is primarily responsible for this situation. The present chapter is meant to acquaint clinicians with important rheumatological mergencies

30.2 Acute Low Back Pain

Acute low back pain (LBP) is the commonest rheumatological emergency in medical practice. Individuals at risk include manual workers, material handlers, weight lifters, porters, gymnasts, etc. The notable thing about acute LBP is its favorable natural history: 40% of cases recover within 1 week, 80% of cases recover within 3 weeks, and 90% of cases recover within 6 weeks. Only 7–10% of the patients continue to experience symptoms for more than 6 months. Since low backache is ubiquitous and most often self-limiting, the clinician's first task should be to rule out/rule in medical emergencies like cauda equina syndrome, epidural abscess, rupture of aortic aneurysm, dissection of the aorta, etc. Clinical pointers toward serious disease include unexplained weight loss, history of malignancy, fever, prolonged corticosteroid use, saddle anesthesia, bladder/bowel involvement, asymmetric loss of deep tendon reflexes, pulse inequality, hypotension, circulatory instability, history of uveitis or arthritis in conjunction with inflammatory back pain, etc. A good history and thorough physical examination are mandatory.

Most (>90%) episodes of LBP are mechanical in origin. The term mechanical is used to designate an anatomical or functional abnormality without an underlying malignant, inflammatory or infective disease. Nearly 85% of these patients cannot be given a precise pathoanatomical diagnosis, and terms like nonspecific LBA, strain, or sprain are widely used. Discrete lesions like herniated disc, spinal stenosis, spondylolysis, spondylolisthesis, etc. are found only in a small minority of patients. Investigations in acute LBP should be kept to a minimum except when red flag signs are present.

All patients where the basic history and physical examination are normal should be subjected to 6 weeks of conservative therapy. This is because LBP's natural history is favorable, and 90–95% of patients improve within 2 months. The catchword should be "restricted physical activity" rather than "absolute bed rest," which is counterproductive. No more than a day or two of bed rest is advisable. Progressive mobilization should follow this as the patient's pain improves. Back exercises are not helpful in the acute phase. They are useful later for preventing recurrences and for treating chronic LBP. Short-term NSAIDs for 2–4 weeks are used in acute LBP unless there are contraindications. Paracetamol (acetaminophen) can be employed as the first-line drug for pain relief in some patients with contraindication to NSAIDs. In case of inadequate relief, a non-benzodiazepine muscle relaxant can be added. Opioid analgesics or tramadol should be used only if the above measures do not yield benefits. The benefit, if any, of alternative therapies like spinal manipulation, acupuncture, massage, etc. is not fully known.

30.3 Acute Gout

Acute gout is a common rheumatological emergency. Patients present with acute pain in one of the lower limb joints. The presentation is usually with monoarthritis (single joint) or oligoarthritis

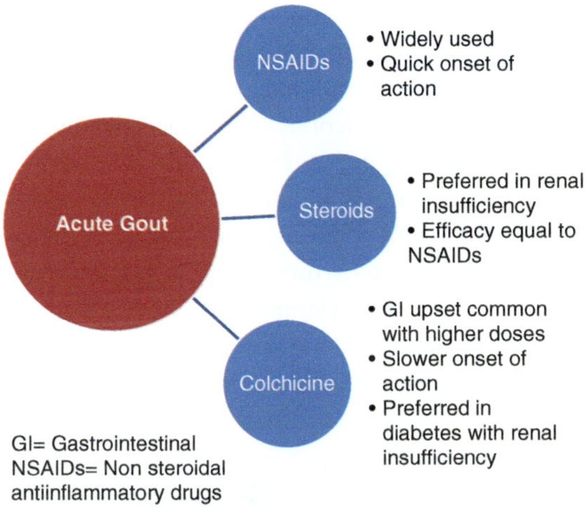

Fig. 30.1 Treatment options in acute gout

(2–4 joints). A polyarticular presentation is rare. All patients presenting with monoarthritis of uncertain etiology should undergo joint aspiration to rule out septic arthritis.

Physical modalities include rest, elevation, and ice. Acute gout can be treated by one of the three agents: NSAIDs, low-dose oral colchicine, or corticosteroids depending on patient co-morbidities and preference (Fig. 30.1). NSAIDs are widely utilized. No one agent is superior to another. The use of NSAIDs has replaced the use of colchicine to treat acute attacks because of GI toxicity associated with the latter and the slower onset of action. Intravenous colchicine is no longer available, and higher doses of colchicine have been abandoned. Treatment is continued till the acute attack subsides over a few days. Corticosteroids (oral, intraarticular, or intramuscular) may be used in patients with contraindications to NSAIDs, e.g., renal failure or congestive cardiac failure. There is no consensus on agent, dose, or route of administration. Oral prednisolone 20–40 mg daily tapered over 2 weeks or intramuscular methylprednisolone 40–120 mg is commonly used. Intraarticular corticosteroids are also effective in acute gout. Allopurinol or febuxostat should not be started during an acute attack of gout as it may precipitate another attack or prolong the duration. Patients already on allopurinol or febuxostat should continue the drug. IL-1 inhibitors (anakinra, rilonacept, or canakinumab) may be considered in refractory patients.

30.4 Acute Arthritis

Acute arthritis may start afresh (de novo) or represent acute exacerbation in a patient with a pre-existing arthritic illness like RA. Several arthritic illnesses resemble each other at the onset, and proper categorization into a specific disease entity may not be possible at the first patient encounter. Symptomatic treatment with close clinical observation is recommended.

The causes of de novo arthritis can be conveniently divided into:

(a) **ACUTE MONOARTHRITIS.**
   Causes: Gout, septic arthritis, trauma, etc.
(b) **ACUTE OLIGO/POLY ARTHRITIS.**
   Causes: Reactive arthritis, viral arthritis, rheumatic fever, disseminated gonococcal infection, etc. Very rarely, RA may have an acute onset.

Acute monoarthritis should be considered a medical emergency. If the etiology is unclear, joint aspiration is carried out to exclude pus in the joint. The synovial fluid should also be subjected to crystal studies, preferably using polarized microscopy. Radiology has a limited role in acute monoarthritis. X-rays are needed in patients with a history of trauma so as to exclude fracture.

The clinical profile of septic (acute bacterial) arthritis includes the rapid onset of severe joint pain, warmth, tenderness, and movement restriction. Usually, it occurs in the setting of an immunocompromised host with diabetes, transplant recipients, or patients with prosthetic joints. Rarely, septic arthritis may afflict normal joints. Usually, the presentation is monoarticular. However, in 10–15% of patients, septic arthritis may be polyarticular. Large joints like the knee and hip are commonly involved. Elderly patients may not manifest fever or other signs of inflammation. Joint drainage is a must to drain the intraarticular pus. This can be achieved by large-bore needle aspiration or lavage, which may be arthroscopic. Surgical arthrotomy is usually required for septic hips/shoulders, if osteomyelitis coexists with septic arthritis and if the joint infection is not controlled by 5–7 days of needle/arthroscopic drainage. Antibiotics form the cornerstone of treatment.

Reactive arthritis (ReA) may be post dysenteric or follow nongonococcal urethritis/cervicitis with chlamydia. The classical triad of Reiter's syndrome, which includes urethritis, conjunctivitis, and arthritis, may not be present in all the patients. In the acute stage, reactive arthritis is managed by NSAIDs. In severe cases of acute ReA, when NSAIDs have been ineffective, a short course of steroids may be used. Short-term antibiotics have virtually no role, although long-term antibiotics have been tried in sexually acquired reactive arthritis. Early antibiotic treatment of urogenital chlamydial infections in endemic areas, with drugs like lymecycline for several weeks, may decrease the subsequent development of ReA. Patients with chronic joint involvement may require methotrexate or sulfasalazine.

Viral arthritides are most often self-limited and managed symptomatically. The clinical profile and treatment of rheumatic fever are well known and will not be discussed here. Human immunodeficiency virus (HIV) is also known to have a variety of rheumatic manifestations, including Reiter's syndrome, psoriatic arthritis, arthralgias as part of acute HIV syndrome, HIV-associated arthropathy, and the "painful articular syndrome."

Triggers of a rheumatoid flare include de-escalation of treatment, high-loading physical activities, weather changes, infections, or stress. Sometimes no provocative factor can be identified. Acute flares of RA are best treated with NSAIDs and/or a short course of corticosteroids with an escalation of disease-modifying antirheumatic drug (DMARD) therapy. Rheumatoid vasculitis is an indication for high-dose corticosteroids (1 mg/KBW/day of prednisolone). Other emergencies in RA may include tendon rupture and finger drop, rupture of Baker's cyst (pseudothrombophlebitis), subluxations in the cervical spine, cricoarytenoid arthritis, and septic arthritis. Cervical spine involvement may require surgical intervention in case of refractory pain, neurologic compromise, or intrinsic spinal cord signal changes on MRI. In RA, septic arthritis can be polyarticular and difficult to differentiate from RA flare. Treatment entails joint drainage and appropriate antibiotics. Ocular complications like corneal melt or scleritis can present as emergencies (Fig. 30.2).

Another common urgency is the sudden worsening of pain in knee osteoarthritis (OA). This may be due to osteoarthritis flare, septic arthritis, rupture of Baker's cyst, pseudogout (CPDD disease), osteonecrosis, or Anserine bursitis (Fig. 30.3). An intraarticular steroid (IAS) injec-

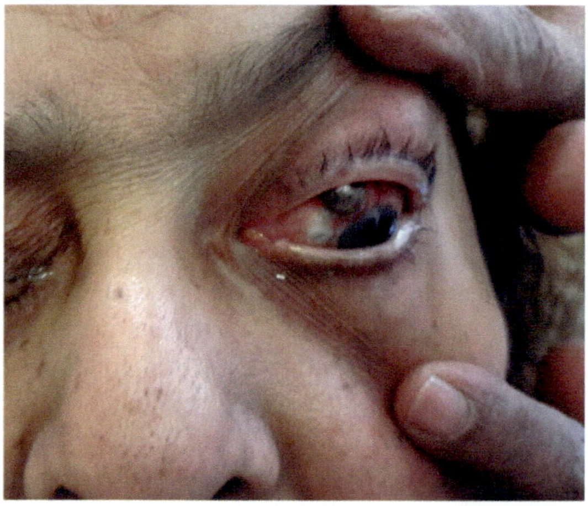

Fig. 30.2 Necrotizing Scleritis in Rheumatoid Arthritis

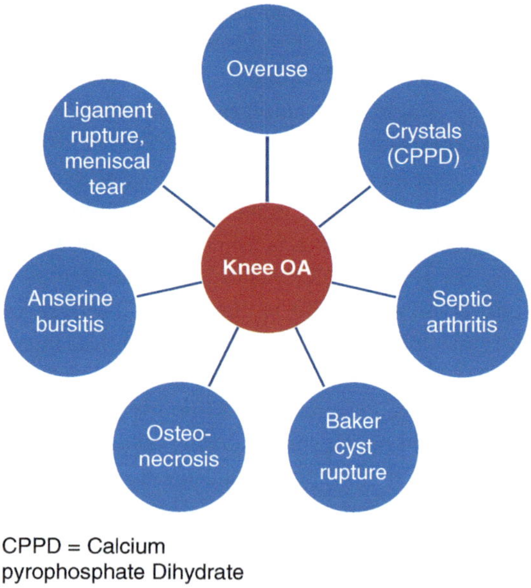

Fig. 30.3 Causes of Flare in Knee OA

tion can provide significant relief in selected patients with flare-up of knee OA. Infected joints should never be injected with steroids. Anserine bursitis requires local steroid injection into the bursa, not intraarticular. IAS does not help osteonecrosis. In fact, high-dose steroids are known to cause osteonecrosis.

30.5 Lupus Flare

Like any other chronic rheumatic disease, the course of SLE is punctuated by exacerbations termed "lupus flare." The features of mild to moderate flare are a new rash or worsening of preexisting rash, photosensitivity, lupus profundus, cutaneous vasculitis, serositis, arthritis, or fever attributable to lupus. The SLE disease activity index (SLEDAI) score increases by 3 or more. Severe flare is defined as new or worse CNS lupus activity, vasculitis, nephritis, myositis, thrombocytopenia <60,000/mL or hemolytic anemia (Hb < 7 gm/dl or decrease in Hb > 3 gm/dl). The SLEDAI score increases by 12 or more. A lupus flare may be precipitated by stress, exposure to sunlight, steroid reduction/withdrawal, pregnancy, infection, etc. Many patients exhibit multiple organ involvement.

A common clinical dilemma is to decide whether fever in a given case is due to increased lupus activity or infection. SLE, being an immunocompromised state, is frequently complicated by infections, especially tuberculosis. In such a setting, the presence of leukocytosis and/or increased CRP is a pointer toward infection. In contrast, leukopenia and/or normal/minimally elevated CRP levels favor a diagnosis of increased lupus activity. However, these are relative points, and bacteriologic isolation or histological confirmation remains the only foolproof method of differentiating between fever due to lupus activity or infection. The two may also coexist!

The management of flare includes identification and removal of triggering cause, if any, and increase of corticosteroid dose (Fig. 30.4). Major flares require the institution of or increase in dosage of cyclophosphamide, azathioprine, methotrexate, or mycophenolate mofetil. Life-threatening or organ-threatening situations are tackled by intravenous methylprednisolone pulses (usually 1 Gm daily X 3 days). Rituximab is also used for major organ lupus.

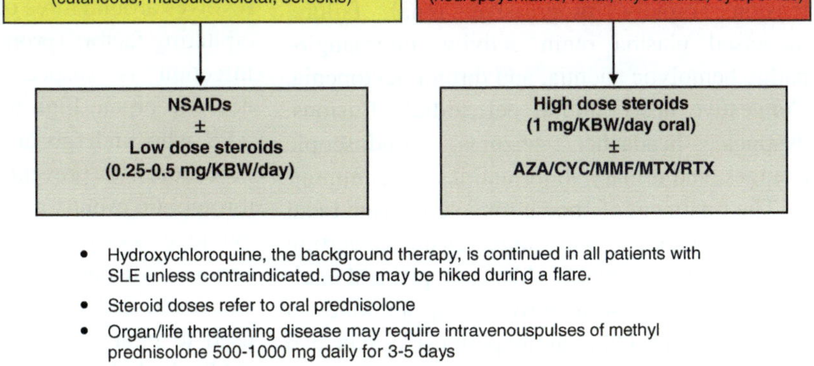

Fig. 30.4 Approach to lupus flare. *AZA* azathioprine, *CYC* cyclophosphamide, *MMF* mycophenolate mofetil, *MTX* methotrexate, *RTX* Rituximab

30.6 Systemic Vasculitides

In general, flares of systemic vasculitides require escalation of immunosuppressive treatment, viz. corticosteroids, azathioprine, cyclophosphamide, etc., depending on the extent of organ involvement and the specific diagnosis. Methylprednisolone may be required in serious situations (vide supra). Like in lupus, rituximab is being increasingly employed in the treatment of antineutrophil cytoplasmic antibody (ANCA)-associated vasculitides. Sometimes, vasculitis may present in an acute fashion with digital ischemia, pulmonary hemorrhage, rapidly progressive renal failure, etc. as the presenting manifestations. These are discussed in detail in the chapter on vasculitides.

30.7 Scleroderma Renal Crisis

This is an uncommon emergency. Approximately 80% of the renal crises occur in patients with diffuse cutaneous systemic sclerosis within the first 4–5 years. The problem is less common in patients with long-standing disease. Also, renal crisis is infrequent in limited scleroderma (<1% patients). Hypertension (HT) is a frequent finding though normotensive renal crisis is also known (11% patients). Risk factors include diffuse skin disease, new unexplained anemia, new cardiac events (like pericardial effusion or congestive cardiac failure), high-dose steroids, and the presence of anti-RNA polymerase III antibody. The syndrome is characterized by accelerated hypertension, rapidly progressive renal failure, increased plasma renin activity, microangiopathic hemolytic anemia, and thrombocytopenia. Congestive heart failure, pericardial effusions, dyspnea, headache, seizures, fundoscopic changes, and urinary abnormalities are common.

The treatment of choice for scleroderma renal crisis is therapy with angiotensin-converting enzyme (ACE inhibitors) like captopril and enalapril. These reverse underlying hyper-reninemia and control HT. Other antihypertensives can also be added if needed. ACE inhibitors are of value, even in the normotensive renal crisis. Nearly one-third to one-half of the patients require permanent dialysis or die. In some patients, renal failure may ensue despite early and vigorous treatment. ACE inhibitors should be continued in these patients. Even in patients on dialytic support, the continuation of ACE inhibitors may lead to enough renal recovery to permit dialysis discontinuation after 6–18 months. No studies on the prophylactic role of ACE inhibitors are available. Plasmapheresis, corticosteroids, and immunosuppressives have no role in the management of scleroderma renal crisis. Renal transplantation may be considered in selected patients only after several months of dialysis because of the chances of recovery in some patients.

30.8 Catastrophic Antiphospholipid Syndrome (CAPS)

The term "CAPS" does not apply to a variant of APS but rather to a time-limited episode. The presentation in CAPS is essentially that of multi-organ failure in a patient with APS. Precipitating factors, seen in one-third of patients, include infections, oral contraceptives, surgical stress, and discontinuation of anticoagulants. Occasionally patients may not give a history of APS, and CAPS may be the first presentation making diagnosis difficult. Pulmonary, gastrointestinal, cardiac, renal, and neurologic involvement is common as in systemic inflammatory response syndrome. Disseminated intravascular coagulation is common. The management revolves around three objectives: to treat any precipitating factors (prompt use of antibiotics if an infection is suspected, amputation for any necrotic organ, high awareness in patients with APS who undergo an operation or an invasive procedure); to prevent and to treat the ongoing thrombotic events; and to suppress the excessive cytokine "storm." Anticoagulation (usually intravenous heparin) corticosteroids, plasma exchange, and intravenous immunoglobulin are used to treat CAPS. Agents tried in refractory CAPS include B cell depletion therapies (rituximab) or complement inhibition therapies (eculizumab). The mortality is high (~60%) and causes include myocardial failure, acute respiratory distress syndrome, renal failure, central nervous system causes, or a combination.

30.9 Erythema Nodosum (EN)

Erythema nodosum is the commonest panniculitis seen in clinical practice. Panniculitides are rare disorders characterized by inflammation of subcutaneous fat. The patient presents with painful, erythematous nodules, mainly on the shin and lower limbs. Joint pains are seen in nearly 50% of the patients with EN. Ankles are the commonest joints affected. Other joints affected include the knees, hips, wrists, fingers, shoulders, and elbows. The condition may be idiopathic. Known triggers include infections (streptococcal pharyngitis, TB, etc.); drugs (sulfonamides, penicillin, oral pills, etc.); sarcoidosis; lymphoma; inflammatory bowel disease; and Behcet's Syndrome. Usually, EN is a self-limiting disease. NSAIDs may be used to give pain relief. If acute pain persists or is unresponsive to NSAIDS, a short course of steroids may be used. For recurrent attacks of unknown cause colchicine, or dapsone may be tried.

30.10 Complex Regional Pain Syndrome (CRPS)

Complex regional pain syndrome or reflex sympathetic dystrophy syndrome (RSDS), as it is also known, is characterized by severe pain affecting a distal extremity. The pain is disproportionate to the inciting event and is accompanied by edema, vasomotor, and sudomotor changes. The clinician should suspect RSDS when a patient presents with sudden onset, severe pain affecting an area like hand or foot, which does not conform to a single nerve distribution. Precipitating factors present in some patients include trauma, nerve injury, entrapment neuropathy, stroke, diabetes, antituberculous drugs, etc. Plain radiographs may show patchy osteopenia while three-phase bone scans reveal asymmetric, usually increased, perfusion, and periarticular uptake in early and delayed phases. Treatment modalities include corticosteroids, gabapentin, sympathetic nerve blockade, etc. Further details may be obtained in the chapter on CRPS.

30.11 Conclusions

Rheumatological emergencies are common and, in most instances, can be handled by the physician himself/herself. Rheumatology referral or orthopedic intervention is needed only in a fraction of the patients. Awareness holds the key to successful management.

Suggested Reading

1. Gutiérrez-González LA. Rheumatologic emergencies. Clin Rheumatol. 2015;34:2011–9.
2. Slobodin G, Hussein A, Rozenbaum M, Rosner I. The emergency room in systemic rheumatic diseases. Emerg Med J. 2006;23:667–71.

31 Joint Aspiration and Injection

31.1 Introduction

Joint aspiration and injection is a commonly performed procedure in Rheumatology. Indeed, it is a skill that is likely to stand every physician in good stead. With guidance and experience, it is not difficult to learn, especially in the case of the knee joint, which happens to be the commonest joint aspirated in clinical practice. The procedure is usually performed in the physician's office/outpatient department without the need for sophisticated equipment. Joints are needled for two reasons—diagnostic and therapeutic. The former is essential when septic arthritis is a diagnostic consideration, or synovial fluid is required for crystal studies. Therapeutic joint or soft tissue injections with steroids are a rewarding, procedure intended to relieve inflammation and provide symptomatic relief in a persistently inflamed joint or a soft tissue problem like a tennis elbow not responding to conservative measures.

31.2 Joint Aspiration (Arthrocentesis)

Joint aspiration is usually done in patients who have joint inflammation of uncertain etiology. This is often a monoarthritis where infection is the prime suspect. The two important differentials of monoarthritis are infection and crystal arthritis. The role of joint aspiration in polyarticular joint disease is limited. When septic or tuberculous arthritis is suspected in a patient with a preexisting joint disease like rheumatoid arthritis (RA), joint aspiration is warranted. The thumb rule often repeated to residents and fellows is "if a joint aspiration is being considered, it should probably be performed." There are more reasons to perform than not to perform arthrocentesis. Overlooking septic arthritis or delayed diagnosis can lead to rapid joint destruction. Repeated aspirations are sometimes a part of treating a septic joint to relieve discomfort and prevent joint damage. Aspiration is occasionally needed in large hemarthrosis to prevent adhesions. Sometimes aspiration is required in suspected prosthetic joint infection. This is best left to the orthopedic surgeons.

31.2.1 Indications

1. Monoarthritis—where septic arthritis/other infections are a consideration.
2. Suspected crystal arthritis.

31.2.2 Contraindications to Joint Aspiration

1. Skin infection/cellulitis overlying the joint.
2. Coagulation disorders or patients on anticoagulants (relative contraindication).
3. Prosthetic joints (relative contraindication).

R. Handa, *Clinical Rheumatology*, https://doi.org/10.1007/978-981-33-4885-1_31

31.2.3 Synovial Fluid Analysis

The synovial fluid should be subjected to a naked eye examination, cell counts (total and differential), Gram and Ziehl–Neelsen stain, cultures (aerobic, anaerobic, fungal, mycobacterial as appropriate), and crystal examination. Polarized microscopy is desirable, if available. It aids crystal recognition. In some situations, the GeneXpert (nucleic acid amplification test for simultaneous rapid tuberculosis diagnosis and identification of rifampicin resistance) is ordered. Synovial fluid PCR for *Mycobacterium tuberculosis* is a notoriously fallacious test, and the diagnosis of TB should not be solely based on this one test.

A white count of 2000/mm^3 is used as a cut off to differentiate inflammatory from noninflammatory fluids. The cell count of normal synovial fluid is <200/ mm^3. A noninflammatory fluid generally has <50% neutrophils while infected fluids (septic arthritis) has >95% neutrophils. Unlike pleural/peritoneal fluids or CSF, the utility of protein and sugar estimation in synovial fluid is limited value. Further information on synovial fluid can be obtained in Chap. 2.

There are practically no complications of joint aspiration save the risk of infection as with any invasive procedure. Uncommonly, vasovagal syncope can occur. Ultrasound guidance is finding an increase in directing joint aspiration and injection.

31.3 Joint/Soft Tissue Injections

Therapeutic joint injections employ corticosteroids in the vast majority of cases. However, joint injection is also used to deliver other agents like hyaluronic acid, platelet-rich plasma (PRP), radionuclides like yttrium, etc. A detailed discussion of this is beyond the purview of this chapter, which focuses on corticosteroids. In general, joint aspiration should be performed immediately before injecting intra-articular corticosteroids to improve efficacy.

31.3.1 Indications for Joint/Soft Tissue Steroid Injections

Joint injections are primarily carried out when one or a few joints continue to exhibit persistent synovitis and do not settle down despite optimum medical management. Here, the recalcitrant joint is injected rather than escalate systemic therapy (Fig. 31.1). Polyarticular flares are best treated by up-titration of medical treatment rather than joint injections. There is no fixed agreement on the number of joints that can be injected in a single sitting. One should reconsider treatment options

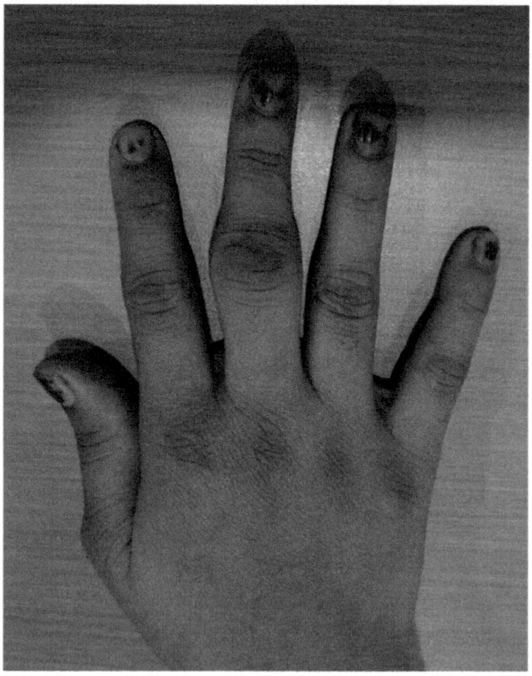

Fig. 31.1 The 3rd PIP joint demonstrates active synovitis with quiescent disease in other joints in this patient with Rheumatoid Arthritis

when multiple joint injections are being contemplated in the same sitting.

Indications of joint injection/soft tissue injection include but are not confined to arthritides (osteoarthritis, gouty arthritis, RA, peripheral spondyloarthritis, etc.); soft tissue lesions (trigger finger, Baker's cyst, adhesive capsulitis, plantar fasciitis, etc.); entrapment syndromes like carpal tunnel syndrome, etc. and ganglion cysts. The major indication is a single inflamed joint that refuses to settle. Trigger point injections and facet joint injections are also commonly carried out in clinical practice.

31.3.2 Contraindications to Joint/Soft Tissue Steroid Injections

- Skin infection overlying joint.
- Joint infection.
- Severe coagulopathy (relative contraindication).
- Uncontrolled severe diabetes (relative contraindication).

Potential side effects of corticosteroid injections include infection, subcutaneous tissue atrophy, skin depigmentation (Fig. 31.2), and tendon rupture. These complications are uncommon, resulting from a faulty technique or superficial location of the lesion like de Quervain's tenosynovitis or too large a volume injected. Post injection flares are rare with steroids but may occur with drugs like hyaluronic acid of avian origin.

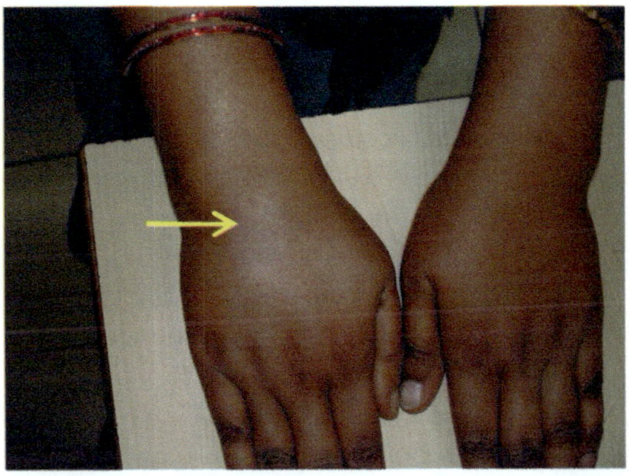

Fig. 31.2 Post steroid Hypopigmentation

31.4 Practical Points

1. Almost any joint can be injected safely, often as a bedside/clinic procedure. The hip joint being a deep-seated joint with adjoining vascular structures, should preferably *not* be injected without radiological guidance. Common soft tissue lesions amenable to local injection treatment (LIT) are—tennis/golfer's elbow, trochanteric bursitis, rotator cuff lesion, bicipital tendinitis, flexor tenosynovitis, etc.
2. The steroid preparations used are either Methylprednisolone (*Depomedrol®*) or Triamcinolone acetonide (*Tricort®*). Doses vary from 80 mg for large joints such as knee/shoulder; 40 mg for medium joints such as ankle/wrist; and 10–20 mg for small joints such as MCP joints: details are given below:

	Joint and dose					
Preparation	Knee	Shoulder	Elbow	Wrist	Ankle	MCP/MTP
Methylprednisolone acetate (Depomedrol®)	80 mg	80 mg	40 mg	40 mg	40 mg	10–20 mg
Triamcinalone acetonide (Tricort®)	40 mg	40 mg	20 mg	20 mg	20 mg	5–10 mg

3. Triamcinolone hexacetonide is the preferred preparation because it is long-acting. It is not available so far in India. Triamcinolone acetonide and hexacetonide are longer acting than methylprednisolone. Methylprednisolone is preferred for soft tissue injections.
4. Local anesthetics used include lignocaine and bupivacaine. Lignocaine has a quicker onset but a shorter duration of action than bupivacaine. It is half as potent as bupivacaine at inducing local anesthesia.
5. A joint can be injected more than once, but preferably should not be injected at intervals of less than 3–4 months.
6. In patients with uncontrolled diabetes and patients on full anticoagulants (or with known coagulation disorders), LIT should be avoided or, if necessary, performed with extreme caution.
7. Mild facial flushing and an occasional increase in joint synovitis may occur very infrequently. It is important to inform the patient about this possibility in advance. Symptomatic treatment usually suffices to deal with this.
8. *The presence of infection, either confirmed or suspected, is an absolute contraindication to LIT.*

31.5 Procedure

A step-wise guide to the actual procedure of performing a LIT is given below. As mentioned above, the procedure can be performed safely by the bedside or in the outpatient clinic. Operation theater is not essential. It is important to ensure that one uses good quality, sterile, disposable syringes, and needles. While many experts in the past injected without sterile surgical gloves using a "no-touch" technique and carefully avoiding touching the skin at the point of injection after it has been cleaned, more and more operators are opting for gloves now. Safe and appropriate disposal of used needles and syringes is essential.

1. Confirm the necessity for the procedure and ensure that there is no contraindication to the injection (such as infection, uncontrolled diabetes, or an extremely unstable joint).

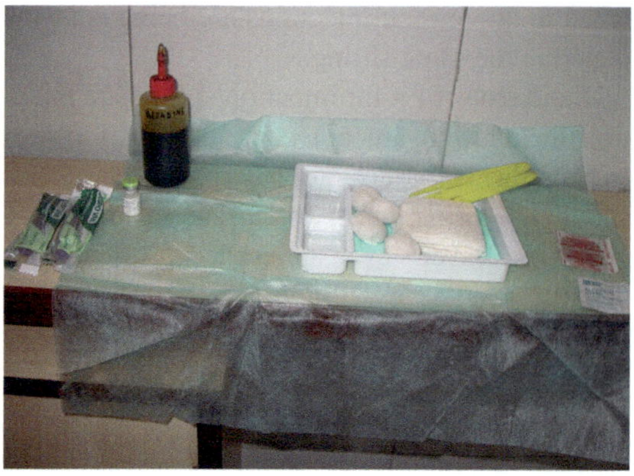

Fig. 31.3 Equipment used for LIT: *Disposable tray, cotton swabs, forceps, syringes, and needles. Betadine; alcohol swab; band-aid; (not shown: local anesthetic, sterile, container for synovial fluid; syringe/needle disposer)*

2. Equipment required is simple and comprises the following: a sterile, disposable tray with sterile cotton, gauze swabs, and forceps; sterile disposable syringes and needles; alcohol swab; betadine solution; band-aid; a sterile, dry container for synovial fluid (if obtained); a local anesthetic (if needed); and a syringe/needle disposal container (Fig. 31.3). It is best to neatly spread out the equipment on a clean and handy surface next to the patient, but avoid opening the syringe or needle until use.
3. Make the patient comfortable and explain the procedure to the patient *before* performing the injection.
4. A full "surgical scrub" is not necessary, but it is prudent to wash hands before each procedure, preferably with antiseptic soap, and dry the hands thoroughly. Most operators now glove themselves.
5. Identify and mark the injection spot over the joint or soft tissue. The injection site is located depending upon the joint/soft tissue to be injected, and the point of injection can be marked by a cross with a ballpoint pen or waterproof marker, such that the actual point of injection falls in the center of the cross, which is left unmarked (as shown). Figure 31.4 demonstrates the markings for injection of the wrist joint.
6. Clean the skin at the injection site with spirit/isopropyl alcohol and then paint with beta-

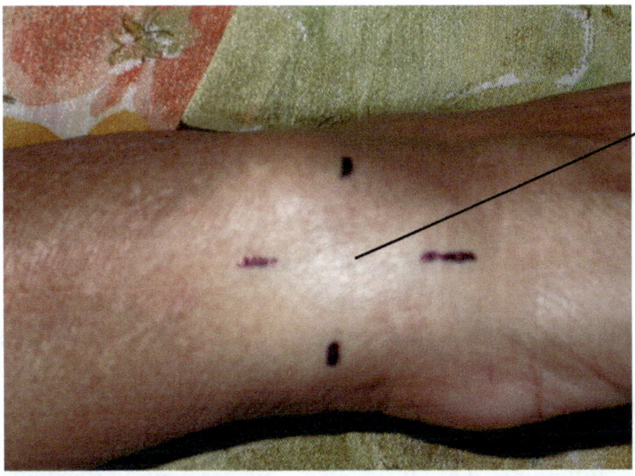

Fig. 31.4 Marking the point of injection

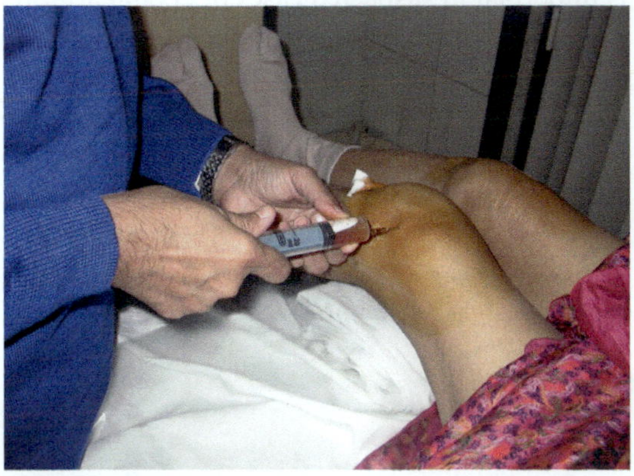

Fig. 31.5 Aspiration of the left knee: a 20-ml syringe with a 19-G needle is being used

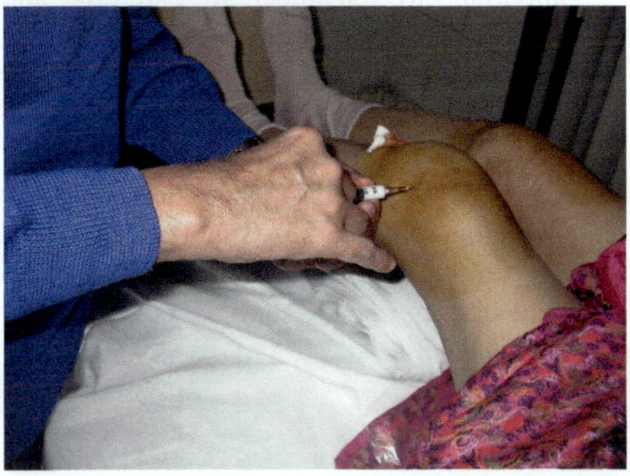

Fig. 31.6 The left knee being injected

dine solution, using sterile cotton or gauze, held by the forceps. Once the skin has been cleaned, load the syringe with the required dose of steroid, with a careful, "no-touch" technique. Corticosteroids and the local anesthetic can be coadministered in the same syringe.

7. Avoid touching the injection spot. First, aspirate any joint effusion present (usually relevant for the knee joint) using an appropriately sized syringe and a fresh needle of adequate size. Figure 31.5 demonstrates aspiration of the left knee: a 20-ml syringe with a 19-g needle is being used. If the synovial fluid looks turbid, is very thick, or is frankly hemorrhagic—making septic arthritis likely—***then do not*** inject the steroid into the joint. In any event, if any synovial fluid is obtained, it should *always* be sent for counts, Gram's stain, and routine culture in an appropriate sterile container.
8. If the joint aspirate looks clear (or no fluid is obtained), then inject the requisite dose of steroid from the preloaded syringe, into the joint, by carefully removing the syringe used for aspiration and changing to the syringe with the steroid, again avoiding touching the needle or connection between needle and syringe, directly. Figure 31.6 demonstrates the left knee being injected.
9. Once the injection has been made, rapidly remove the syringe and needle, simultaneously pressing down (with the other hand) on the puncture site with sterile gauze for a minute or two—this would avoid any steroid tracking into the soft tissue and also prevent any oozing of blood. Then use a sterile band-

aid or similar dressing to seal the puncture site temporarily. Strapping or immobilizing the area or joint is *not* required. The patient is advised to remove the band-aid the following day. Carefully dispose the used syringe and needle(s) in puncture-proof containers.

10. Aftercare following the intra-articular injection: The patient should be advised to "take it easy" for a few days following the injection. If a large joint such as the knee is injected, then the injection response is better if the patient rests the affected knee as far as possible, for about 1–2 days. The band-aid can be removed the following day. It is also important to remember to carefully and safely dispose of all sharps (needles) and syringes used in the procedure.

Providing the above guidelines are followed, intra-articular injections can provide considerable symptomatic benefit by relieving synovitis. In many situations, LIT can therefore help to avoid the use of systemic steroids, besides being the treatment of choice, for most soft tissue problems. In inflammatory joint diseases, the effect of an intra-articular injection can often last for several weeks and months, thereby protecting the joint from the sequelae of continued synovitis and providing symptom control while waiting for disease-modifying drugs to work.

31.6 Conclusions

Joint aspiration for diagnostic purposes is most often required in the setting of monoarthritis, where septic arthritis is a prime consideration. It is important in suspected cases of crystal arthritis where the diagnosis cannot be established by other means. Joint and soft tissue steroid injections provide rapid symptomatic relief and are an invaluable adjunct in the management of arthritis and soft tissue rheumatism.

Acknowledgments The author acknowledges the invaluable contribution of Dr. SJ Gupta to this chapter.

Pregnancy, Lactation, Contraception, and Fatherhood in Rheumatic Diseases

32

32.1 Introduction

Autoimmune rheumatic diseases (ARD) like rheumatoid arthritis (RA), systemic lupus erythematosus (SLE), and spondyloarthritides (SpA) afflict young individuals with many women belonging to the childbearing age group. Contraception, pregnancy, lactation, fatherhood, and allied issues often figure prominently during patient consults. The girl child with a chronic illness like SLE is especially vulnerable to social stigma in addition to medical hardships in male-dominated societies like India. Patient, and equally important, "family" education goes a long way in mitigating this negativism prevalent in society. The therapeutic nihilism so pervasive in non-rheumatologists needs to be acknowledged and addressed rather than brushed under the carpet. The lack of interdisciplinary dialog only compounds this problem. Instances of young girls with lupus being instructed (*by doctors*) not to marry or conceive are remarkable not for their rarity, but their commonality. This chapter aims to address these issues.

As a general rule, sexual relations, marriage, pregnancy, and fatherhood are eminently feasible in most situations. Fertility is not compromised in the majority of cases with ARD. Pregnancy is advised when the rheumatic disease has been quiescent for several months. Ideally, pregnancy should be a planned pregnancy. Contraceptive measures depend on the underlying disease. Some drugs are proscribed during pregnancy. In the case of males, current drug recommendations have been relaxed considerably. For example, methotrexate and leflunomide are no longer withheld in males wishing to father a child. Gonadal preservation strategies are available and may need specialist consultation. Breastfeeding should be undertaken only on drugs that are deemed safe for the baby.

32.2 Risk Categories of Drugs

The United States Food and Drug Administration (FDA) drug categories were in widespread use earlier (Table 32.1) and are widely cited in the literature. These letter categories, in use since 1979, inaccurately implied increased risk as one went from category A to B to C to D to X. However, the categories were actually determined not by risk but by assessing the reliability and type of data available (adequate or not, well-controlled or observational, human or animal studies). The risk-to-benefit ratio was based on this. Another short-

Table 32.1 FDA Drug Pregnancy Categories (Initiated in 1979. Phased out on December 3, 2014. No longer in use now)

Category	Interpretation
A	Human studies show no risk
B	No evidence of risk in studies
C	Risk cannot be ruled out
D	Positive evidence of risk
X	Contraindicated in pregnancy

R. Handa, *Clinical Rheumatology*, https://doi.org/10.1007/978-981-33-4885-1_32

coming that became apparent was that these categories did not take into account any risks from pharmaceutical agents or their metabolites in breast milk. This information was found in the section "Use in Specific Populations" in the drug product label. Over the years it was felt that the system had outlived its utility because it was overly simplistic, led to misinformation, and did not adequately address the available information. The FDA, therefore, changed this format for labeling medications after it published the Content and Format of Labeling for Human Prescription Drug and Biological Products; Requirements for Pregnancy and Lactation Labeling referred to as the "Pregnancy and Lactation Labeling Rule" (PLLR or final rule) on December 3, 2014. This system, being implemented from mid-2015, provides a discussion of the available data regarding a particular drug's safety in pregnancy and lactation, as well as information regarding the risk of untreated disease (Table 32.2).

There is limited information regarding the toxicity and teratogenic potential of many drugs. The limited evidence comes from animal studies or registry data. Dissecting out iatrogenic risk from the background risk is not always possible. Readers are advised to always check the manufacturer inserts for updated prescribing information.

Evaluation of risk during breastfeeding entails calculating the relative infant dose (RID), which is the dose administered to the infant through breast milk in mg/kg/day divided by the maternal dose in mg/kg/day. A value of less than 10% of the maternal dose is generally considered safe.

Table 32.2 Current FDA Labeling (in use since 2015)

Pregnancy (includes labor and delivery): • Pregnancy exposure registry • Risk summary • Clinical considerations • Data
Lactation (includes nursing mothers) • Risk summary • Clinical considerations • Data
Females and males of reproductive potential • Pregnancy testing • Contraception • Infertility

32.3 Nonsteroidal Anti-Inflammatory Drugs (NSAIDs)

Low-dose aspirin can be continued throughout pregnancy. NSAIDs should be avoided from the third trimester onward because of the risk of premature closure of the ductus arteriosus. Cyclooxygenase-2 (COX-2) inhibitors are avoided during pregnancy because of insufficient data. Ibuprofen is the preferred NSAID during lactation because of its long-term track record and because only small amounts pass into breast milk.

32.4 Corticosteroids

If required during pregnancy, corticosteroids may be used. However, the dose of steroids should be kept as low as required by the disease activity. Abrupt cessation of long-term steroids is not recommended. In such patients, the dose may need to be hiked up during surgery. Negligible amounts of prednisolone cross the placenta. However, dexamethasone and betamethasone cross the placenta and are best avoided unless there are specific reasons like heart block in the fetus. The earlier reports of cleft lip and cleft palate with steroids were discounted in subsequent studies. Maternal risks of steroids include increased risk of premature rupture of the membranes, intrauterine growth restriction, pregnancy-induced hypertension, gestational diabetes, and osteoporosis. Steroids are compatible with breastfeeding (Table 32.3).

Table 32.3 Drugs deemed safe in pregnancy and lactation

Drugs with minimal maternal and fetal risk	Drugs compatible with breastfeeding
Hydroxychloroquine	Hydroxychloroquine
Sulfasalazine	Sulfasalazine
Azathioprine	Azathioprine
Colchicine	Colchicine
Low-dose corticosteroids	Low-dose corticosteroids

32.5 Disease-Modifying Antirheumatic Drugs (DMARDs)

Hydroxychloroquine (HCQ), sulfasalazine (SSZ), and azathioprine are compatible with pregnancy and lactation (Table 32.3). Folate supplementation is recommended for all patients on SSZ during pregnancy. SSZ should not be used while breastfeeding premature infants and infants with hyperbilirubinemia.

Methotrexate (MTX), mycophenolate mofetil (MMF), and leflunomide (LEF) are contraindicated during pregnancy and lactation. MTX should be discontinued 3 months and MMF 6 weeks before a planned pregnancy. While the half-life of LEF is only 15 days, its major metabolite teriflunomide undergoes extensive enterohepatic circulation and may remain detectable in serum for up to 24 months. LEF should be stopped 24 months before planned pregnancy or drug elimination accelerated by cholestyramine washout (8 gm orally three times daily for 11 days). This should ideally be confirmed by measuring drug levels that should be lower than 0.02 mg/L on two tests performed 2 weeks apart. Plasma levels >0.02 mg/L require retreatment with cholestyramine and deferment of pregnancy.

The calcineurin inhibitors, cyclosporine and tacrolimus, can be used during pregnancy and lactation if warranted by the maternal disease. Cyclophosphamide (CYC) is contraindicated in pregnancy and lactation unless there is a life-threatening disease with no better alternative options.

32.6 Biologics and Targeted Synthetic DMARDs

Data accumulated over the last two decades suggests that tumor necrosis factor inhibitors (TNFi) can be continued during pregnancy if warranted by the disease activity. Certolizumab has minimal or no placental transfer compared with other TNFi because it lacks the antibody Fc region responsible for the placental transfer of immunoglobulins. Infants exposed to TNFi in utero should avoid live vaccines like BCG. TNFi are compatible with breastfeeding because very little of these large molecules find its way in breast milk. Table 32.4 summarizes the data available with respect to non-TNF biologics and the JAKi.

Table 32.4 Non-tumor necrosis factor (non-TNF) biologics and targeted synthetic DMARDs in pregnancy and lactation

Rituximab	Because of the IgG1 component, placental transfer in the first trimester negligible. Can be continued through conception. Stop when pregnancy is confirmed.	Can be used during lactation (conditional recommendation)
Tocilizumab		Can be used during lactation (conditional recommendation)
Secukinumab		Can be used during lactation (conditional recommendation)
Belimumab		No data to inform use during lactation
Anakinra		Probably safe during lactation
Abatacept		Can be used during lactation (conditional recommendation)
Ustekinumab		No data to inform use during lactation
Sarilumab		No data to inform use during lactation
Tofacitinib	Contraindicated in pregnancy. Stop 2 months before pregnancy.	Avoid during lactation. Being a small molecule likely to be transferred into breast milk
Barictinib	Insufficient data. Best avoided during pregnancy and lactation	
Upadacitib		
Apremilast		

Rituximab can be used during pregnancy in life-threatening conditions

32.7 Intravenous Immunoglobulin (IVIG)

IVIG is considered compatible with pregnancy and lactation.

32.8 Specific Rheumatic Diseases

32.8.1 Systemic Lupus Erythematosus (SLE)

Continued treatment with pregnancy compatible drugs is vital in SLE. Discontinuation of medications to control disease activity like HCQ increases the risk of flare and pregnancy complications. Pregnancy in lupus patients should be a planned affair when the disease has been quiescent for at least 6 months. Relative contraindications to pregnancy include active disease, recent stroke, significant cardiac involvement, pulmonary hypertension, severe interstitial lung disease, and advanced renal insufficiency.

The maternal and fetal complications of SLE are tabulated in Table 32.5. Flares are common during pregnancy and the postpartum period. Flare rates vary from 25 to 50% (background rate of lupus flare is ~25% per year). Factors predictive of increased risk of SLE flare during pregnancy include active disease during the 6 months prior to conception, history of lupus nephritis, HCQ withdrawal, and primigravidas. Physiological changes of pregnancy may mimic disease flare. Mild anemia, mild thrombocytopenia, elevated erythrocyte sedimentation rate (ESR), and proteinuria up to 300 mg in 24 h are commonplace in normal pregnancy. Complement levels may rise by 10–50% in normal pregnancy. The decline in C3/C4 due to lupus activity may not be discernible due to this. It is, therefore, important to monitor trends rather than a single value. Lupus nephritis flares during pregnancy may mimic preeclampsia making distinction difficult. The differentiating features are set out in Table 32.6. Active lupus nephritis and preeclampsia can coexist. Evidence of lupus activity in other organs is more suggestive of a lupus flare.

Table 32.5 Possible complications during lupus pregnancy

Obstetric complications	Disease-related complications in mother	Fetal complications
Preterm labor Unplanned cesarean Preeclampsia Eclampsia	Disease flare Hypertension Thrombosis Infection Increased mortality	Miscarriage Fetal growth restriction Heart block Stillbirth Neonatal lupus Complications related to prematurity

Table 32.6 Differentiation between lupus nephritis and preeclampsia

	Lupus nephritis	Preeclampsia
Onset	Any time	After 20 weeks
Proteinuria	Present	Present
Active urine sediment	Present	Absent
Complement (C3 and C4)	Low	Normal or increased
dsDNA	Increased	Normal
Transaminases (AST/ALT)	Normal	Elevated
Serum uric acid	Normal	Elevated
Worsening	Gradual	Rapid, over days
Remission after pregnancy	No	Yes

Preterm birth (before 37 weeks) is the most common obstetric complication in lupus women seen in 15–50% cases against 5–18% in the general obstetric population. This may be medically warranted due to preeclampsia or maternal disease. Preeclampsia is seen in 15–30% of lupus patients compared to <5% in the general obstetric population. Risk factors include active nephritis, past history of lupus nephritis, falling complement levels, and thrombocytopenia.

The autoantibodies that are required in a woman planning pregnancy are outlined in Table 32.7. Congenital complete heart block (CHB) occurs in approximately 1–2% of children born to women with anti-Ro/SSA antibodies. The mother may be totally asymptomatic. In women who have had one child with CHB, the risk

Table 32.7 Autoantibodies required in women with ARD planning pregnancy

aPLs: (a) Lupus anticoagulant (LA) (b) Anticardiolipin (aCL) IgG and IgM (c) β2 glycoprotein I (GPI) IgG and IgM
Anti-Ro/SSA and anti-La/SSB antibodies
For lupus patients: dsDNA C3 and C4

increases to several folds in subsequent pregnancies (~15%). Congenital heart block develops between 18 and 24 weeks of gestation. Fetal echocardiography is required for detection.

The treatment of active SLE during pregnancy is governed by the severity and degree of organ involvement. Therapy should not be initiated or escalated based on serologic findings alone. Hydroxychloroquine should be continued in all patients unless there are cogent reasons to withhold this drug. Current guidelines recommend low-dose aspirin in all women with SLE, beginning 12 weeks gestation, to reduce the risk of preeclampsia and its sequelae like fetal growth restriction, irrespective of aPL status. This approach is in keeping with the approach adopted for women at higher risk of preeclampsia. The use of other pregnancy compatible drugs like prednisolone, azathioprine, or calcineurin inhibitors depends on the disease attributes. Antihypertensive drugs employed in pregnancy include nifedipine, methyldopa, hydralazine, and labetalol. Angiotensin-converting enzyme (ACE) inhibitors and angiotensin II receptor blockers are contraindicated during pregnancy. The pregnancy outcome is favorable in >80% of cases.

32.8.2 Systemic Sclerosis (SSc)

Women with SSc usually have successful pregnancies despite some studies showing increased frequency of preterm delivery, intrauterine growth restriction, and low birth weight babies compared to the general population. The skin involvement of SSc is not exacerbated by pregnancy. Increased abdominal pressure in pregnancy may aggravate dyspepsia and reflux. Raynaud's may diminish because of the vasodilatation in pregnancy. It is difficult to differentiate renal dysfunction due to SSc from preeclampsia and eclampsia. Data on whether the pregnancy is associated with an increased incidence of renal crisis in scleroderma patients is limited, and no firm conclusions can be drawn.

The biggest challenge is pulmonary artery hypertension (PAH). Significant pulmonary hypertension is a contraindication to pregnancy in SSc and other ARD. Severe PAH (defined as mean pulmonary artery pressure ≥ 50 mmHg) may be associated with increased mortality. For women who choose to become pregnant or develop pulmonary hypertension when pregnant, the clinical course can be tumultuous with the emergence of life-threatening issues during pregnancy. These include worsening dyspnea and hypoxemia, progressive PAH, cardiovascular collapse, and death. The first 24–48 h after delivery constitute the gravest period when death is common. Chronic maternal hypoxemia increases the risk of fetal growth restriction.

Endothelin receptor antagonists (ERAs) like bosentan, ambrisentan, macitentan, and guanylate cyclase stimulants like riociguat should be discontinued since they are contraindicated in pregnancy because of their teratogenic potential. The current European Society of Cardiology/European Respiratory Society guidelines recommend that women with PAH who choose to continue with pregnancy should either be treated with (or continue treatment with) PAH-specific therapies except for ERAs. Calcium channel blockers, prostacyclin and its analogs, and phosphodiesterase type-5 inhibitors like sildenafil and tadalafil have been used.

32.9 Contraception

This issue is particularly important in diseases like lupus that disproportionately affect young women more than any other group. Pregnancies in lupus should ideally be planned when the disease has been in remission for at least 6 months.

During active nephritis or pulmonary hypertension, pregnancy is associated with high maternal morbidity and mortality and poor fetal outcome. Contraceptive choice in lupus is governed by disease activity, presence or absence of antiphospholipid antibodies (aPL); and patient preference. It is important to point out that medications like warfarin, cyclosporine, MMF, steroids, and anticonvulsants may have potential interactions with estrogen-containing contraceptives.

In general, long-acting reversible contraceptives (LARCs) like intrauterine devices (IUDs) are considered the most reliable form of contraception compared to barrier methods like condoms, diaphragms, spermicides, etc. which are less reliable due to inconsistent or improper use. The two common IUDs used in India are levonorgestrel (LNg)-containing IUD and copper IUD. The latter is more commonly used because of the lesser cost. LNg-IUD may reduce menstrual blood loss, which may be a benefit in patients on anticoagulants. In contrast, copper IUDs may be associated with heavier bleeding.

SLE patients without aPLs do not appear to be at increased risk for thrombosis or disease flare when taking the present-day low-dose oral pills. Lupus patients with high disease activity and those with positive aPLs are advised against the use of estrogen-containing contraceptives because of concerns of thromboembolic risk and risk of a disease flare. Progestin-only contraceptives are advised although they may have higher rates of discontinuation due to unscheduled "break-through" bleeding. Second-generation progestins may cause androgenic side effects like acne, hirsutism, and weight gain compared to third-generation progestins. The latter may have a slightly higher risk of venous thrombosis. For long-term protection, IUDs are a safe and effective option for most SLE patients, including patients with positive aPLs. Table 32.8 mentions the various contraceptive options available. A consult with the gynecologist may help the lupus patient choose the best available alternative. If required, emergency contraception may be used by patients with SLE, including those with positive aPLs.

Table 32.8 Contraceptive choices in lupus

Clinical setting	Contraceptive choice
Lupus patients with low disease activity and negative aPLs	• Oral hormonal contraceptives—The estrogen–progestin pill with ethinyl estradiol doses of 30 mcg or lower. [transdermal patch gives higher estrogen exposure]. • Intrauterine devices (IUDs).
Lupus patients with high disease activity and positive aPLs	• Progestin-only contraceptives. • Intrauterine devices (IUDs).
aPLs with or without lupus	• Progestin-only contraceptives. • Intrauterine devices (IUDs).

Note: Barrier methods (female and male condoms) are not a very effective contraceptive method and may be used if the above options are not exercised/refused

32.10 Fertility Preservation in Autoimmune Rheumatic Diseases

The use of drugs like CYC may lead to permanent sterility. However, at times their use is unavoidable because of the requirement of the underlying disease. In such a scenario, women desiring fertility preservation should be referred to an expert for cryopreservation techniques. Gonadotropin-releasing hormone (GnRH) agonists like leuprolide, despite frequent use, have uncertain results. The resumption of menses is not considered a reliable marker of fertility because women may remain infertile despite the resumption of menses. Anti-müllerian hormone (AMH) levels are employed as markers of ovarian reserve. Preservation of fertility in men is technically less difficult and can be achieved by semen cryopreservation. GnRH agonists to reversibly suppress the hypothalamic–pituitary–testicular axis are not recommended because of uncertain benefits.

32.11 Male Fertility and Fatherhood Issues

Spermatogenesis is much more affected by drugs than testosterone production. The effect varies according to the drug used and is dose- and duration-dependent. SSZ and CYC adversely affect spermatogenesis. SSZ causes reversible azoospermia or oligospermia, while CYC can cause irreversible sterility. Libido is uninfluenced by these drugs.

MTX, LEF, azathioprine, MMF, TNFi, and most biologics can be continued in males wishing to father a child. CYC and thalidomide should be stopped by males wishing to embark on fatherhood. A waiting period of 3 months is recommended to allow for a full spermatogenesis cycle before attempting conception.

32.12 Conclusions

Most autoimmune rheumatic diseases provide a window of opportunity for motherhood when the disease is quiescent. Drug prescriptions during pregnancy and lactation should be carefully reviewed to optimize benefit and minimize risk. Contraceptive options need shared decision making. Patients and their families should be educated, reassured, and involved in all aspects of their disease management. Pregnancy, even when planned, can throw up challenges that require interdisciplinary dialog and care.

Suggested Reading

1. Micu MC, Ostensen M, Villiger PM, Micu R, Ionescu R. Safety of anti- rheumatic drugs in men trying to conceive: a systematic review and analysis of published evidence. Semin Arthritis Rheum. 2018;48:343–55.
2. Sammaritano LR, Bermas BL, Chakravarty EE, Chambers C, Clowse MEB, Lockshin MD, et al. American college of rheumatology guideline for the management of reproductive health in rheumatic and musculoskeletal diseases. Arthritis Rheumatol 2020. 2020;72:529–56.
3. Flint J, Panchal S, Hurrell A, van de Venne M, Gayed M, Schreiber K, et al. BSR and BHPR standards, guidelines and audit working group. BSR and BHPR guideline on prescribing drugs in pregnancy and breastfeeding-Part I: standard and biologic disease modifying anti-rheumatic drugs and corticosteroids. Rheumatology (Oxford). 2016;55:1693–7.
4. United States Food and Drug Administration. https://www.fda.gov/drugs/labeling-information-drug-products/pregnancy-and-lactation-labeling-drugs-final-rule. Accessed 6 September 2020.

33 Immunisation in Autoimmune Rheumatic Diseases

33.1 Introduction

Patients with autoimmune rheumatic diseases (ARD), such as rheumatoid arthritis (RA), systemic lupus erythematosus (SLE), etc. are at a greater risk for infections because of disease-related factors as well as drugs used to treat the disease. Several of the infections, such as influenza and *Streptococcus pneumoniae* pneumonia, are vaccine-preventable. The vaccine uptake in patients, especially in India, is not high. Reasons include, but are not limited to, recurring cost, physician and rheumatologist unfamiliarity, vaccine nonavailability, safety and efficacy concerns, a paucity of data regarding cost–benefit in low-income countries, overworked clinics, patient reluctance, and inadequate documentation. Most guidelines now urge rheumatologists to incorporate assessment of immunisation status at the time of the initial encounter. While pretreatment vaccination (before starting immunosuppressives) is ideal because the likelihood of developing a protective immune response is highest at this point of time without attenuation of efficacy by immunosuppressives, vaccination should be offered whenever practically feasible. Also, live vaccines can be given safely in the pretreatment period.

The immune response to vaccination in ARD patients on immunosuppressive treatments has been best studied for pneumococcal and influenza vaccinations. Despite lower seroprotection rates and blunted immune response, the existing literature suggests that vaccination in this patient population is likely to confer adequate protection. Rituximab is associated with the greatest blunting of the immune response to vaccinations, followed by methotrexate and abatacept. Tumor necrosis factor inhibitors (TNFi) are less likely to dampen the immune response except for response to hepatitis B virus (HBV) vaccination.

As a general rule, live vaccines like measles, yellow fever, or the older zoster vaccine should be administered ≥4 weeks before the start of immunosuppression. This is especially important for drugs like rituximab. In situations where live vaccines need to be used (e.g., yellow fever), immunosuppressive medication is temporarily stopped 4 weeks prior to vaccination and resumed only 4 weeks post vaccination. Live vaccines like Bacillus Calmette Guerin (BCG) and measles, mumps, and rubella (MMR) should be avoided during the first 6 months of life in children of mothers treated with biologics during the second half of pregnancy.

The vaccine-preventable diseases include:

- Influenza
- Invasive pneumococcal disease
- Herpes zoster
- Hepatitis B
- Papillomavirus

R. Handa, *Clinical Rheumatology*, https://doi.org/10.1007/978-981-33-4885-1_33

33.2 Influenza Vaccine

This is administered yearly. As the influenza virus constantly mutates, a new batch is prepared every year based on the advice of the World Health Organization (WHO). A single dose of 0.5 ml is given intramuscularly into the deltoid muscle. The vaccine becomes effective in 2 weeks after administration. The timing of administration depends on the location. In most parts of India, it is just before the onset of monsoon months (around May–June). It is administered just before the onset of winter months (September–October) in the extreme north and south of the country. The various types available include inactivated influenza vaccine, recombinant influenza vaccine, or live attenuated influenza vaccine. Live attenuated vaccine delivered by nasal spray is avoided in ARD. Both trivalent (three-component) and quadrivalent (four-component) flu vaccines are available. No preference is expressed for any influenza vaccine over another. This vaccine can be given along with the pneumococcal vaccine in the same session but at a different site.

33.3 Pneumococcal Vaccine

Pneumococcal vaccine is available in two forms:

1. *P*neumococcal *P*oly*S*accharide *V*accine (PPSV23).
2. *P*neumococcal *C*onjugate *V*accine (PCV13).

PPSV contains polysaccharides from 23 serotypes. This vaccine is less immunogenic because it stimulates B cells mainly and provokes poor immunological "memory." Boosters are needed every 5 years. Revaccination recommendations may vary among experts. Generally, two booster doses of PPSV23 can be injected during the life of an individual. After the age of 65, only one booster dose is given. The PCV 13 is conjugated to diphtheria protein as a carrier to stimulate T cells. A single dose is good for life. Both vaccines should be given to achieve high prevention rates.

For patients who have not received pneumococcal vaccine previously, a single dose of PCV13 should be given first, followed by a dose of PPSV23 $\geq$ 8 weeks later. In those who have received PPSV23 earlier, this should be followed by PCV13 after an interval of $\geq$1 year. Revaccination can be done with PPSV23 at least 5 years after the first dose. Patients aged <65 years are given two doses at an interval of 5 years and the third dose (the last dose) after crossing 65 years (total 3 doses). After the age of 65 years, only one dose of PPSV23 is administered. Thus, a patient starting vaccination series at 50 years is given PCV13 followed by PPSV23 after at least 8 weeks. The first booster of PPSV23 is given after 5 years of the first dose of PPSV23. The second (and final booster) is given after the patient crosses the age of 65.

33.4 Zoster (Shingles) Vaccines

Vaccination against herpes zoster (HZ) is recommended in patients with ARD who are $\geq$50 years old. Two vaccines are available for herpes zoster: The live attenuated vaccine (Zostavax) and the new recombinant (non-live) HZ subunit vaccine (Shingrix). The subunit vaccine combines a key surface VZV glycoprotein (E) with a T cell boosting adjuvant (AS01B). The live vaccine is administered as a single dose and should only be used in patients not on immunosuppressives (before the start of treatment if conditions permit). It carries a risk of dissemination in patients on immunosuppressants. The immunity induced by the live vaccine decreases markedly within 10 years. A booster has not yet been approved. In contrast, the recombinant vaccine is much more effective, and there is no risk of developing the disseminated disease. It, however, requires two doses spaced 4 weeks apart. This should be followed by a 2-week interval prior to the start of immunosuppressants. In unvaccinated patients already on immunosuppressants, it is prudent to wait for at least one dosing interval or 1 month (depending on the half-life of the immunosuppressant) before giving the vaccine and then subsequently deferring any additional immunosuppressants for at least 1 month.

33.5 Hepatitis B Virus (HBV) Vaccine

Hepatitis B vaccination has been integrated into the Universal Immunization Program (UIP) in India. India's national policy recommends that children receive three doses of Hepatitis B vaccine administered concurrently with diphtheria, pertussis, tetanus (DPT), and trivalent oral polio vaccine at 6, 10, and 14 weeks. Besides, a birth dose is recommended for all newborns (within 24 h of delivery) for all institutional deliveries. If immunization status is not known, serologic testing is obtained. The interpretation of Hepatitis B serology is listed in Table 33.1. Susceptible individuals are offered vaccination with 3 doses: 0, 1 to 2 months, and 4 to 6 months. For patients who fail to seroconvert, repeat vaccination may be needed. Whether standard- or higher dose HBV vaccine should be used in ARD is uncertain.

33.6 Other Inactivated Vaccines

Other inactivated vaccines (like tetanus, diphtheria, pertussis [Tdap]; tetanus, diphtheria [Td]; human papillomavirus; and meningococcal vaccine) should be given per the indications and schedules in the general adult population.

Table 33.1 Interpretation of serologic tests employed for Hepatitis B

Tests	Results	Interpretation
HBsAg	Negative	Susceptible
Anti-HBc	Negative	
Anti-HBs	Negative	
HBsAg	Negative	Immune due to natural infection
Anti-HBc	Positive	
Anti-HBs	Positive	
HBsAg	Negative	Immune due to hepatitis B vaccination
Anti-HBc	Negative	
Anti-HBs	Positive	

33.7 Postexposure Prophylaxis

Postexposure prophylaxis (PEP) may be needed in case of situations like rabies after an animal bite. Inactivated vaccines can be used in such situations. In severely immunocompromised patients, rabies immune globulin can be used alongside the rabies vaccine.

33.8 Conclusions

Vaccination should be included in the routine management of ARD. Pneumococcal vaccination and influenza vaccination should be offered to all patients, while the zoster vaccine is offered to patients over 50 years of age. Live vaccines should be used with caution in this patient population.

Suggested Reading

1. Furer V, Rondaan C, Heijstek MW, Agmon-Levin N, van Assen S, Bijl M, et al. Update of EULAR recommendations for vaccination in adult patients with autoimmune inflammatory rheumatic diseases. Ann Rheum Dis 2020. 2019;79:39–52.
2. Kumar S, Rath P, Malaviya AN. A practical guide to adult vaccination for patients with autoimmune inflammatory rheumatic diseases in India. Indian J Rheumatol. 2017;12:160–8.

Coronavirus Disease (COVID-19) and the Rheumatologist

34

34.1 Introduction

The pandemic of the century, COVID-19, has impacted all nations and all spheres of life. Medical specialties are no exemption. Apart from a slew of front-line disciplines like infectious diseases, pulmonary and critical care, microbiology, intensive care, radiology, etc. involved in direct care, the other so-called "unrelated" disciplines too have been impacted by this virus in myriads of ways. Rheumatology is one of them. Rheumatologists have been willy nilly sucked into the vortex of this life-changing disease.

Rheumatologists handle a variety of autoimmune diseases and use dozens of immunomodulatory therapies. The primary questions that need to be addressed are the impact of COVID-19 on autoimmune rheumatic diseases (ARD) and continuation or initiation of corticosteroids, immunosuppressives, biologics, or other disease-modifying antirheumatic drugs (DMARDs) by our patients. Rheumatic manifestations of acute COVID-19 infection or post-recovery is an evolving area. Rheumatologists also lead the way in the adoption and adaptation of technology like telemedicine to provide uninterrupted patient care in these difficult times. Last but not the least, rheumatologists with years of experience in using drugs like hydroxychloroquine (HCQ), tocilizumab, etc. and given their familiarity with hyper inflammation and cytokine storms, are uniquely placed to share experience and expertise with colleagues from other specialties.

This chapter discusses some of the clinically pertinent issues relevant to a rheumatologist. Telemedicine and the repurposing of drugs like HCQ and tocilizumab for use in COVID-19 is beyond the scope of this chapter. The rapid advances in this new disease will inevitably result in changing concepts that no textbook can keep pace with. Readers are, therefore advised, to check for updated information through journals or other scientific websites. Also, recommendations may need to be modified according to disease type, patient characteristics, geographic location, and resource availability. General guidance is not meant to be a substitute for individualized treatment decisions.

34.2 COVID-19 and Autoimmune Rheumatic Diseases

At present, there is little evidence to suggest that patients with rheumatic diseases are more susceptible to infection with COVID-19 or worse outcomes. Data from COVID-19 Global Rheumatology Alliance registry that looked at 600 cases of COVID-19 in patients with rheumatic diseases from 40 countries revealed that the majority of patients with rheumatic diseases recover from COVID-19. Factors associated with higher odds of COVID-19 hospitalization com-

R. Handa, *Clinical Rheumatology*, https://doi.org/10.1007/978-981-33-4885-1_34

prise older age, comorbidities, and higher doses of prednisolone (≥10 mg/day). More important than the rheumatic disease per se are factors like age > 65 years, smoking, obesity, diabetes mellitus, hypertension, chronic lung disease, cardiovascular disease, chronic kidney disease, etc. General measures like a healthy diet and exercise to maintain fitness, social distancing, frequent hand washing, and masks should be universally recommended. Elective surgeries like joint replacements may be deferred in accordance with patient desires. The role of medication is discussed below.

Patients with ARD without symptoms of COVID-19 should be advised to update their vaccination status, especially pneumococcal and influenza vaccines. Patients on cyclophosphamide or steroids should be offered *Pneumocystis jiroveci* pneumonia prophylaxis.

34.3 Antirheumatic Drugs During COVID-19

Patients with ARD are on a variety of drugs like nonsteroidal anti-inflammatory drugs (NSAIDs), corticosteroids, DMARDs, biologics, Janus kinas (JAK) inhibitors, cyclophosphamide (CYC), etc.

34.3.1 Treatment Continuation

Patients with ARD should be urged to continue their medicines as treatment interruptions can lead to a flare. Drugs like NSAIDs, HCQ, sulfasalazine (SSZ), methotrexate (MTX), leflunomide (LEF), mycophenolate mofetil (MMF), azathioprine, and calcineurin inhibitors can be continued without change. For drugs like CYC, dose de-escalation may be considered if permitted by the underlying disease condition. Corticosteroid doses should be tapered if feasible. However, steroids should not be abruptly stopped even if there is exposure to or infection with SARS-CoV-2. Biologics and JAKi may be continued if required by the underlying disease. If stable, dose reduction or increase in dosing interval may be contemplated. In the case of intravenous drugs, subcutaneous alternatives may be explored. Notwithstanding any of the above, suboptimal dosing or dose reductions are to be avoided in patients with life-threatening or organ-threatening disease.

There have been reports of QT prolongation and risk of ventricular arrhythmia due to Hydroxychloroquine-Azithromycin treatment for COVID-19. While chloroquine and HCQ prolong the QT interval, the risk of arrhythmic death from an individual or concurrent use of these medications is exceedingly low. Patients admitted with COVID-19 are likely to have longer baseline QTc and have higher potential arrhythmic risks as a result of the metabolic and physiologic sequelae of their illness, and a typically greater burden of comorbid disease. HCQ is the anchor drug for ARD like lupus, and rheumatologists have extensively used it for decades. While exercising due to pharmacovigilance, patients and doctors alike should be reassured about the safety of HCQ and its important role in the management of ARD.

Concomitant medication like angiotensin-converting enzyme (ACE) inhibitors or angiotensin receptor blockers (ARBs) may be initiated or continued as required.

34.3.2 Treatment Initiation

This is primarily influenced by the ARD diagnosed and its activity. Drug initiation should factor in the underlying disease, and treatment should not be compromised for fear of COVID-19. Corticosteroid initiation and biologic initiation can be undertaken if warranted by the ARD.

34.4 Patients with ARD Who Develop COVID-19

In such a scenario, the control of infection gets precedence over the ARD. While drugs like HCQ and NSAIDs may be continued, it is prudent to temporarily stop MTX, LEF, biologics, and JAK inhibitors. NSAIDs are best withheld in those who develop severe respiratory symptoms.

Corticosteroids should be tapered if permitted by the underlying condition, but not abruptly stopped. The opinion regarding SSZ is divided among experts. Some experts feel that adverse effects of SSZ like gastrointestinal upset, transaminitis, and cytopenias, should they occur, may cause confusion with signs of COVID-19. Hence, temporary withdrawal is recommended by some.

The withheld drugs can be restarted 7–14 days after symptom resolution. For asymptomatic patients with a positive RT-PCR test for SARS-CoV-2, withholding treatment for 10–17 days is recommended. Those with post-COVID-19 sequelae may defer treatment as necessitated by their individual condition.

34.5 COVID-19 Testing Before Biologic Infusions

This practical issue lacks consensus. Guidance issued by local authorities or professional societies may be followed. The Infectious Disease Society of America recommends SARS-CoV-2 testing in asymptomatic individuals prior to immunosuppressive procedures, even in the absence of known exposure to SARS-CoV-2. These procedures include long-acting biologic therapy, high-dose steroids, cytotoxic chemotherapy, solid-organ or stem-cell transplantation, and cellular immunotherapy. Some hospitals require SARS-CoV-2 testing conducted 2–3 days prior to hospitalization for any reason.

34.6 Musculoskeletal (MSK) Manifestations of COVID-19

MSK pains are fairly common in viral illnesses. Data on this aspect of severe acute respiratory syndrome coronavirus 2 (SARS-CoV-2) is sparse. Arthralgias have been reported in nearly 15% of patients and myalgias in 40–45% of patients with COVID-19. The severity of musculoskeletal symptoms does not parallel the severity of COVID-19. A study from Spain reported muscle and joint pains in 26.4% of the 306 patients admitted with COVID-19. None of the patients had frank arthritis at admission, but four (1.3%) developed acute arthritis while in hospital. These patients had a previous history of arthritis, and the flares were due to crystals (monosodium urate and calcium pyrophosphate dehydrate). Synovial fluid testing for SARS-CoV-2 by RT-PCR in three out of the four patients was negative. Joint symptoms may persist in as many as 25% of patients after recovery from COVID-19 for a variable period of time.

34.7 SARS-CoV-2 Vaccination in Patients with Rheumatic Diseases

Several countries have started national vaccination programs. All vaccines that are presently being used for COVID-19 are non-live vaccines and can be used in patients with rheumatic diseases. Vaccination should preferably be given when the rheumatic disease is in a quiescent phase and before planned immunosuppression, if feasible. There is no data to support the choice of any one vaccine over the other.

34.8 Conclusions

The risk for infection and outcome of SARS-CoV-2 in patients with ARD is influenced more by factors such as age, cardiopulmonary disease, and other comorbidities rather than primary disease. Masks, frequent hand washing, and physical distancing remain the cornerstone of prevention strategies. Individual circumstances govern antirheumatic drug initiation and continuation. Given the rapid pace with which this field is evolving, readers need to continually update themselves.

Suggested Reading

1. Mikuls TR, Johnson SR, Fraenkel L, Arasaratnam RJ, Baden LR, Bermas BL, et al. American college of rheumatology guidance for the management of rheu-

matic disease in adult patients during the COVID-19 Pandemic: Version 3. Arthritis Rheumatol. 2020 Dec 5. doi:10.1002/art.41596. Online ahead of print.

2. Gianfrancesco M, Hyrich KL, Al-Adely S, Carmona L, Danila MI, Gossec L, et al. Characteristics associated with hospitalisation for COVID-19 in people with rheumatic disease: data from the COVID-19 Global Rheumatology Alliance physician-reported registry. Ann Rheum Dis. 2020;79:859–66.
3. Tam LS, Tanaka Y, Handa R, Chang CC, Cheng YK, Isalm N, et al. Care for patients with rheumatic diseases during COVID-19 pandemic: a position statement from APLAR. Int J Rheum Dis. 2020;23:717–22.
4. Landewé RB, Machado PM, Kroon F, Bijlsma HW, Burmester GR, Carmona L, et al. EULAR provisional recommendations for the management of rheumatic and musculoskeletal diseases in the context of SARS-CoV-2. Ann Rheum Dis. 2020;79:851–8.
5. Schett G, Manger B, Simon D, Caporali R. COVID-19 revisiting inflammatory pathways of arthritis. Nat Rev. Rheumatol. 2020;16:465–70.
6. López-González MD, Peral-Garrido ML, Calabuig I, Tovar-Sugrañes E, Jovani V, Bernabeu P, et al. Case series of acute arthritis during COVID-19 admission [published online ahead of print, 2020 May 29]. Ann Rheum Dis 2020; annrheumdis-2020-217,914
7. Carfì A, Bernabei R, Landi F. Gemelli against COVID-19 post-acute care study group. persistent symptoms in patients after acute COVID-19. JAMA. 2020;324:603–5.

35 Web Resources in Rheumatology

35.1 Introduction

The rapid pace of medical advancements has led to a considerable time lag between what is published in books and what is new. The internet has bridged the gap between the availability of information and its dissemination. It is an important means for physicians to update knowledge. It is also vital for patient education that holds the key to patient empowerment. This chapter aims to list some useful websites and online resources that provide reliable information about rheumatic musculoskeletal diseases. It is by no means a comprehensive or complete listing of all online resources. The biomedical journals and pharmaceutical company websites are not included in this compilation. Listing here is also not meant to be an endorsement by the author or publishers. Readers are urged to check the veracity of information available online with other sources. The information is for general guidance and is not meant to be a substitute for medical advice. Not all the content on all the websites is available free of charge.

35.1.1 American College of Rheumatology (ACR)

https://www.rheumatology.org

The website features several resources like clinical practice guidelines, ACR position statements, patient information sheets, videos in English and Spanish, etc. The ACR's Guideline and Criteria App is free to download and features interactive tools to inform treatment decisions, including algorithms, scores, calculators, full guidelines and criteria content, etc.

35.1.2 European League against Rheumatism (EULAR)

https://www.eular.org

The website features EULAR recommendations for the treatment of various rheumatic disorders. The EULAR also provides a lay summary version, in English, and encourages the translation of these lay versions into different languages.

35.1.3 Asia Pacific League of Associations for Rheumatology (APLAR)

http://www.aplar.org/

APLAR comprises nearly 30 member national organizations from the Asia Pacific. Training modules in English, Japanese, and Chinese are available along with a host of other useful information.

R. Handa, *Clinical Rheumatology*, https://doi.org/10.1007/978-981-33-4885-1_35

35.1.4 British Society for Rheumatology

https://www.rheumatology.org.uk

A useful site for clinical guidelines that support evidence-based clinical practice in rheumatology

35.1.5 Indian Rheumatology Association

https://www.indianrheumatology.org/

This website features several useful things like an image bank, Fellows corner, etc. Some features are available only to members. The e-newsletter is freely accessible.

35.1.6 Osteoarthritis Research Society International (OARSI)

https://www.oarsi.org/

The focus is on all aspects of osteoarthritis. The OARSI Resource Library contains the speaker slides from the World Congresses on Osteoarthritis as well as guidelines, outcome, and physical measures and white papers.

35.1.7 Disease Activity Score (DAS) Website

https://www.das-score.nl/das28/en/

This provides all information about the DAS-28, an instrument to measure the disease activity in people with Rheumatoid Arthritis. Various DAS calculators are available.

35.1.8 RheumaHelper

https://rheumahelper.com/

A mobile app offering several essential tools for daily clinical practice. The app is free to download, has been translated into 6 languages, and is active in more than 120 countries

35.1.9 Assessment of SpondyloArthritis international Society (ASAS)

https://www.asas-group.org/

As the name indicates, the focus is on Spondyloarthritis (SpA). The ASAS slide library offers more than 400 freely downloadable slides and an ASAS handbook. The ASAS app offers a calculator for the Ankylosing Spondylitis Disease Activity Score (ASDAS), a calculator for the Bath Ankylosing Spondylitis Disease Activity Index (BASDAI) as well as information on classification, diagnosis, outcome assessment, and treatment of SpA.

35.1.10 Spondyloarthritis Research and Treatment Network (SPARTAN)

https://www.spartangroup.org

SPARTAN is a network of health care professionals in North America dedicated to research, awareness, and treatment of spondyloarthritis.

35.1.11 Group for Research and Assessment in Psoriasis and Psoriatic Arthritis (GRAPPA)

https://www.grappanetwork.org/

The website offers GRAPPA's interactive learning modules focused on the treatment of PsA. Many are accessible to all users. "A Patient's Guide to Treatments for Psoriatic Arthritis" in booklet format is available.

35.1.12 Pediatric Rheumatology INternational Trials Organisation (PRINTO)

https://www.printo.it

The website primarily deals with pediatric rheumatic diseases. Only some parts are open to nonmembers.

35.1.13 Lupus Foundation of America

https://www.lupus.org

Dealing with Systemic Lupus Erythematosus (SLE) primarily, the website offers much information for the patients and caregivers. Besides, *Lupus Science & Medicine*™, the first lupus-specific open access journal in the world, is owned by the Lupus Foundation of America and published by BMJ.

35.1.14 Antinuclear Antibody (ANA) Patterns

https://www.anapatterns.org/index.php

The official website for the International Consensus on ANA Patterns (ICAP). ICAP was initiated as a workshop aiming to thoroughly discuss and to promote consensus regarding the richness in nuances of morphological patterns observed in the indirect immunofluorescence assay on HEp-2 cells. The ICAP initiative was implemented at the 12th International Workshop on Autoantibodies and Autoimmunity (IWAA) by members of the Autoantibody Standardization Committee (ASC), a subcommittee of the International Union of Immunological Societies (IUIS) Quality Assessment and Standardization Committee and affiliated with the Centers for Diseases Control and Prevention (CDC).

35.1.15 The Sjögren's Foundation

https://www.sjogrens.org

The Sjögren's Foundation is dedicated to providing the most up-to-date information about Sjogren's Syndrome to patients and healthcare providers.

35.1.16 Scleroderma Foundation

https://www.scleroderma.org

A reliable source of information about systemic sclerosis for patients.

35.1.17 The Myositis Association

https://www.myositis.org

This provides credible information on myositis in several languages, including many Indian languages like Hindi, Tamil, Bengali, Gujarati, Punjabi, etc.

35.1.18 International Osteoporosis Foundation (IOF)

https://www.iofbonehealth.org/

The website provides a wealth of scientific updates about osteoporosis as well as information for patients.

35.1.19 The Fracture Risk Assessment Tool (FRAX®)

https://www.sheffield.ac.uk/FRAX/

This provides full information about the *FRAX*® tool developed to evaluate the fracture risk of patients. It is available in several languages.

35.1.20 The International Society of Clinical Densitometry (ISCD)

https://www.iscd.org/

This provides a central resource for several scientific disciplines with an interest in the assessment of skeletal health.

35.1.21 The Rare Diseases Clinical Research Network

https://www.rarediseasesnetwork.org

This is an NIH-funded research network of 23 active consortia or research groups—teams of researchers, patients, and clinicians—each focused on a group of rare disorders. Rheumatic diseases include Behcet's syndrome, vasculitis amongst others.

35.1.22 The COVID-19 Global Rheumatology Alliance

https://rheum-covid.org/

This provides authentic information about Coronavirus Disease (COVID-19) in reference to rheumatic diseases.

35.1.23 UpToDate

https://www.uptodate.com

Apart from physician resources that require a subscription, UpToDate offers two levels of authentic patient information. **The Basics** are short overviews. They are written in accordance with plain language principles and answer the four or five most important questions a person might have about a medical problem. **Beyond the Basics** are longer, more detailed reviews. They are best for readers who want detailed information and are comfortable with some medical terminology.

35.1.24 Drugs and Lactation Database (LactMed)

https://www.ncbi.nlm.nih.gov/books/NBK501922/

The LactMed® database, produced by the National Library of Medicine, contains information on drugs and other chemicals to which breastfeeding mothers may be exposed. It includes information on the levels of such substances in breast milk and infant blood and the possible adverse effects in the nursing infant. Suggested therapeutic alternatives to those drugs are provided, where appropriate. All data are derived from the scientific literature and fully referenced. A peer review panel reviews the data to assure scientific validity and currency. The LactMed apps for Android and iOS devices are being retired. Current users of the LactMed apps are encouraged to continue accessing LactMed via Bookshelf. Alternatively, the dataset can be downloaded from NLM's Data Distribution site and through the NLM Open Access subset.

35.1.25 Sex and U

https://www.sexandu.ca/

An initiative of the Society of Obstetricians and Gynaecologists of Canada. This provides information on sexually transmitted infections, contraception and various methods of birth control, lifestyle choices, and healthy sexuality for teens, adults, parents, teachers, and health professionals.

GPSR Compliance

The European Union's (EU) General Product Safety Regulation (GPSR) is a set of rules that requires consumer products to be safe and our obligations to ensure this.

If you have any concerns about our products, you can contact us on ProductSafety@springernature.com

In case Publisher is established outside the EU, the EU authorized representative is:

Springer Nature Customer Service Center GmbH
Europaplatz 3
69115 Heidelberg, Germany

Batch number: 10731385

Printed by Printforce, the Netherlands